# BASIC UROLOGICAL SCIENCES

# BASIC UROLOGICAL SCIENCES

Edited by

## Karl H. Pang
Specialist Registrar in Urological Surgery
Yorkshire and Humber Deanery
Honorary Clinical Lecturer
University of Sheffield

## Nadir I. Osman
Consultant Urological Surgeon
Sheffield Teaching Hospitals NHS Foundation Trust
Honorary Senior Lecturer
University of Sheffield

## James W.F. Catto
Professor of Urological Surgery
University of Sheffield
Honorary Consultant Urological Surgeon
Sheffield Teaching Hospitals NHS Foundation Trust

## Christopher R. Chapple
Consultant Urological Surgeon
Sheffield Teaching Hospitals NHS Foundation Trust
Honorary Professor
University of Sheffield
Visiting Professor
Sheffield Hallam University

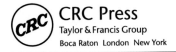

**CRC Press**
Taylor & Francis Group
Boca Raton  London  New York

CRC Press is an imprint of the
Taylor & Francis Group, an **informa** business

First edition published 2021
by CRC Press
6000 Broken Sound Parkway NW, Suite 300, Boca Raton, FL 33487-2742

and by Taylor & Francis Group
2 Park Square, Milton Park, Abingdon, Oxon, OX14 4RN

# Contents

# Contributors

**Omar Aboumarzouk**
Consultant Urological Surgeon
Queen Elizabeth University Hospital
NHS Greater Glasgow and Clyde
Glasgow, UK

**Pedro Abreu-Mendes**
Assistant Professor and Resident in Urological Surgery
Faculty of Medicine of Porto and Hospital São João
i3S: Institute for Investigation and Innovation in Health
Porto, Portugal

**Hashim Ahmed**
Professor and Chair of Urology
Imperial College London
Consultant Urological Surgeon
Imperial College Healthcare NHS Trust
London, UK
Chair, NCRI Prostate Clinical Studies Group
Chair, NHS England Prostate Clinical Expert Group
London, UK

**Sam H. Ahmedzai**
Emeritus Professor
The University of Sheffield
NIHR CRN National Specialty Lead for Cancer - Supportive Care and Community-Based Research
Co-chair of NCRI Living With and Beyond Cancer Research Group
Chair of NIHR Cancer & Nutrition Collaboration Steering Committee
Chair of British Pain Society Education Committee
Sheffield, UK

**Ased Ali**
Consultant Urological Surgeon
Pinderfields Hospital
The Mid Yorkshire Hospitals NHS Trust
Wakefield, UK

**Ibrahim Ali**
Specialist Registrar in Nephrology and General Internal Medicine
Salford Royal Hospital
Salford Royal NHS Foundation Trust
Salford, UK

**Tarik Amer**
Consultant Urological Surgeon
University Hospital Monklands
NHS Lanarkshire
Glasgow, UK

**Eleni Anastasiadis**
Consultant Urological Surgeon
Croydon University Hospital
Croydon Health Services NHS Trust
Honorary Consultant
Department of Urology
St Georges Hospital
London, UK

**Ken Anson**
Consultant Urological Surgeon
St George's University Hospitals NHS Foundation Trust
and St George's University of London
London, UK

**Roger Bayston**
Professor of Surgical Infection
Head of Biomaterials-Related Infection Group
Chief Investigator
NIHR CAUTI Trial
School of Medicine
University of Nottingham
London, UK

**Katherine Belfield**
Research Fellow
Queen's Medical Centre
University of Nottingham
Nottingham, UK

**James W.F. Catto**
Professor of Urological Surgery
Department of Oncology and Metabolism and Academic Urology Unit
University of Sheffield
Honorary Consultant Urological Surgeon
Royal Hallamshire Hospital
Sheffield Teaching Hospitals NHS Foundation Trust
Sheffield, UK

**Christopher R. Chapple**
Honorary Professor
University of Sheffield
Consultant Urological Surgeon
Section of Functional and Reconstructive Urology
Royal Hallamshire Hospital
Sheffield Teaching Hospitals NHS Foundation Trust
Visiting Professor
Sheffield Hallam University
Sheffield, UK

**Francisco Cruz**
Full Professor and Consultant Urological Surgeon
Faculty of Medicine of Porto and Hospital São João
i3S: Institute for Investigation and Innovation in Health
Porto, Portugal

**Elizabeth Day**
Specialist Registrar in Urological Surgery
West of Scotland
Scotland, UK

**Ian Eardley**
Consultant Urological Surgeon
St James's Hospital
The Leeds Teaching Hospitals NHS Trust
Leeds, UK

**Jason A. Efstathiou**
Consultant in Radiation Oncology and Professor of Radiation Oncology
Department of Radiation Oncology
Harvard Medical School
Massachusetts General Hospital
Boston, Massachusetts, USA

**Judith Hall**
Reader in Molecular Urology
Faculty Medical Sciences
Institute for Cell and Molecular Biosciences
Newcastle University
Newcastle, UK

**Christopher K. Harding**
Consultant Urological Surgeon
Freeman Hospital
The Newcastle upon Tyne Hospitals NHS Foundation Trust
Senior Lecturer
Translational and Clinical Research Institute
Newcastle University
Newcastle, UK

**Jade Harrison**
Specialist Registrar in Urological Surgery
St George's University Hospitals NHS Foundation Trust
London, UK

**Hashim Hashim**
Consultant Urological Surgeon and Honorary Professor of Urology
Bristol Urological Institute
North Bristol NHS Trust
Bristol, UK

**Allan Johnston**
Specialist Registrar in Urological Surgery
Ninewells Hospital
NHS Tayside
Dundee, UK

**Ibrahim Jubber**
PhD Research Fellow and Specialist Registrar in Urological Surgery
Department of Oncology and Metabolism and Academic Urology Unit
University of Sheffield
Royal Hallamshire Hospital
Sheffield Teaching Hospitals NHS Foundation Trust
Sheffield, UK

**Philip A. Kalra**
Professor of Nephrology and Consultant Nephrologist
Salford Royal Hospital
Salford Royal NHS Foundation Trust
Salford, UK

**Sophia C. Kamran**
Consultant in Radiation Oncology and Assistant Professor of Radiation Oncology
Department of Radiation Oncology
Harvard Medical School
Massachusetts General Hospital
Boston, Massachusetts, USA

**Oliver Kayes**
Consultant Urological Surgeon
St James's Hospital
The Leeds Teaching Hospitals NHS Trust
Honorary Senior Lecturer
University of Leeds
Leeds, UK

**Andrei Kozan**
Specialist Registrar in Urological Surgery
St James's Hospital
The Leeds Teaching Hospitals NHS Trust
Leeds, UK

**Alexander Kutikov**
Professor and Chair in Urology and Urologic Oncology
Division of Urologic Oncology
Department of Surgical Oncology
Fox Chase Cancer Center
Temple University Health System
Philadelphia, Pennsylvania, USA

**Michael Laffan**
Professor of Haemostasis and Thrombosis
Faculty of Medicine
Department of Immunology and Inflammation
Imperial College London and Hammersmith Hospital
Imperial College Healthcare NHS Trust
London, UK

**Weida Lau**
Consultant Urological Surgeon
Khoo Teck Puat Hospital
Singapore

**Hing Leung**
Professor of Urology and Surgical Oncology
Institute of Cancer Sciences
Beatson Institute
University of Glasgow
Consultant Urological Surgeon
NHS Greater Glasgow and Clyde
Scotland, UK

**Sanjeev Madaan**
Consultant Urological Surgeon
Darent Valley Hospital
Dartford and Gravesham NHS Trust
Visiting Professor
Canterbury Christ Church University
Kent, UK

**Altaf Mangera**
Consultant Urological Surgeon
Royal Hallamshire Hospital and the Princess Royal
Spinal Cord Injuries Centre
Sheffield Teaching Hospitals NHS Foundation Trust
Sheffield, UK

**Selma Masic**
Society of Urologic Oncology Fellow
Division of Urologic Oncology
Department of Surgical Oncology
Fox Chase Cancer Center
Temple University Health System
Philadelphia, Pennsylvania, USA

**Sarah McClelland**
Senior Lecturer and Group Leader
Queen Mary University of London
Barts Cancer Institute
London, UK

**Saiful Miah**
Consultant Urological Surgeon
Buckinghamshire Healthcare NHS Trust
Oxford University Hospitals NHS Foundation Trust
Oxford, UK

**Masood Moghul**
Specialist Registrar in Urological Surgery and Research
Fellow
Barts Cancer Institute
Queen Mary University of London
London, UK

**Asif Muneer**
Associate Professor in Urological Surgery and
Consultant Urological Surgeon
Institute of Andrology
University College London Hospital
NIHR Biomedical Research Centre UCLH and Division
of Surgery and Interventional Science
University College London
London, UK

**Jonathon Olsburgh**
Consultant Transplant Urological Surgeon
Guy's Hospital
Guy's and St Thomas' NHS Foundation Trust
London, UK

**Nadir I. Osman**
Consultant Urological Surgeon
Section of Functional and Reconstructive Urology
Royal Hallamshire Hospital
Sheffield Teaching Hospitals NHS Foundation Trust
Honorary Clinical Senior Lecturer
University of Sheffield
Sheffield, UK

**Fausto Palazzo**
Professor and Consultant in Endocrine Surgery
Hammersmith Hospital
Imperial College Healthcare NHS Trust
London, UK

**Karl H. Pang**
Specialist Registrar in Urological Surgery
Yorkshire and Humber Deanery
Honorary Clinical Lecturer
Department of Oncology and Metabolism and
Academic Urology Unit
University of Sheffield
Sheffield, UK

**Sanjeev Pathak**
Consultant Urological Surgeon
Royal Hallamshire Hospital
Sheffield Teaching Hospitals NHS Foundation Trust
Honorary Clinical Senior Lecturer
University of Sheffield
Sheffield, UK

**Thomas Powles**
Professor of Genitourinary Oncology
Barts Experimental Cancer Medicine Centre
Barts Cancer Institute
Queen Mary University of London
Consultant Medical Oncologist
St Bartholomew's Hospital
Barts Health NHS Trust
London, UK

**Stephen Radley**
Consultant Urogynaecologist
Royal Hallamshire Hospital
Sheffield Teaching Hospitals NHS Foundation Trust
Honorary Professor
University of Sheffield
Sheffield, UK

**Prabhakar Rajan**
Clinical Senior Lecturer
Barts Cancer Institute
Queen Mary University of London
Consultant Urological Surgeon
University College London Hospitals and Barts Health
NHS Trusts
London, UK

**Sabrina H. Rossi**
PhD Researcher
Academic Urology Group
Department of Surgery
University of Cambridge
Specialist Registrar in Urological Surgery
Addenbrooke's Hospital
Cambridge University Hospitals NHS Foundation Trust
Cambridge, UK

**Maria Satchi**
Consultant Urological Surgeon
Darent Valley Hospital
Dartford and Gravesham NHS Trust
Kent, UK

**Majid Shabbir**
Consultant Urological Surgeon
Guy's Hospital
Guy's and St Thomas' NHS Foundation Trust
Honorary Senior Lecturer
King's College London
London, UK

**Joanna Shepherd**
Specialist Registrar in Obstetrics and Gynaecology
Royal Hallamshire Hospital
Sheffield Teaching Hospitals NHS Foundation Trust
Sheffield, UK

**João Silva**
Invited Professor and Consultant Urological Surgeon
Faculty of Medicine of Porto and Hospital São João
i3S: Institute for Investigation and Innovation in Health
Porto, Portugal

**Seshadri Sriprasad**
Consultant Urological Surgeon
Darent Valley Hospital
Dartford and Gravesham NHS Trust
Professor of Urological Surgery
Canterbury Christ Church University
Kent, UK

**Abhishek Srivastava**
Society of Urologic Oncology Fellow
Division of Urologic Oncology
Department of Surgical Oncology
Fox Chase Cancer Center
Temple University Health System
Philadelphia, Pennsylvania, USA

**Grant D. Stewart**
Professor of Surgical Oncology
Academic Urology Group
Department of Surgery
University of Cambridge
Honorary Consultant Urological Surgeon
Addenbrooke's Hospital
Cambridge University Hospitals NHS Foundation Trust
Cambridge, UK

**Paul Sturch**
Specialist Registrar in Urological Surgery
Darent Valley Hospital
Dartford and Gravesham NHS Trust
Kent, UK

**Lynne Sykes**
Specialist Registrar in Nephrology and General
Internal Medicine
Salford Royal Hospital
Salford Royal NHS Foundation Trust
Salford, UK

**Bernadett Szabados**
Consultant Urological Surgeon
University College London Hospital
Clinical Research Fellow
Barts Experimental Cancer Medicine Centre
Barts Cancer Institute
Queen Mary University of London
London, UK

**Joseph Tam**
Clinical Research Fellow
Imperial College London
Imperial College Healthcare NHS Trust
London, UK

**Nicholas A. Watkin**
Consultant Urological Surgeon
St George's Hospital
St George's University Hospitals NHS Foundation Trust
Professor of Urology
St George's University of London
London, UK

**Thomas E. Webb**
Specialty Doctor in Urological Surgery
Airedale Hospital
Airedale NHS Foundation Trust
Yorkshire, UK

**Rhana H. Zakri**
Consultant Transplant Urological Surgeon
Guy's Hospital
Guy's and St Thomas' NHS Foundation Trust
London, UK

# Abbreviations

| | | | |
|---|---|---|---|
| 5AR (i) | 5-alpha-reductase (inhibitor) | EPN | emphysematous pyelonephritis |
| Ab | antibody | EPO | erythropoietin |
| ABU | asymptomatic bacteriuria | ER | endoplasmic reticulum |
| AC | adenylyl cyclase | ERAS | enhanced recovery after surgery |
| ACTH | adrenocorticotrophic hormone | ESBL | extended-spectrum beta-lactamases |
| AD | autonomic dysreflexia | ESRF | end-stage renal failure |
| ADH | anti-diuretic hormone | ESSIS | European Society for the Study of Interstitial Cystitis |
| ADT | androgen deprivation therapy | | |
| AFP | alpha-fetoprotein | FAD | flavin adenine dinucleotide |
| Ag | antigen | FDA | Food and Drug Administration |
| AKI | acute kidney injury | FGF | fibroblast growth factor |
| AMH | anti-Müllerian hormone | FSH | follicle stimulating hormones |
| AML | angiomyolipoma | GAG | glycosaminoglycan |
| ANP | atrial natriuretic peptide | GBM | glomerular basement membrane |
| APC | antigen presenting cells | GFR | glomerular filtration rate |
| ARDS | acute respiratory distress syndrome | GN | glomerulonephritis |
| ATN | acute renal tubular necrosis | GnRH | gonadotrophin releasing hormone |
| ATP | adenosine triphosphate | GTP | guanosine triphosphate |
| BC | bladder cancer | hCG | human chorionic gonadotropin |
| BCG | Bacillus Calmette–Guérin | HIF | hypoxia-inducible factor |
| BEC | bladder epithelial cells | HLA | Human Leucocyte Antigen |
| BMI | body mass index | HPV | Human Papilloma Virus |
| BNF | British National Formulary | IARC | International Agency for Research on Cancer |
| BOO | bladder outlet obstruction | | |
| BPH | benign prostatic hyperplasia | ICSI | intracytoplasmic sperm injection |
| cAMP | cyclic adenosine monophosphate | IELT | intravaginal ejaculation latency time |
| CDK | cyclin dependent kinase | IFN | interferon |
| CFU | colony forming units | IIEF | International Index of Erectile Function |
| cGMP | cyclic guanosine monophosphate | IL | interleukin |
| Chm | chromosome | IMDC | International Metastatic RCC Database Consortium |
| CIT | cold ischaemia time | | |
| CKD | chronic kidney disease | IMRT | intensity modulated radiation therapy |
| CKD EPI | Chronic Kidney Disease Epidemiology Collaboration | IS | immunosuppression |
| | | IP3 | inositol triphosphate |
| CNS | central nervous system | IRI | ischaemic reperfusion injury |
| CPPS | chronic pelvic pain syndrome | ISUP | International Society of Urological Pathology |
| CRP | C reactive protein | | |
| DBD | donation after brain death | IPSS | International Prostate Symptom Score |
| DCD | donation after circulatory death | IVC | inferior vena cava |
| DCT | distal convoluted tubule | LDH | lactate dehydrogenase |
| DGF | delayed graft function | LH | luteinising hormone |
| DHT | dihydrotestosterone | LMP | last menstrual period |
| DNA | deoxyribonucleic acid | LOH | loop of Henle |
| DSD | detrusor-sphincter-dyssynergia | LUT | lower urinary tract |
| EAU | European Association of Urology | MDR | multidrug-resistant |
| EBRT | external beam radiation therapy | MDRD | modification of diet in renal disease |
| ECM | extracellular matrix | MHC | major histocompatibility complex |
| ED | erectile dysfunction | MIS | müllerian inhibitory substance |
| EMT | epithelial-mesenchymal transition | MLC | myosin light chain |
| EORTC | European Organisation for Research and Treatment of Cancer | MMR | mismatch repair |
| | | mRNA | messenger RNA |

| | |
|---|---|
| mTOR | mammalian Target of Rapamycin |
| NAD | nicotinamide adenine dinucleotide |
| NICE | National Institute for Health and Care Excellence |
| NK | natural killer cells |
| NO | nitric oxide |
| NOS | nitric oxide synthase |
| PCR | polymerase chain reaction |
| PCT | proximal convoluted tubule |
| PDE5i | phosphodiesterase 5 inhibitors |
| PDGF | platelet-derived growth factor |
| PD-1 | programmed cell death protein 1 |
| PD-L1 | programmed cell death ligand 1 |
| PET | positron emission tomography |
| PLC | phospholipase C |
| PMC | pontine micturition centre |
| PTH | parathyroid hormone |
| qSOFA | quick sequential organ failure assessment |
| RAA | renin-angiotensin-aldosterone |
| RE | retrograde ejaculation |
| RNA | ribonucleic acid |
| RT | radiation therapy |
| SHBG | sex hormone binding globulin |
| SIRS | systemic inflammatory response syndrome |

| | |
|---|---|
| SM | smooth muscle |
| SRY | sex-determining region Y gene |
| TB | tuberculosis |
| TCA | tricarboxylic acid (also termed citric acid or Krebs cycle) |
| TCGA | The Cancer Genome Atlas |
| TGF | transforming growth factor |
| THP | Tamm-Horsfall protein |
| TLR | toll-like receptor |
| TNF | tumour necrosis factor |
| TRUS | transrectal ultrasound |
| TSG | tumour suppressor gene |
| TURBT | transurethral resection of bladder tumour |
| UCC | urothelial cell carcinoma |
| UDT | undescended testis |
| UICC | Union for International Cancer Control |
| UP | uroplakin |
| UPEC | uropathogenic *Escherichia coli* |
| UTI | urinary tract infection |
| UTUC | upper urinary tract urothelial carcinoma |
| VEGF | vascular endothelial growth factor |
| VHL | von Hippel-Lindau |
| WIT | warm ischaemia time |

# Preface

Surgeons should understand biology, pathology, and the interaction of both in the organism they work with. We should know when and how to intervene and, just as importantly, when not to. At the most elemental level, basic science covers the biology of these systems and forms the fundamental basis of surgery. Whilst readers may use this information to pass exams, we believe this biology is fascinating and offers many insights to improve patient care. For example, common evolutionary pressures drive bacteria to develop antibiotic resistance, and prostate cancer cells to escape androgen deprivation, whilst there are disparate distinct physiologies that arise from upper and lower urinary tract obstruction.

We wrote this book with candidates taking the theoretical component of postgraduate Urology examinations in mind. Exit examinations are required at the end of specialist Urology training in most countries to ensure that trainees meet the required competencies to become independent practitioners. Basic science is invariably assessed, usually in the form of a written exam. This part is often challenging for trainees as the subjects encountered may have last been studied during undergraduate medical education.

A synopsis of the scientific basis of urological practice is provided, including embryology, anatomy, physiology, microbiology, immunology, pharmacology, and the pathogenesis of disease processes. These are subjects that underpin clinical practice and are important in understanding the clinical features of diseases and the basis of treatment. We have written and formatted the text in bullet points that covers the essential areas in an easy-to-access format. The text is not intended as a substitute for the larger, more comprehensive textbooks.

Each chapter was led by an expert in the field and we thank all authors for their hard work in putting this book together. We hope you enjoy this book and find it helpful, and good luck to those sitting examinations.

**Karl H. Pang**
**Nadir I. Osman**
**James W.F. Catto**
**Christopher R. Chapple**

# Foreword

In general, the quantity of scientific information in the health and the life sciences sector doubles every nine years. Not all of it represents a step-change in how we think about disease processes and physiology; often, it is incremental. Nevertheless, some of what we are taught in medical school soon becomes out-of-date and, over a working lifetime, much of this knowledge is either incomplete or frankly, sometimes even wrong. Keeping up-to-date is a key attribute for a doctor, alongside with the humility to acknowledge that the wrong type of care will be provided unless we work within our capacity, knowledge, and expertise.

A working knowledge of the basic sciences that underpin mechanisms of disease and the body's response is widely recognised to be a critical part of urological training and is assessed towards the end. Some urologists will contribute through their academic work to increase our knowledge base in specific areas that will impact on the treatments and modes of management that we offer to patients. Others spend much of their time working with patients and also contribute to teaching and training in highly significant ways. All require an understanding of the basic sciences as they are applied to urology.

The authors of this book have gathered an impressive group of clinicians and scientists to distil complex knowledge into excellent summaries of their particular field. The chapters cover anatomy and physiology, the basic principles of immunology and oncology, and particular diseases. This book is aimed at trainees to ensure they are up-to-date with this breadth of knowledge and will be used to revise the basic sciences component of final assessments for urological trainees. The authors are largely based in the UK and bring a succinctness and clarity to the topics that will enable all to get the latest summary of the field. The book deserves to get a wider acceptance globally and I can strongly recommend it.

**Professor David E. Neal**
CBE, FMedSci, FRCS
Professor Emeritus of Surgical Oncology
Nuffield Department of Surgical Sciences
University of Oxford

# Section I

## BASIC MECHANISMS

# 1 Cellular and Immunobiology

*Masood Moghul, Sarah McClelland, and Prabhakar Rajan*

## Cell Structure

- The cell contains fluid (cytoplasm) and intracellular structures enclosed by a lipid membrane (Figure 1.1).
- *Cytoplasm:* gel-like substance which forms majority of the cellular volume (90%).
  - Contains specialised subunits (organelles), cytoskeletal fibres, free molecules, proteins, carbohydrates, lipids, and DNA/RNA.

## Cell (Plasma) Membrane

- Phospholipid bilayer derived from fatty acids with a hydrophobic core and a hydrophilic exterior.
- Impermeable to water; fully permeable to gases and lipophilic molecules.
- Acts as the first barrier to protect the cell from the external environment.
- Proteins are found within the membrane and can freely move within it. Important roles of these proteins include:
  - Transport receptors, enzymes, and adhesion molecules.

## Cytoplasmic Organelles
### Nucleus

- Contains the genetic information of the cell and is surrounded by a double membrane nuclear envelope.
- Contains DNA arranged in a double helix structure, grouped in 23 chromosome pairs.
  - *Chromosomal DNA:* condensed form of tightly wound DNA with associated histone proteins which allow DNA coiling and packaging into a superhelix (a helix within another helix).
    - One pair of sex chromosomes (XX, XY) and 22 pairs of autosomes.
- Contains subnuclear structures (nucleoplasm, nucleoli, cajal bodies, and speckles).
  - Contain a variety of proteins and nucleic acids involved in gene regulation and signalling.

- Has pores (nuclear pores) for the active transport of large molecules.

## Endoplasmic Reticulum (ER)

- There are two types of ER (rough and smooth) - both are formed by flattened membranous sheets.
- The *rough ER* has ribosomes on its surface and is key in protein manufacture.
  - Ribosomes are molecular machines—sites of *protein synthesis*.
- *Smooth ER*
  - Involved in lipid synthesis.
  - Contains the enzyme p450 in the liver, which breaks down lipid-soluble drugs.

## Golgi Apparatus

- Similar structure to ER.
- Accepts protein-containing vesicles from the rough ER.
- Sorts, modifies, and packages proteins for secretion.

## Mitochondria

- Power plant of the cell; producing energy in the form of adenosine triphosphate (ATP).
- Has a double membrane enclosing a matrix which contains hundreds of enzymes.

## Intracellular Molecules
### Proteins

- Biomolecules made from variable length chains of amino acids.
- The 20 different amino acids can combine to make an unlimited number of proteins.
  - Some amino acids are indispensable (*essential*).
    - Cannot be synthesised within humans.
    - Required through diet (lysine, threonine, and tryptophan).
- Some amino acids can be synthesised (*non-essential*), but often not quickly enough to meet

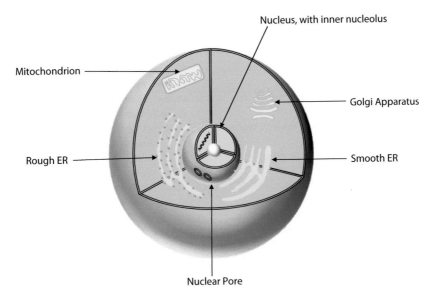

**Figure 1.1** Diagram of a human cell.

bodily demands. These may be included in the essential category.

- Proteins can be classified depending on the function:
- *Structural proteins* (e.g., collagen, keratin)
  - Provide form and structure both within and between cells.
- *Enzymes*
  - Catalysts for chemical reactions.
- *Gene expression* (e.g., transcription factors)
- *Intercellular communication* (e.g., growth factors and hormones)

- *Primary* structure: amino acid sequence.
- *Secondary* structure: amino acid chains organised into α-helix, β-strand, or β-sheets.
  - Held together by hydrogen bonds.
  - A single protein can contain multiple secondary structures.
- *Tertiary* structure: three-dimensional folding of the secondary structures.
  - Utilises weak bonds which make the tertiary structure malleable.
- *Quaternary* structure: multiple protein interaction which forms a new structure.

## Lipids

- Lipids are made from fatty acids which form a chain—the longer the chain, the less water soluble it is.
- *Saturated* fatty acids: no double bonds between carbon atoms in hydrocarbon chain.
- *Unsaturated* fatty acids: double bonds are present.
- *Lipophilic ligands* (e.g., steroids)

- Bind to cytoplasmic receptors and can freely diffuse the cell membrane.
- Once activated, receptors pass into the nucleus to induce gene transcription.

## Deoxyribonucleic Acid (DNA) and Ribonucleic Acid (RNA)

- Both are nucleic acids made from organic molecules called nucleotides, consisting of:
  - A *nitrogenous base* (thymine or uracil in RNA, cytosine, adenine, guanine).
  - A *5-carbon sugar* (ribose or deoxyribose).
  - One or more *phosphate* groups (acid).
- DNA is formed as an H-shape spiral (double helix).
- The nucleotides attach to each other via phosphodiester bonds.
- The bases of each nucleotide interact with the opposing base on the other side of the chain (forming the horizontal bar).
- Each nucleotide base can only bond with one type of base (base pairing):
  - G⇔C
  - A⇔T/A⇔U in RNA
- A *codon* is a three sequence of base pairs.
  - Codes for a specific amino acid.
- Chromosomes contain genetic information that codes for protein formation.
- Areas that code for proteins are used by RNA polymerase enzymes to form messenger RNA (mRNA).
  - mRNAs are found in the nucleus and cytoplasm and are involved in the next stage of protein formation.

- mRNA also acts as a cellular messenger (non-coding RNA).

## Others

- *Carbohydrates:* major source of energy for the cell.
- *ATP:* utilised by all cells to transfer energy from the breakdown of glucose.
  - ATP → ADP: releases a phosphate group and energy.
- *Free Ions:* sodium, potassium, calcium, chloride, and magnesium are all found within cells.
  - *Sodium and Potassium:* maintain electric balance at the cell membrane and play key roles in generating nerve cell action potential.
  - *Calcium:* involved in signal transduction and muscle contraction.
  - *Chloride:* involved in action potential.
  - *Magnesium:* catalyst for enzymes and activates ATP.

## Cellular Processes

## Cell Cycle

- *Cells*
  - Constant cycling through different phases of the cell cycle.
  - Continuously being lost via programmed cell death (apoptosis).

- Different cells have different replication rates.
- Certain cells cannot divide and can still be damaged and lost (e.g., neuronal cells and skeletal muscle fibres).
- Phases of the cell cycle include (Figure 1.2):
  - *Interphase*
    - *G1 phase* (Gap): some cells enter *G0* (rest) phase.
    - *S Phase* (Synthesis): DNA/chromosome replication.
    - *G2 Phase:* rest.
  - *Mitosis (M phase)*
    - *Prophase:* chromosome condensation.
    - *Prometaphase:* kinetochores form upon centromeres and attach to spindle fibres.
    - *Metaphase:* chromosomes align at the centre of cell.
    - *Anaphase:* spindle fibres separate chromosomes, pulling them towards spindle poles.
    - *Telophase:* nuclear membrane reforms.
    - *Cytokinesis:* cytoplasm separates in half.
  - *Checkpoints* at *G1/S, G2/M,* and *metaphase* control entry prior to the next phase to
    - Check whether the cell is big enough,
    - Confirm if the environment is favourable enough.
    - Check the DNA integrity (G2) and chromosomal alignment on spindles (metaphase).

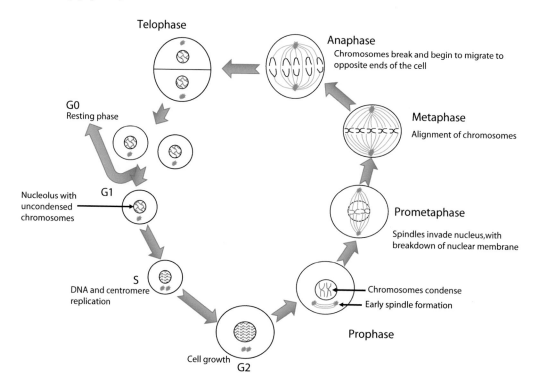

**Figure 1.2** Mitosis and the cell cycle.

- Cells need to be able to replicate accurately without coding errors, which can affect cellular function.
  - Replication requires the DNA to become unwound at 'replication forks'.
  - Many forks simultaneously replicate each chromosome.
  - DNA polymerases act on both strands to copy DNA.
- Replication errors can occur due to incorrect base insertion or incorrect number of nucleotides.
  - Errors are normally repaired by nucleotide excision enzymes or repair enzymes.
  - Unrepaired errors give rise to cell dysfunction and mutations and are involved in cancer development.

## Cell Death

- Death occurs when the cell has aged or has suffered an insult, rendering it unable to function.
- Balance between cell growth and cell death is important in disease development.
- Programmed cell death (PCD).
- The cell is destroyed without causing inflammation in an energy-dependent process
  - Two types of PCD—overlapping pathways. The cell is removed by macrophages.

*Apoptosis/Type I Death*
- Mechanisms:
- *Extrinsic*: activation of transmembrane proteins (e.g., TNFR or tumour necrosis factor receptor).
- *Intrinsic*: caused by ionising radiation or chemotherapy.
- Activation of intracellular proteins (BCL2 family) to permeate the mitochondrial membrane and activate proteolytic enzymes.
- Cell shrinks with organelle breakdown.
- DNA condenses while permeability of the cell membrane increases.

*Autophagic/Type II Death*
- Intracellular products are surrounded by a cell membrane.
- New structure is termed as *autophagosome*.
- Fuses with lysosomes where enzymes destroy the contents.

*Necrosis/Type III Death*
- Cell is destroyed due to damage.
- Causes cell swelling and leakage of intracellular contents, causing inflammation.

## Cell Metabolism

- Metabolic pathways are continuously active to generate energy and carry out designated functions.
- Catalysed by enzymes.

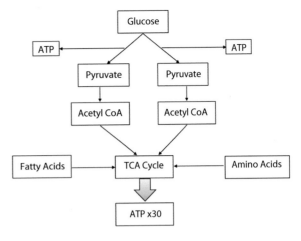

Figure 1.3 An overview of cell metabolism.

- *TCA (tricarboxylic acid, citric acid, or Krebs) cycle* is the main source of cellular energy from aerobic metabolism (Figure 1.3).
- Glucose is the most common energy source, but fats and proteins can also be used.
- Glucose undergoes glycolysis in the cytoplasm and releases two ATP molecules.

- *TCA (Krebs) cycle* takes place within the mitochondria.
  - As acetyl CoA is oxidised, it de-oxidises (reduces) electron carriers NAD and FAD → NADH, FADH$_2$.
  - NAD and FAD pass their electrons into the electron transport chain—oxidative phosphorylation.
  - As electrons pass along the chain, they lose energy, which is used to pump hydrogen ions into inter-membrane space of mitochondria, causing an electrochemical gradient.
  - Hydrogen flows back down the electrochemical current and through membrane enzyme *ATP synthase*, producing ATP.
    - This process is called *chemiosmosis* and yields the most ATP from glucose.
- At times of cellular stress
  - Proteins are broken down into amino acids for energy source and enter the TCA cycle.
  - Ammonia, a highly toxic byproduct of amino acid breakdown, must be excreted.
    - The conversion of ammonia into urea (urea cycle) takes place in the liver (and to a lesser extent, in the kidneys).

## Vesicle Trafficking

- Small molecules and ions can pass freely.
- Larger molecules require specialised transport processes—endocytosis and exocytosis.

## Endocytosis

- A cell absorbs external material through phagocytosis and pinocytosis.

- *Phagocytosis*: the absorption of *large particles* or *cells*.
  - Important immune mechanism to remove dead tissue.
  - Phagocytic cells activated by antibodies cause cell-cell adhesion with the cell, engulfing its target.
  - Conducted by the Rho-family GTPases.

- *Pinocytosis*: the absorption of *liquid* into the cell.
  - Invagination of cell membrane.
  - *Larger* molecules trigger projections from the cell membrane—crumpling and fusing with it.
  - *Smaller* molecules absorbed after binding with receptors in small pits are contained in the cell membrane and are dependent on specialist proteins (calveolin or clathrin).

## Exocytosis

- Golgi apparatus receives proteins from the ER and packages them for exocytosis.
  - Stored in vesicles until signals are received, triggering their transport to the cell membrane.
  - Fusion of vesicle to the cell membrane triggered by SNARE proteins.
  - Exocytosis may be calcium-dependent (regulated) (e.g., nerve cells) or -independent (unregulated).
  - Exocytosis also expels messages outside the cell to communicate with the environment.

## Gene Regulation/Expression

- Gene expression is the conversion of genetic information from DNA into proteins.
- Its stages include transcription and translation.

## Transcription (Nucleus)

- Double helix DNA
  - One strand to code for a protein during transcription.
  - Another strand is for *non-coding*.
- *Initiation:* RNA polymerase attaches to DNA.
  - Attaches upstream to the gene (5′) at specialised DNA sequences (promoters).
- *Elongation:* as DNA unwinds, RNA polymerase adds nucleotides, forming pre-mRNA.
- *Termination:* RNA polymerase stops, pre-mRNA is released, and the two DNA strands reform the double helix.
- Start and stop codons indicate where RNA polymerase begins and ends.
- Pre-mRNA is matured to form mRNA.

- *5′ capping* protects degradation by RNase by adding a methylated guanine cap.
- *Polyadenylation* stabilises RNA by adding a poly(A) tail to the 3′ end.
- *Splicing* is where non-coding introns are removed by spliceosome excision. Coding exons are joined together by ligation.

## Translation (Cytoplasm)

- mRNA exits the nucleus and attaches to ribosomes.
- Ribosomes consist of 60S and 40S subunits.
- *Initiation:* initiation factor proteins bind to the smaller ribosomal subunit and attach at the start (mRNA AUG) codon, forming the initiation complex. Larger subunits bind later.
- Transfer RNA (tRNA) is formed when amino acids bind to mRNA codons.
- *Elongation:* as ribosome complex reads each codon, tRNA molecules attach reciprocally, forming peptide bonds and the peptide chain.
- mRNA open reading frame (ORF) are translated into proteins.
- mRNA 5′ and 3′ ends have untranslated regions (UTR).
- *Termination:* stop codons (UAG, UGA, UAA) end the sequence and peptide is released.
- Post-translational modifications modify existing proteins by adding/removing molecules.
  - Can change both structure and function of proteins.
  - Common methods include phosphorylation, ubiquitylation, and sumoylation.

## Control of Gene Expression and Epigenetics

- Different cells within the human body contain the same DNA.
  - Functionally very different due to differences in the genes they express.
- Epigenetic processes are reversible as opposed to genetic processes. Affect gene expression mainly in transcription, but can also affect translation.
- Epigenetic processes can be inherited by cells after mitotic division. Processes include:
  - Cytosine methylation.
  - Post-translational modification of histone proteins and remodelling of chromatin.
  - Transcription factors binding to specific DNA sequences to promote/inhibit gene expression.
  - MicroRNA binds to specific mRNA sequence, inhibiting gene expression.

## Signal Transduction

- Activated receptors perform an action or trigger a chain of events to fulfil their function.

- *Intracellular pathways* carry out receptors' function within the cell.
  - Some lipid rich molecules such as hormones (e.g., testosterone, progesterone) pass directly into the cell and bind to receptors.
  - Most cannot, and require binding with transmembrane receptors (e.g., G protein-coupled and receptor tyrosine kinases).
  - These, then, require second messengers (e.g., cyclic AMP and GMP) to further propagate the signal within the cell.

# DNA Damage and Repair
## Nucleotide Excision Repair

- Damage to the genetic code must be promptly recognised and repaired.
- Ultraviolet radiation damages DNA by causing cyclobutane pyrimidine dimers and 6-4 photoproducts lesions on the DNA.
  - Alters DNA structure, impeding correct replication and transcription.
  - Lesions are excised with the recognition, removal, and replacement of the damaged DNA—*'nucleotide excision repair'*.
  - *Base excision repair* occurs with localised damage (from free radicals).
- Cancer cells (many mutation errors) inhibit repair enzymes (e.g., Poly (ADP-ribose) polymerase, PARP) and lead to their death.
  - Implicated in developing new therapies.

## Homologous Recombination (HR) and Non-Homologous End Joining (NHEJ)

- Repairs double-stranded breakages in DNA.
- NHEJ is more frequently used as it acts throughout the cell cycle.
  - HR occurs in the late S or G2 phases.
- HR is more accurate at repair than NHEJ as it uses a DNA template.
  - NHEJ repairs damaged DNA ends and has a higher tolerance for errors.

## DNA Mismatch Repair (MMR)

- Focuses on DNA errors in replication and prevents its propagation in daughter cells.
- Focuses on base pair mismatching or insertion/deletion errors.
- Can result in arrest of cell cycle or apoptosis.

## Migration/Movement

- Cell movement needed for wound healing, immunity, development, and maintenance of the human body.

- Involves extracellular factors which act as chemoattractive agents.
  - Cause polymerisation of actin cytoskeleton at the leading edge of the cell.
- Filament projections from cell membrane attach to extracellular matrix (ECM) or other cells, which provide traction and contractility.
- Simultaneously on opposite end of the cell, reverse occurs with retraction of adhesional structures (polarisation of the cell).
- Various oncogenes increase cell motility or dissociate the cell from its surrounding tissues.

# Intracellular Connections/Cell Adhesion

- Cells require adhesional structures to keep them in specific arrangements required for different tissues.
- These connections are to surrounding cells and ECM.

## Cadherins

- Transmembrane receptors dependent on calcium.
- Binds cadherin molecules in adjacent cells (adherens junctions).
- Binds cytoplasmic actin cytoskeleton, increasing adhesional strength.
- E-Cadherin is important in epithelial adhesion and suppresses epithelial tumour invasion.

## Desmosomal Junctions

- Rely on cadherin receptors.
- Tether cells to intermediate filament cytoskeletal network.
  - Less motile than actin filaments.
  - Provide an overriding structural integrity to epithelial and cardiac tissue.

## Tight Junctions

- Formed from the fusion of plasma membranes of adjacent cells with the transmembrane proteins claudin and occludin.

## Gap Junctions

- Hydrophilic pores between cells.
- Composed of protein connexin, which allows diffusion of small molecules and ions.

# Immunology
## Inflammation

- This is a response to injury in living tissue with a local increase of plasma and phagocytic cells.
  - Protective.

- Designed to limit damage and remove non-viable tissue.
- Inappropriate activity occurs in autoimmune conditions.
- *Mechanisms* of injury:
  - Mechanical, infective, chemical, radiation, ischaemic.
- *Physical characteristics:* calor (heat), dolour (pain), rubor (redness), and tumour (swelling).

- *Mechanisms:*
1. Changes in *microcirculation*
   - Vasodilation and increased permeability of vessels → calor, rubor.
   - Exudation → oedema (tumour).
   - Loss of water, electrolytes, and proteins into the interstitium.
   - Increased intravascular hydrostatic pressure.
   - Decreased plasma oncotic pressure.

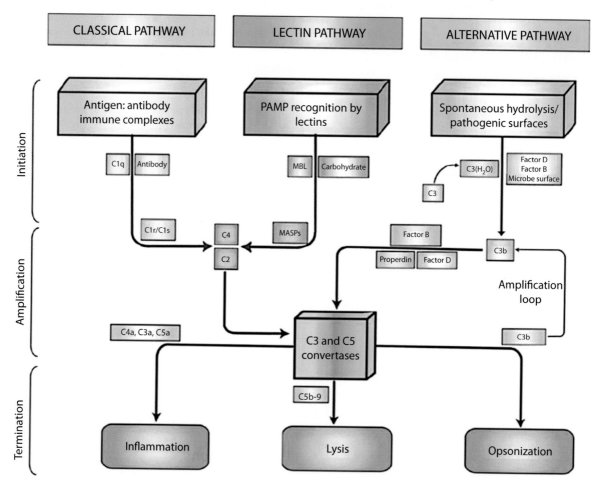

**Figure 1.4** The complement pathway. The *Classical Pathway* is activated when C1q binds to antibody attached to antigen, activating C1r and C1s, which cleave C4 and C2. The *Lectin Pathway* is activated when Mannose-binding Lectin (MBL) encounters conserved pathogenic carbohydrate motifs, activating the MBL-associated Serine Proteases (MASPs) and again cleaving C4 and C2. C4 and C2 cleavage products Form the classical and lectin pathway C3 convertase, C4bC2a, which cleaves C3 into C3b and C3a. A second molecule of C3b can associate with C4bC2a to form the C5 convertase of the classical and lectin pathways, C4bC2aC3b. The *Alternative Pathway* (AP) is activated when C3 undergoes spontaneous hydrolysis and forms the initial AP C3 convertase, C3(H$_2$O)Bb, in the presence of factors B and D, leading to additional C3 cleavage and eventual formation of the AP C3 convertase (C3bBb) and AP C5 convertase (C3bBbC3b). Properdin facilitates AP activation by stabilising AP convertases. All three pathways culminate in the formation of the convertases, which in turn generate the major effectors of the complement system: anaphylatoxins (C4a/C3a/C5a), the Membrane Attack Complex (MAC) and opsonins (e.g., C3b). Anaphylatoxins are potent proinflammatory molecules derived from the cleavage of C4, C3 and C5. The MAC is a terminal assembly of complement components C5b through C9, which can directly lyse targeted surfaces. C3b induces phagocytosis of opsonized targets and also serves to amplify complement activation through the AP. (Reprinted by permission from Springer Nature [12])

2. *Leucocyte activation* and *chemotaxis* towards inflammation
   - Initially mediated by neutrophils.
   - Later activation of monocytes → macrophages
   - Different to neutrophils:
     - Longer life span can undergo cell division.
     - Reciprocal activation with T- and B-lymphocytes.
   - Phagocytosis of dead tissue/microorganisms
     - The coating of designated cells with proteins (IgG or complement) is required.
     - The membrane of the phagocyte engulfs the cell (phagosome), then passes into the cytoplasm.
     - The formation of hydrogen peroxide to kill the phagosome.
- Endogenous mediators of inflammation:
   - *Complement:* coats microorganisms with proteins (opsonisation).
   - TNF-α and IL-1.
   - Secreted by activated macrophages, providing a positive feedback loop for the inflammatory response.

## Innate Immunity

- Found in all organisms due to its ancient origins compared to acquired immunity.
- Fast-acting, non-specific response to pathogens without the development of clonal expansion seen in adaptive immunity.
- Overlaps with inflammatory pathways.
- *First-line* includes barriers (e.g., skin, mucus, and stomach acid).

- Initiation of innate immunity begins with pattern recognition receptors:
   - *C-type lectin receptors:* activated by sugars on yeast, bacterial, and fungal cell walls.
   - *Toll-like receptors:* results in the activation of NFκβ, causing transcription of immune genes.
   - *NOD-like receptors:* involved in intracellular pattern recognition (when the pathogen infiltrates host cells).
   - *Retinoid acid-inducible gene 1 like receptors:* produces cytokine IFN-β.
- *Complement proteins* are involved in enzyme cascades and cause cell damage via a membrane attack complex (Figure 1.4):
   - Classical pathway
     - C1 ← → IgM/G → C3 + C5 production
   - Alternative pathway
   - Lectin pathway
- Once cells have been activated, they attack pathogens
   - *NK cells*
     - Kill cells infected by viruses.
     - Recognise MHC Class 1 and prevent the destruction of healthy cells.
   - *Phagocytes* (e.g., neutrophils, macrophages)
   - *Dendritic cells*
     - Phagocytic cells connect innate and adaptive immunity.
     - Break proteins into small chains; presented to T-cells via MHC.

## Acquired/Adaptive Immunity

- *Second line* of defence if pathogens survive innate immunity responses.

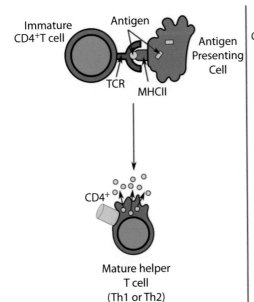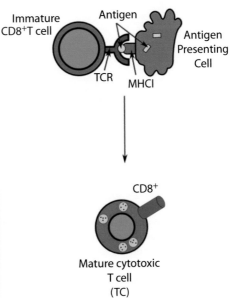

Figure 1.5 Antigen presentation and activation of T-cells.

- Involves antigen presentation and activation of T-cells (Figure 1.5).
- Cells characterised by the response are produced in the bone marrow.
- Stored in lymph nodes for rapid activation.
- Adaptive immune cells retain a memory and enable rapid activation in case of re-infection.
- Once activated, cells undergo clonal expansion.
  - Each activated cell produces over one thousand clones—each with the same specific antigen activity.
- *Major histocompatibility complex (MHC):*
  - Group of glycoproteins.
  - Bind foreign peptides; presented for T-cell activation.
  - *Two MHC classes* (chromosome 6):
    - *Class 1*
      - Seen on most cells.
      - Approximately nine amino acids.
      - Binds to intracellular proteins.
      - Activate CD4 cells.
  - *Class 2*
    - Seen on certain immune cells (e.g., dendritic cells).
    - Up to 25 amino acids.
    - Binds to extracellular proteins.
    - Activate CD8 and dendritic cells (viral breakdown products from virally infected cells).
- *Lymphocytes*—main cells of adaptive immunity.
- *T lymphocytes*—produced in the bone marrow, with a random production of receptors on each cell.
  - Continuously recirculate between lymphatics and blood.
  - Activated by antigens bound to MHC.
  - *Types:*
    - *CD4* (Th, helper cells)
      - Binds to MHC 2 during activation of the T-cell receptor.

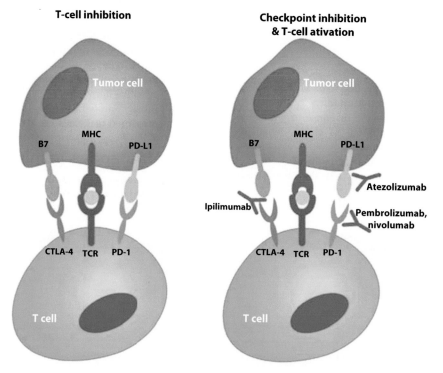

**Figure 1.6** T-Cell coinhibitory receptor expression and checkpoint inhibition. Tumour cells and antigen presenting cells (APCs) express a specific antigen that is presented to cytotoxic T-cells in a peptide major histocompatibility complex (MHC). T-cells recognise this presented antigen with their t-cell receptor (TCR) and, together with binding of costimulatory receptors (e.g., CD28); this leads to T-cell activation and subsequently elimination of the (tumour) cell. Interaction of coinhibitory receptors on T-cells with their ligands on APCs or tumour cells inhibits T-cell activation. Known coinhibitory receptors are PD-1 (that interacts with its ligand PD-L1) and CTLA-4. Blocking antibodies against these coinhibitory receptors or their ligands can prevent their interaction and the subsequent inhibition of T-cell activity. CTLA-4, cytotoxic T lymphocyte-associated protein 4; PD-1, programmed cell death 1; PD-L1, programmed cell death receptor ligand 1. (Reprinted with permission from Elsevier [14])

- Recruit other cells by cytokine production (IL, IFN-y, TGFB).
- *CD8* (Tc, cytotoxic cells)
  - Binds to MHC 1 during activation of the T-cell receptor.
  - Once activated, they kill cells with specific MHC 1.
- *B-lymphocytes* recognise specific antigens and secrete antibodies (immunoglobulins).
  - Glycoproteins interact with antigens, triggering a variety of responses.
  - B-cells also express MHC 2 complexes, enabling them to activate CD4 cells.
- Types of *antibodies* include:
  - IgM: first antibody produced by B-cells post-infection; activates complement.
  - IgG: produced second, and yields a much bigger response.
  - IgA: only seen in mucosal sites.
  - IgD: antigen recognition in B-cells.
  - IgE: found on mast cells and involved in allergic responses.

## Immune Checkpoints

- If left unchecked, immune reactions would propagate, causing sustained damage.
- Checkpoints inhibit immune response, preventing overactivity.
- Checkpoints are the target of cancer treatments or immunotherapies (Figure 1.6).
- Tumours may utilise these pathways in cancer development and hasten tolerance to immunotherapies.

## Recommended Reading

1. Lodish H, Berk A, Zipursky SL, Matsudaira P, Baltimore D, Darnell J. Molecular Cell Biology. 4th ed. New York: W. H. Freeman; 2000.
2. Pray L. DNA replication and causes of mutation. Nat Educ. 2008;1(1):214.
3. Clancy S. DNA transcription. Nat Educ. 2008;1(1):41.
4. Clancy, S. & Brown W. Translation: DNA to mRNA to protein. Nat Educ. 2008;1(1):101.
5. Gibney ER, Nolan CM. Epigenetics and gene expression. Heredity (Edinb). 2010 May 12;105:4.
6. Simmons D. Epigenetic influences and disease. Nat Educ. 2008;1(1):6.
7. Clancy S. DNA damage & repair: Mechanisms for maintaining DNA integrity. Nat Educ. 2008;1(1):103.
8. Lieber MR. The mechanism of human nonhomologous DNA end joining. J Biol Chem. 2008 Jan;283(1):1–5.
9. Mao Z, Bozzella M, Seluanov A, Gorbunova V. Comparison of nonhomologous end joining and homologous recombination in human cells. DNA Repair (Amst). 2008/08/20. 2008 Oct 1;7(10):1765–71.
10. Li G-M. Mechanisms and functions of DNA mismatch repair. Cell Res. 2007 Dec 24;18:85.
11. Janeway CA, Medzhitov R. Innate immune recognition. Annu Rev Immunol. 2002 Apr 1;20(1):197–216.
12. Dunkelberger JR and Song WC. Complement and its role in innate and adaptive immune responses. Cell Res. 2010;20(1):34–50.
13. Pardoll DM. The blockade of immune checkpoints in cancer immunotherapy. Nat Rev Cancer. 2012 Mar 22;12:252.
14. Rijinder M, de Wit r, Boormans JL et al. Systematic review of immune checkpoint inhibition in urological cancers. Eur Urol. 2017;72(3):411–23.

# 2 Genetics

*Karl H. Pang and Saiful Miah*

## Chromosomes

- Genes are the basic physical unit of inheritance.
- Humans have ~20,000–25,000 genes.
- Every person has two copies (alleles) of each gene — inherited from each parent.
- Genes are found on chromosomes.
- There are 46 chromosomes (23 pairs) in each cell (Figure 2.1):
  - 22 pairs are numbers (autosomes).
  - The 23rd pair is made up of X and Y sex chromosomes.
  - XY = male, XX = female.
- Each chromosome has a *short* arm (p) — 'petite' meaning 'small' in French — and a *longer* arm (q) — 'q' being the letter after 'p' or 'queue' which means 'tail' in French.

## Chromosomes Abnormality

- *Numerical* or *structural* (rearrangements) abnormalities exist.
- *Causes:* error in cell division (mitosis or meiosis).
- *Risk factors:*
  - Maternal age.
  - Teratogens (e.g., tobacco smoking, alcohol, medical/recreational drugs, radiation).

## Numerical Abnormality

- *Aneuploidy* is an abnormal number of chromosomes.
- Missing a chromosome – monosomy (e.g., Turner syndrome, 45XO).
- More than two chromosomes – trisomy (e.g., Down's syndrome or trisomy 21, Klinefelter syndrome or 47XXY).

## Chromosomal Rearrangements

- Structural changes can cause problems with growth, development, and function.
- Clinical and phenotypic effects depend on their size, location, or gain/loss of genetic material.
- Structural changes include (Figure 2.2):
  - *Deletion:* loss of genetic material.
- *Duplication:* genetic material is copied.
- *Inversion:* DNA breaks in two places and the resulting piece of DNA is reversed and reinserted.
- *Isochromosomes:* two identical arms, instead of one short (p) and one long (q) arm.
- *Translocation:* a piece of chromosome breaks off and attaches to another chromosome:
  - *Balanced:* no gain/loss of genetic material.
  - *Unbalanced:* gain/loss of genetic material.

## Gene Expression

- DNA *transcription* to RNA (nucleus)
  - Initiation, elongation, termination (Figure 2.3).
  - Mediated by RNA polymerase.
  - Pre-messenger RNA (mRNA) matures to form mature mRNA (see Chapter 1).
- RNA *translation* to protein (cytoplasm)
  - Mediated by transfer RNAs (tRNAs).
  - *mRNA* are 'coding' RNAs – translated into proteins.
  - *microRNA* are 'non-coding' RNAs– *not* translated → modulate protein expression by annealing to mRNA:
    - The 5' end of miRNA binds to the 3' end of mRNA.
    - miRNA-mRNA pair recruits a silencing complex: RNA induced silencing complex (RISC) → the fate of mRNA depends on the complementation.
    - '*Perfect* complementation'→ mRNA degradation.
    - '*Imperfect* complementation' → altered translation of mRNA (may lead to oncogenesis).

## Patterns of Inheritance

- This describes traits that are passed by genetics from parents to child.
- *Dominant* mutation: DNA variation in only one of the pair of genes.
- *Recessive* mutation: DNA variation in both copies of the gene.

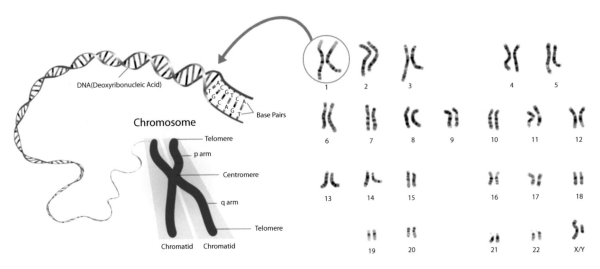

Figure 2.1 Chromosome picture (Karyotype) from a male 46XY. Chromosomes consist of DNA arranged in double helix structures with associated histones. A chromosome has a short arm (p) and a long arm (q). Courtesy: National Human Genome Research Institute, https://www.genome.gov/.

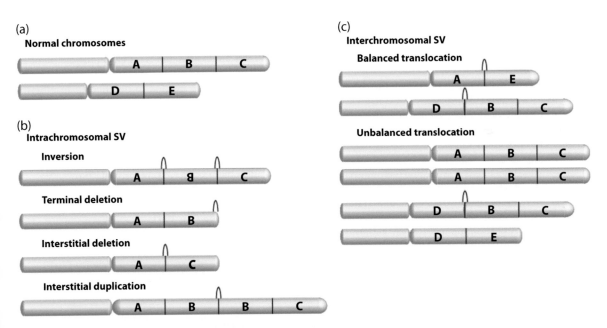

Figure 2.2 Simple chromosome rearrangements. (a) Two nonhomologous chromosomes shown in blue and pink. Segments are labelled with letters A -E. Black arches indicate structural variation (SV) breakpoint junctions; (b) Intrachromosomal rearrangements include inversions, interstitial and terminal deletions, and interstitial duplications; (c) Simple translocations between two different chromosome ends. Balanced translocations do not result in copy-number variation (CNV), but unbalanced translocations have partial monosomy (segment E) and partial trisomy (segments B,C). (Reprinted with permission from Elsevier [1])

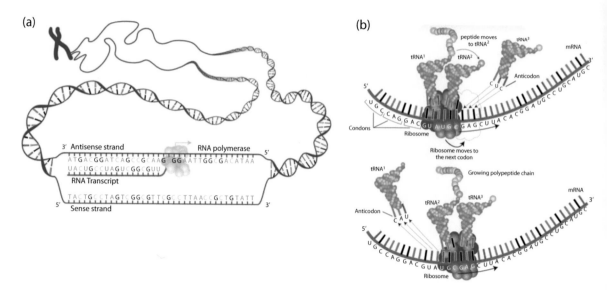

**Figure 2.3** Gene expression and protein synthesis. (a) Transcription: RNA polymerase attaches to DNA 3' end (ATG start codon). Elongation occurs via base pairing (A-U, T-A, C-G, G-C); (b) Translation: tRNA carries an amino acid and binds to mature mRNA. tRNA 1 transfers the peptide chain to tRNA 2 and exits the ribosome. tRNA 3 binds the mRNA, tRNA 2 transfers the peptide chain to tRNA 3 and exits the ribosome. The process repeats (elongation) until the stop codon is reached. Courtesy: National Human Genome Research Institute, https://www.genome.gov/.

## Autosomal Dominant Inheritance

- Affects autosomal genes on chromosome pairs 1 to 22.
- One copy is needed to be affected to inherit the disease (Table 2.1).
  - One affected; other copy not = *Heterozygous.*
  - Both copies affected = *Homozygous* (severe form of disease).
- *Examples:*
  - Von Hippel-Lindau syndrome (chromosome 3p).
  - Hereditary papillary renal cell carcinoma (7q).
  - Hereditary leiomyomatosis and renal cell cancer (1q).
  - Autosomal dominant polycystic kidney disease (16p, 4q).
  - Tuberous sclerosis (9q, 16p).
  - Birt-Hogg-Dubé syndrome (17p).
  - Noonan syndrome (~50% associated with 12q).

## Autosomal Recessive Inheritance

- Affects autosomal genes on chromosome pairs 1 to 22.
- Two copies are needed to be affected to inherit the disease (Table 2.2).
  - One affected; other copy not = *Heterozygous* (carriers).
  - Both copies affected = *Homozygous.*
- *Examples:*
  - Congenital adrenal hyperplasia (6p).
  - Autosomal recessive polycystic kidney disease (6p).
  - Cystinuria (2p, 19q).
  - Cystic fibrosis (7q).
  - Kartagener's syndrome.
  - 5-alpha reductase type 2 deficiency (2p).
  - Sickle cell disease (11p).

**Table 2.1 Punnett Squares Showing Patterns of Autosomal Dominant Inheritance**

| a | | | b | | | c | | |
|---|---|---|---|---|---|---|---|---|
| | **A** | **a** | | **A** | **a** | | **A** | **a** |
| **A** | AA | Aa | **A** | AA | Aa | **a** | Aa | aa |
| **a** | Aa | aa | **A** | AA | Aa | **a** | Aa | aa |

*Notes:* (a) Heterozygous (Aa) parents: 25% homozygous (AA) affected, 50% heterozygous (Aa) affected, 25% (aa) unaffected; (b) one heterozygous (Aa) and one homozygous (AA) parent: 50% homozygous (AA) affected, 50% heterozygous (Aa) affected; (c) one heterozygous (Aa) parent and one unaffected (aa) parent: 50% heterozygous (Aa) affected, 50% (aa) unaffected.

**Table 2.2 Punnett Squares Showing Patterns of Autosomal Recessive Inheritance**

| a |  |  | b |  |  | c |  |  |
|---|---|---|---|---|---|---|---|---|
|   | **A** | **a** |   | **A** | **a** |   | **A** | **a** |
| **A** | AA | Aa | **A** | AA | Aa | **a** | Aa | aa |
| **a** | Aa | aa | **A** | AA | Aa | **a** | Aa | aa |

*Notes:* (a) Heterozygous (Aa) parents: 25% homozygous (AA) unaffected, 50% heterozygous (Aa) carriers, 25% affected (aa) recessive; (b) one heterozygous (Aa) and one homozygous (AA) parent: 50% homozygous (AA) unaffected, 50% heterozygous (Aa) carriers; (c) one heterozygous (Aa) parent and one affected (aa) parent: 50% heterozygous (Aa) carriers, 50% affected (aa) recessive.

## X-Linked

- Affects genes on sex chromosome X.
- More prone than Y-linked because the X chromosome is larger, containing more genes.
- *X-linked dominant* – one copy is needed to be affected to inherit the disease.
  - *No* male-to-male transmission.
  - In females, the effect of the mutation may be masked by the second normal copy of the X chromosome.
- *X-linked recessive* – both copies are needed to be affected to inherit the disease.
  - *No* male-to-male transmission.
- *Examples:*
  - Lesch-Nyhan syndrome (recessive).
  - Kallman syndrome (recessive).
  - Haemophilia (recessive).
  - Alport's syndrome (dominant).

## Y-Linked

- Affects genes on sex chromosome Y.
- Affects only males.

- Mutation can only be transmitted from father to son.

## Mitochondrial Inheritance

- Also known as maternal inheritance.
- Applies to genes in mitochondrial DNA.
- Only female ova contribute mitochondria to the developing embryo; therefore, only females can pass on mitochondrial mutations.
- *Example*: Leber hereditary optic neuropathy (LHON).

## Recommended Reading

1. Weckselblatt B, Rudd MK. Human structural variation: Mechanisms of chromosome rearrangements. Trends Genet. 2015 Oct 1;31(10):587–99.
2. Clancy, S, Brown W. Translation: DNA to mRNA to protein. Nat Edu. 2008 1(1):101.
3. Nussbaum, R L, McInnes, R. R. Thompson & Thompson. Genetic in Medicine. 8th Edition. Philadelphia: Elsevier. 2015.

# 3 Oncogenesis and Metastasis

*Elizabeth Day and Hing Leung*

## Oncogenesis

### Cancer

- Cancer results from uncontrolled cell proliferation.
- Cells avoid normal homeostatic mechanisms and multiply in an unregulated manner → results in local invasion and distant metastasis.
- *Normal cells* may undergo *reversible* pathophysiological processes:
  - *Hypertrophy* (increase in size).
  - *Hyperplasia* (increase in number).
  - *Metaplasia* (changes in cell type/trans-differentiation).
- *Malignant growth* is unregulated and *irreversible*. Therefore, solid tumours are surgically removed or destroyed non-surgically (e.g., radiation-based therapy).
- *Oncogenesis* (or carcinogenesis):
  - A dynamic process whereby normal cells transform into cancerous cells.
  - Multiple rounds of genetic and epigenetic alterations occur.
  - Results in microscopic (morphological or structural) and molecular abnormalities.
  - Normal cells → precursor lesions → invasion and cancer.
- *Cancer cells characteristics:*
  - Pleomorphic (varied appearance).
  - Necrotic or ulcerated.
  - Edges are not well-demarcated.
  - Contain abnormal DNA (aneuploidy).
  - High cell division/mitotic rate (may be abnormal and unequal).

### Clinical Relevance of Cancer Cells Characteristics: Precursor Lesions

- Bladder carcinoma *in situ (CIS)* is a high-risk precursor lesion.
- High-grade cells exist within transitional epithelium.
- No invasion through the basement membrane into the lamina propria.
- CIS demonstrate some hallmarks of cancer:
  - Resist cell death.

- Sustain proliferative signals.
- Evade growth suppressor.
- Induce angiogenesis.
  - But *no* invasion beyond basement membrane or metastasis.
- *Other examples of precursors include*:
  - Penile intraepithelial neoplasia (PeIN) in penile cancer.
  - Atypical small acinar proliferation (ASAP) and high-grade prostatic intraepithelial neoplasia (HGPIN) in prostate cancer.
  - Germ cell neoplasia in situ (GCNIS) in testicular cancer.

## Cell Populations and Stroma

- There are ~200 cell types in the human body.
  - Some have no renewal/differentiation capability (neurones and myocytes).
  - Some divide conditionally (hepatocytes).
  - Others divide and differentiate continually (intestinal epithelium).
- The *'Degree of differentiation'* is how different a cancer appears from its cell of origin.
  - Used to classify tumour grades.
    - *High-grade tumours* are poorly or undifferentiated and do not resemble the cell of origin.
    - *Example:* The *Gleason score* (Donald Gleason, 1960s) reflects prostate glandular architecture.
- Cell are supported by surrounding connective tissue—*stroma*.
  - Stroma has a structural and supportive role.
  - Connects different cell populations.
  - Source of nutrients—vascular network.
  - Allows immune cells to weave through to their target.
- Cancer cells and tumour *microenvironment:*
  - Cancer cells resist inhibitory effects of stromal interactions on abnormal cell growth.
  - Paradoxically condition the stroma to support growth by paracrine signalling.
  - Recruit additional vasculature (or 'neo-angiogenesis').
  - Inhibit action of local immune cells.

## Invasion and Metastasis

- *Micro-metastasis:* colonisation of the new microenvironment before developing into a macroscopic tumour.
- Alteration of cell-to-cell and stromal connections.
- Cancer cells spread outside their usual confines and seed into distant locations.
- The 'mesenchymal' multipotent stem cells develop from the mesoderm into epithelial structures during organogenesis.
- This process is reversed in the first step of metastasis:
  - *Epithelial-mesenchymal transition* (EMT).
  - Cells lose polarity/contact with the basement membrane.
  - Cells migrate from the epithelium from which they arose.
- Once spread, metastatic cancer cell reverses the process again:
  - Mesenchymal to epithelial cell to establish metastatic deposits.

## The Cell Cycle

- Cell replication is governed by the cell cycle.
- Four stages with three intervening checkpoints (Figure 3.1).

- *Checkpoints* control cell cycle progression.
  - Inappropriate passage causes errors within the cell and its genetic content.

## Cell Cycle

1. *G1-phase* (Gap 1): cell prepares to replicate its genetic content.
2. *S-phase* (Synthesis): DNA replication into two copies of the cell's genome.
3. *G2 phase* (Gap 2): prepares for cell division.
4. *M phase* (Mitosis): cell splits into two daughter cells.

## Checkpoints

1. *G1-S-phase:* ensures correct timing of DNA replication.
2. *G2-M phase:* ensures correct DNA replication.
3. *Anaphase:* controls mitosis, where chromosomes are split and incorporated into two daughter cells.

## Cyclins and Cyclin-Dependent Kinases (CDKs)

- *Checkpoints* are governed by the interaction between cyclins and CDKs.

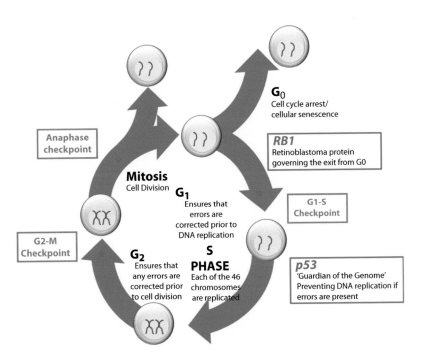

Figure 3.1 The mitotic cell cycle. The cell cycle controls the replication of cellular DNA and contents to produce two identical daughter cells. It is formed of four phases. There are 3 key checkpoints: G1-S, G2-M, and the anaphase checkpoint (marked*).

- *Cyclins:* expressed in a cyclical manner throughout the cycle - interacts with the respective CDK for downstream signalling.
- *Kinase:* an enzyme responsible for catalysing phosphorylation - can alter the activity of the target protein.

## Tumour Protein (TP53)

- Cells respond to errors within their genome/ cellular machinery.
- DNA damage must be repaired before genome replication.
- *TP53* – 'Guardian of the Genome', tumour suppressor gene (TSG).
- Prevents replication of damaged DNA and avoids incorporating genomic errors.
- Short half-life present at low concentrations → stabilises and increases level during DNA damage.
- Functions as a transcription factor:
  - Regulates expression of cell cycle control genes.
  - Transcriptionally activates p21 → p21 protein inhibits CDKs.
  - Despite cyclins being present, CDKs cannot activate downstream pathways.
  - Cell will not progress through G1/S checkpoint.
  - Cell cycle is 'stalled' until genetic repair is completed.
  - If DNA damage is irreparable, prolonged TP53 activation may trigger cell death.
- Normal TP53 function is lost in >50% of all cancers.
  - Cells survive and replicate with DNA damage.
  - Leads to genetic instability.
  - Mutations are propagated and potentially lead to the activation of cancer genes.

## Growth Factors and Signalling Pathways

- *Growth factors*
  - Function in extrinsic control of cell cycle through signalling pathways.
  - *Examples:* epidermal growth factor (EGF) and fibroblast growth factor (FGF).
  - Bind cell surface receptors.
  - Drive cell proliferation.
- *Steroid hormones*
  - Diffuse into the cell and interact with receptor within the cytosol.
  - *Example:* dihydrotestosterone (active metabolite of testosterone) binds to androgen receptors.
  - Receptors translocate to the nucleus to function as transcription factors.

## Signalling

- A single kinase can phosphorylate many other proteins, amplifying signals.

- *Tyrosine kinases:* subgroup (family) of protein kinases.
  - Alterations can upregulate growth factor pathway activities → promote tumorigenesis.
  - *Examples:* FGFR3 (Fibroblast Growth Factor Receptor 3) is upregulated and/or mutated in bladder cancer, while Pan-FGFR inhibitor (FDA approved Erdafitinib) is used to treat advanced bladder cancer.
- *PI3 kinase (PI3K/AKT)* and *MAP kinase (RAS/ MAPK)* pathways activate *mTOR (mammalian target of rapamycin)* and downstream effectors of *MAPK* (e.g., ERK1/2), respectively.
  - These pathways form signalling networks.
  - Errors lead to inappropriate activation of downstream pathways.
- Cancers may evade chemotherapeutic control by selecting mutations to bypass particular signalling pathways being inhibited by therapy (*tumour plasticity*).
  - *Example: Bevacizumab* is a recombinant humanised monoclonal antibody against VEGF-A (vascular endothelial growth factor A) in renal cancer.
    - Resistance occurs through upregulation of parallel components of the signalling network.
    - Cancer cells induce stromal cells to express pro-angiogenic factors (e.g., platelet-derived growth factor (PDGF) and FGF), bypassing the inhibited VEGF receptor.

## Immortality and Quiescence

- Cells not actively dividing are held in cellular quiescence in *G0 phase.*
  - This occurs in response to the lack of nutrition/ growth signals.
- Cells must re-enter the cell cycle in appropriate circumstances.
  - Controlled in part by *Retinoblastoma 1* (TSG).

## Retinoblastoma 1 (RB1)

- RB1 binds transcription factor E2F and prevents it from influencing gene expression.
- When RB1 is phosphorylated → E2F is released.
- E2F activates downstream pathways → signals release from G0.

## Telomerase and the Hayflick Limit

- Every time the genome is replicated, chromosome length decreases.
  - DNA replication machinery cannot read to the very end of a length of DNA.
  - The section that is not read is not replicated and is lost to the next generation of cell.

- *Telomeres* are DNA 'buffers' at the end of each chromosome.
  - Stretches of repetitive DNA sequences that protect against degeneration.
  - In rapidly dividing cells, telomeres may be 'worn down' and become insufficient to protect cells.
  - At this critical length, cell division will cease—this is called the *'Hayflick limit'*.
- Cancer cells overcome the *Hayflick limit* to obtain replicative immortality by:
  1. Bypassing cell cycle checkpoints → continue replication despite critically short telomeres.
  2. Using *telomerase*.
     - Usually only active in stem cell populations.
     - Works by extending repetitive DNA sequences in the telomeres.

## Cell Death

- Can occur through necrosis, programmed cell death (apoptosis), and autophagy.
- Divided into *programmed* and *unprogrammed* cell death.
- *Unprogrammed* cell death:
  - Occurs as a result of injury/infection and necrosis.

## Apoptosis

- Programmed cell death.
- Dying cell shrinks, chromosomes condense, and cytoplasm blebs.
- Cellular components partitioned into apoptotic bodies → engulfed by immune cells.
- This occurs through a cascade of sequential enzymatic activation that culminates in active caspase function—a family of protease enzymes which breakdown proteins.
- Triggered by intrinsic and extrinsic signals:
  - Coalesce on a common pathway → activate caspase proteins.
- *Intrinsic* pathway is triggered by DNA damage and prolonged TP53 activation.
- *Extrinsic* signals are transmitted by FAS (First Apoptosis Signal) or TNFα receptors.
- *Caspases*
  - BCL-2 (B-cell lymphoma 2) family of proteins signal effector caspases (Caspases 3, 6, 7).
  - Destroy proteins within the cell and execute cell death programme.
  - Members of BCL-2 family can be pro- and anti-apoptotic.

## Autophagy (Autophagocytosis)

- Vacuoles destroy (unnecessary/dysfunctional) cellular contents from 'the inside'.

- A response to nutrient deprivation or a survival mechanism following treatment.

## Clinical Relevance of Triggering Cell Death

- *Radiotherapy* induced DNA damage.
- In untransformed dividing cells, damage will overwhelm repair mechanisms, leading to apoptosis.
- Tumours that have inactivated *TP53* (do not trigger apoptosis) may be resistant to radiotherapy.

## Oncogenesis is a Step-Wise Process

- To overcome 'natural' barriers—these are the hallmarks of cancer.
- Accumulation of mutations in cancer genes.
  - Propagated if DNA repair/apoptotic mechanisms are impaired.
- *Darwinian evolution:* if a mutation provides a survival advantage, it will outgrow and outlive its neighbouring cells, with increasing opportunity to gain additional growth promoting mutations.
- *Carcinogens* can cause DNA mutations:
  - *Direct* (e.g., UV-induced crosslinking)
  - *Indirect* (e.g., aromatic amines such as naphthylamine).
- DNA double-stranded breaks are repaired by homologous recombination.
  - *BRCA1* and *BRCA2* genes are integral to this pathway.
  - Mutations result in hereditary breast, ovarian, and prostate cancer.
- Cancer may promote mutations and respond to selective pressures.
  - *Example:* hormone-sensitive prostate cancer may become castrate resistant with mutations of the androgen receptor.

## Cancer Genes

- Cancer genes are normal genes which cause oncogenesis if functionally altered.
- Categories: *tumour suppressor genes* and *oncogenes* (Figure 3.2, Table 3.1).
  - *TSG:* negatively regulate cell cycle progression; inactivation promotes oncogenesis.
  - *Proto-oncogenes:* provide positive growth signals.
    - *Oncogenes*: abnormal/sustained activity of proto-oncogenes.
    - Result in tumour promoting effects.

## Tumour Suppressor Genes (TSG)

- Human genome (except chromosomes X and Y in men) is diploid.

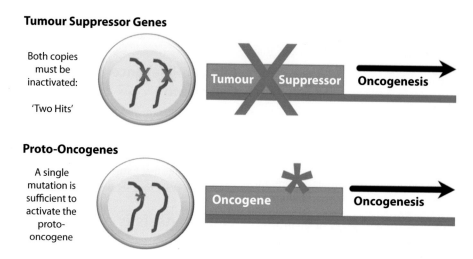

**Figure 3.2** Tumour suppressor gene vs oncogene. TSGs are 'activated' by loss of function of both copies; 'Two Hits' must occur to sufficiently release its control and promote oncogenesis. Proto-oncogenes may be activated by a single mutation that sufficiently alters the genes regulation or function to promote oncogenesis. This mutation may be a single point mutation, but can also include overexpression through epigenetic mechanisms, amplification or abnormal splicing that generates activated gene products.

- Contains two copies of each gene.
- Each copy termed an *allele*.
- Each allele is inherited from one parent.
- *TSG* act in a recessive manner.
  - *Oncogenesis* – both copies must be inactivated through DNA mutation, deletion, or loss of control.
- Alfred Knudsen, 1971 – '*Two Hit Hypothesis*'
  - Children with inherited retinoblastoma inherited one mutation, but only required an additional or 'second hit' before a tumour developed.
  - Those with non-inherited tumours needed to acquire inactivation mutations or deletion of *both* alleles, signifying *RB* as a TSG.

## Clinical Relevance of Tumour Suppressor Gene Activation

- *Example:* mutations in the *VHL* gene lead to Von-Hippel Lindau Syndrome.
- Born with a single normal copy of *VHL*.
- Second copy lost through mutation.
  - *Mutation:* sporadic (during embryogenesis) or inherited (familial cases).
  - Loss of 2nd *VHL* copy → increases the risk of tumour formation (e.g., renal cell carcinoma).
  - 'Second hit' can occur at any point from childhood through late adulthood.

## Oncogenes

- *Oncogenesis:* single copy of a mutated gene is sufficient.

- *Activation mechanisms:*
  1. A *point mutation* in *RAS* prevents its inactivation through the hydrolysis of GTP.
  2. Gene *amplification:* upregulate its expression (e.g., *EGFR*, *C-MYC* can be present in hundreds of copies).

## Hallmarks of Cancer

- Fundamental properties of cancer were conceptualised in the six 'Hallmarks of Cancer' by Hannahan and Weinburg in 2000.
- Subsequently updated with four additional (two emerging and two enabling) hallmarks in 2011 (Figure 3.3).

1. **Sustaining proliferative signalling**
- Upregulated expression of growth factor pathway components.
- Increased cell turnover can be used in diagnostic tests.
  - NMP22 (Nuclear Matrix Protein 22) – marker of cell division.
    - Non-invasive detection tool for bladder cancer using urine analysis.
    - (Alere NMP22® BladderChek® Test, Scarborough, ME, 04074 USA).

2. **Evading growth suppressors**
- *RB1:* inhibitory role at G1/S-phase checkpoint.
- *TP53:* role in cell cycle and apoptosis.
- *PTEN:* negatively regulates PI3 kinase pathway.
- Alterations in all three *TP53/RB/PTEN* TSGs are required for the transformation from low grade to high-grade bladder cancer.

**Table 3.1** Selected Cancer Genes, (a) Oncogenes; (b) Tumour Suppressor Genes

| | Function | Cancer Hallmark | Clinical Relevance |
|---|---|---|---|
| **(a) Oncogenes** | | | |
| **VEGF**<br>*Vascular endothelial growth factor*<br>Chr 6p21 | A tyrosine kinase receptor that stimulates angiogenesis | Angiogenesis | VEGF inhibitors used in renal cancer: Sunitinib, Sorafenib, and Bevacizumab |
| **FGFR3**<br>*Fibroblast growth factor receptor Chr 4p16* | A tyrosine kinase receptor signalling in growth factor pathways | Sustaining proliferative signalling | Frequently mutated in bladder cancer |
| **EGFR/HER2**<br>*Epidermal Growth Factor receptor. (HER2 is a subclass)*<br>Chr 17q12 | A tyrosine kinase receptor signalling in growth factor pathways | Sustaining proliferative signalling | Frequently mutated in bladder cancer |
| **PI3 kinase and mTOR**<br>*Phosphatidylinositol 3-kinase and Mammalian target of rapamycin* | Critical cell signalling pathway | Sustaining proliferative signalling | Frequently mutated in renal cell cancer |
| **NR3C4 (AR)**<br>*Androgen Receptor*<br>Chr Xq12 | Activated by androgenic hormones, testosterone, and dihydrotestosterone | Sustaining proliferative signalling | Mutated and amplified hormone resistance in prostate cancer |
| **c-myc**<br>Chr 8q24 | A transcription factor activating a number of pro-proliferative and anti-apoptotic genes | Sustaining proliferative signalling<br>Resisting cell death | Amplified in advanced prostate cancer |
| **c-met**<br>Chr 7q31 | A receptor tyrosine kinase involved in multiple signalling pathways | Sustaining proliferative signalling<br>Angiogenesis | Mutated in hereditary papillary renal cell cancer |
| **(b) Tumour Suppressor Genes** | | | |
| **p53**<br>*'Guardian of the Genome'*<br>Chr 17p13 | Activates p21 to inhibit cell cycle progression and initiate apoptosis in response to DNA damage | Resisting cell death<br>Genome instability | Normal p53 function is lost in at least 50% of all cancers |
| **RB1**<br>*Retinoblastoma protein*<br>Chr 13q14 | Retinoblastoma protein interacts with E2F, a transcription factor, to prevent passage through G1-phase | Evading growth suppressors | |
| **CDKN2A**<br>*Cyclin-dependent kinase inhibitor 2A*<br>Chr 9p21 | A cyclin-dependent kinase inhibitor, stalling cell cycle progression | Evading growth suppressors | One of the mutations identified in the UroVysion assay for bladder cancer |
| **BRCA 1/2**<br>*Breast cancer susceptibility proteins*<br>Chr 17q21, 13q13 | Responsible for sensing and triggering repair of double-strand breaks by homologous recombination | Genome instability | Mutated in familial breast, ovarian, and prostate cancer |

(*Continued*)

**Table 3.1** (Continued)

| | Function | Cancer Hallmark | Clinical Relevance |
|---|---|---|---|
| **VHL**<br>*Von-Hippel Lindau protein*<br>Chr 3p25 | VHL regulates HIF (hypoxia-inducible factor). In its absence, HIF activates growth factors such as VEGF | Angiogenesis | Mutated in Von-Hippel Lindau Disease. Multi-organ autosomal dominant disease resulting in renal cell carcinomas and pheochromocytoma |
| **PTEN**<br>*Phosphatase and tensin homolog*<br>Chr 10q23 | Negative regulator of the PI3 kinase pathway | Evading growth suppressors | Lost in up to 70% of prostate cancers |
| **TSC 1/2**<br>Also known as hamartin and tuberin<br>Chr 9q34 and 16p13 | Controls the mTOR signalling pathway, downregulating signalling to prevent cell growth | Evading growth suppressors | Mutated in tuberous sclerosis. Multi-organ autosomal dominant disease resulting in renal cysts and angiomyolipoma |
| **CDH1 (E-cadherin)**<br>Epithelial-Cadherin<br>Chr 16q22 | A cell adhesion protein with roles regulating cell adhesion and motility | Activating invasion and metastasis | |

3. **Resisting cell death**
- *TP53* function lost in >50% of all cancers allow cells to survive with DNA damage and evade apoptosis.
- The *Human Papilloma Virus* (HPV) implicated in ~65% of penile cancers.
  - Viral proteins E6 and E7 interact with *TP53* and *Rb*, respectively.
  - Evade growth suppression and apoptosis.
  - Encourages progression through the cell cycle.

4. **Enabling replicative immortality**
- *Telomerase* prevents shortening of chromosomes following multiple rounds of replication.
  - Avoids cellular senescence.
  - TERT (telomerase reverse transcriptase) enables telomerase to lengthen telomeres.
  - TERT activity is increased in most cancers.

5. **Inducing angiogenesis**
- Neo-vascularisation is needed to maintain an adequate supply of nutrients.
- VEGF and FGF stimulate/sustain (neo-) angiogenesis.
- *Tumour vasculatures:*
  - Often abnormal — leaky, convoluted, and branching excessively.
  - *Example:* renal tumours stimulating increased supply from accessory vessels.
- Bevacizumab (VEGF-A inhibitor) is used to treat metastatic renal cancer.

- *VHL* gene inhibits *hypoxia-inducible factors* (HIF).
  - In normoxic condition, VHL targets HIFs for destruction.
  - When VHL function is lost, HIFs are constitutively activated.
    - Stimulates angiogenesis even in the presence of oxygen ('pseudo-hypoxia').

6. **Activating invasion and metastasis**
- Tumour spread via blood, lymphatics, or directly down anatomical spaces (ureter).
- Epithelial-mesenchymal transition (EMT) - loss of connectivity.
  - 'Freely' allow cancer cells to spread.
  - The inactivation/functional loss of cell adhesion molecule *E-cadherin* plays a key role in EMT.
- Natural history of metastasis varies (surrounding stroma implicated):
  - Some tumours progress rapidly with macro-metastasis.
  - Others shed micro-metastasis.
    - May lay dormant or grow upon removal of the primary.

## Enabling Hallmarks

1. **Genetic instability and mutation**
- Oncogenesis relies on the accumulation of mutations.
- Instability occurs because cells evade apoptosis.

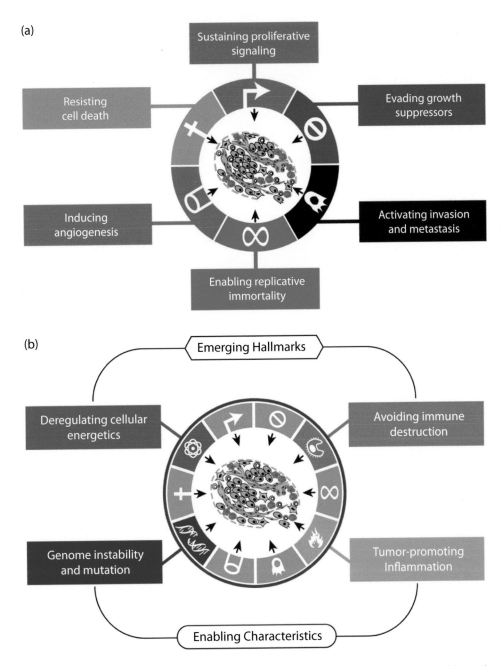

(a)

Sustaining proliferative signaling

Resisting cell death

Evading growth suppressors

Inducing angiogenesis

Activating invasion and metastasis

Enabling replicative immortality

(b)

Emerging Hallmarks

Deregulating cellular energetics

Avoiding immune destruction

Genome instability and mutation

Tumor-promoting Inflammation

Enabling Characteristics

**Figure 3.3** Cancer hallmarks. (a) Six 'original' hallmarks of cancer; (b) demonstrates the four additional properties added later. The Cancer Hallmarks are six properties defining malignant cells. Since their proposal in 2000, four additional properties have been added—two emerging hallmarks and two enabling features. (Reprinted with permission from Elsevier [4] and [5])

- Cells propagate with DNA damage or are unable to repair damage.
- Defects in DNA repair pathways.
- *Example:* mutations/deletion of BRCA1 and BRCA2 genes (breast, ovarian and prostate cancers).

2. **Tumour promoting inflammation**
- Immune cell infiltrate can be pro-tumorigenic.
- Supports cancer growth, angiogenesis, invasion, and metastasis.
- Immune cells generate reactive oxygen species (ROS) → accelerate cancer evolution by mutagenesis.

- Systemic inflammatory markers (e.g., C-reactive protein) have been researched as prognostic tools.
- Anti-inflammatory drugs (e.g., NSAIDs) have a protective role in some cancers.

## Emerging Hallmarks

1. **Reprogramming energy metabolism**
- Cancer cells undergo anaerobic metabolism (glycolysis).
- *Warburg Effect* (aerobic glycolysis) first described by Otto Warburg in 1920s.
- Increased uptake of glucose forms the basis of using the synthetic glucose $^{18}$F-fluorodeoxyglucose (FDG) as a radioactive tracer for PET imaging.
  - FDG does not get fully metabolised.
  - It is retained in cancer cells which exhibit enhanced glycolysis as a 'hot' signal on PET.

2. **Evading immune destruction**
- The immune system is thought to prevent carcinogenesis.
  - Immunocompromised patients have increased cancer incidence.
- Bacillus Calmette–Guérin (BCG) intravesical immunotherapy is a non-specific activator to augment host immune response to bladder cancer.
  - Recruit CD8+ cytotoxic T-cells and natural killer cells to the tumour.
- Immune checkpoint blockade forms the basis of immunotherapy.
  - *PD-L1* (programmed cell death protein ligand 1) on tumour cells.

- *PD-1* (programmed cell death protein 1) on T-cells.
- PD-L1 and PD-1 binding results in T-cell deactivation.
  - PD-L1 and/or PD-1 inhibitor are used in metastatic bladder/renal cancers.
- *CTLA-4* (cytotoxic T-lymphocyte associated protein 4).
  - Expressed by regulatory T-cells.
  - CTLA-4 inhibitors are used in metastatic renal cancer.
- Inhibitors restore tumour-specific T-cell immunity.

## Recommended Reading

1. Loges S, Schmidt T, Carmeliet P. Mechanisms of resistance to anti-angiogenic therapy and development of third-generation anti-angiogenic drug candidates. Genes Cancer. 2010;1(1):12–25.
2. Hayflick L, Moorhead P.S. The serial cultivation of human diploid cell strains. Exp Cell Res. 1961;25(3):585–621.
3. Knudson AG. Mutation and cancer: statistical study of retinoblastoma, Proc Natl Acad Sci U S A. 1971;68(4):820–823.
4. Hanahan D, Weinberg RA. Hallmarks of cancer. Cell. 2000; 7;100(1):57–70.
5. Hanahan D, Weinberg RA. Hallmarks of cancer: the next generation. Cell. 2011;4(5):646–674.
6. Zhou L, Cai X, Liu Q, et al. Prognostic role of C-reactive protein in urological cancers: a meta-analysis. Sci Rep. 2015;5:12733.
7. Zhao X, Xu Z, Li H. NSAIDs use and reduced metastasis in cancer patients: results from a meta-analysis. Sci Rep. 2017;7(1):1875.
8. Ghatalia P, Zibelman M, Geynisman DM, and Plimack E. Approved checkpoint inhibitors in bladder cancer: which drug should be used when? Ther Adv Med Oncol. 2018;10:1–10.

# Microbiology

*Katherine Belfield and Roger Bayston*

## Classification of Bacteria

- *Bacteria* are divided into two groups based on gram stain (Hans Christian Gram method).
  - *Gram-positive* bacteria: blue-black on staining (crystal violet stain).
  - *Gram-negative* bacteria: red (safranin counterstain).

- *Staining:*
  - Bacterial smear stained on a slide with crystal violet for 1–2 minutes.
  - The contents are poured. Gram's iodine is added for 1–2 minutes, then poured off.
  - Acetone is added for 2–3 seconds to wash and decolourise the stain.
  - The slide is washed with water and safranin counterstain is added for two minutes.
  - The slide is washed with water and dried for microscopy.

- *Gram-positive* bacteria have a thick cell wall – retains purple-violet stain (gram-negatives have a thin cell wall and does not retain violet stain).
- Bacteria can be differentiated by morphology:
  - Spherical cells – *cocci* (pair: diplococci).
  - Tubular cells – *bacilli.*

- Urinary tract bacteria include (Table 4.1):
  - *Gram-positive cocci: Staphylococci* and *Enterococci.*
  - *Gram-negative bacilli: Escherichia coli, Klebsiella pneumoniae,* and *Proteus mirabilis.*
  - The latter group are main members of the family Enterobacteriaceae (or enterobacteria), denoting their usual habitat in the large bowel.
  - Other members of Enterobacteria are seen less often in urinary tract infections (UTI).
  - *Enterococci* also inhabit the large bowel.
  - *Staphylococci* are ubiquitous and found in the bowel and on the skin.
  - All bacteria can grow either in air (aerobic) or in its absence (anaerobic).
  - Anaerobic bacteria do not play a significant part in UTI.

## Bacteria Structure

- Cocci and Bacilli are typically 1 micron ($\mu$) in diameter.
- Bacilli can be many $\mu$ in length.
- Bacteria have a rigid cell wall — peptidoglycan (branched aminosugar).
  - Maintains structural integrity of the cell.
  - Phospholipid bilayered *inner* membrane (inside cell wall) have regulatory and synthetic functions to maintain biochemistry of the cytoplasm (Figure 4.1).

- Gram-negative cells have an additional *outer* bilayer membrane (Figure 4.2).
- Gram-negative cells have hair-like appendages.
  - *Flagella* are used to swim in fluid environments.
  - Short ones (*pili*) are involved in the transfer of drug-resistance genetic material and adherence to cells and surfaces.

- Distinct from the outer capsule, both gram-negative and gram-positive bacteria synthesise and exude a mucoid polysaccharide → used to construct biofilms.
  - A *biofilm* is a community of bacteria which behave differently from free-living bacterial cells and from those grown in the laboratory.
  - Their constituent cells are much less susceptible to antibiotics.

- Bacteria synthesise cell wall materials inside the cell.
  - Exported to the cell wall to repair or extend it during growth and multiplication.
- Bacteria synthesise enzymes and other proteins, including toxins.
  - Transported out of the cell through phospholipid membrane(s).
  - Other enzymes are also synthesised to control DNA replication.
  - Most syntheses are carried out in ribosomes — protein synthesis organelles consisting mainly of RNA.

**Table 4.1** Classification of Bacteria and Other Organisms Associated with Urinary Tract Infections

| Gram-positive | Aerobes | Cocci | Streptococcus |
|---|---|---|---|
| | | | Non-haemolytic: *E. faecalis* |
| | | | Haemolytic: |
| | | | β-haemolytic *streptococcus* |
| | | | α-haemolytic *S. viridans* |
| | | | *Staphylococcus* |
| | | | *S. aureus* (coagulase +ve) |
| | | | *S. epidermidis* (coagulase -ve) |
| | | | *S. saprophyticus* |
| | | Bacilli | *Corynebacteria: C. urealytium* |
| | | | *Mycobacteria* (acid fast): *M. tuberculosis* |
| | Anaerobes | Bacilli | *Lactobacillus* (vaginal commensals): |
| | | | *L. crispatis, L. jensenii* |
| | | | *Clostridium: C. perfringens* |
| Gram-negative | Aerobes | Cocci | *Neisseria: N. gonorrhoea* |
| | | Bacilli | *Enterobacteriacaeae* |
| | | | *Escherichia coli* |
| | | | *Proteus mirabilis* |
| | | | *Klebsiella* spp. |
| | | | Non-fermenters: *Pseudomonas aeruginosa* |
| | Anaerobes | Bacilli | *Bacteroides: B. fragilis* |
| Others | | | *Chlamydia trachomatis* |
| | | | *Mycoplasma hominis* |
| | | | *Ureaplasma urealyticum* |
| | | | *Candida albicans* |

- These syntheses are major targets for common antibiotics (Figures 4.3 and 4.4).

# Infection in the Catheterised Patients

- Catheters facilitate entry of bacteria into the bladder by:
  - Inoculating meatal bacteria into the bladder at insertion.
  - Bacteria migrating up the catheter lumen during use.
  - The interface between the catheter and urethra.
- The longer the catheter is in place, the more likely colonisation occurs.
- Catheters may lead to bladder infection or catheter-associated UTI (CAUTI).
- Indwelling catheters will be colonised after 10–28 days.
- A catheter urine sample is likely to indicate bacteriuria, even in the absence of UTI.
  - In the absence of symptoms of infection, it's unnecessary and unwise to examine a urine sample.
  - Asymptomatic bacteriuria (ABU) should not be treated with antibiotics except for high-risk groups (e.g., in pregnancy).
- Causative bacteria of CAUTI are the same as those causing UTI even without a catheter.
  - *E. coli* predominates; others include Enterobacteria, Enterococci, and *Pseudomonas*.
- When bacteria gain access to the catheter:
  - They attach to its inner or outer surface by using surface receptors.

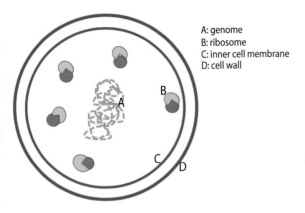

A: genome
B: ribosome
C: inner cell membrane
D: cell wall

Figure 4.1 Gram-positive bacterial Cell (e.g., *Staphylococcus*). (A) Genome. No nuclear membrane, unlike mammalian cells. (B) Ribosome. Where new peptides are produced. (C) Inner Cell Membrane. Consists of phospholipid bilayer. It is an electrochemical 'gate-keeper' for the cell and is also the site of important syntheses. (D) Cell Wall. Consists of a grid of aminosugars (peptidoglycan). Gram-positive cell wall is much thicker than the gram-negative one. Able to contain the high osmotic pressure inside the cell.

- They proliferate and proceed to develop a biofilm.
- Not all biofilms in the catheter will cause CAUTI.
  - In some, one or more of the biofilm bacteria will reach the bladder and may instigate inflammatory processes and UTI.
- CAUTI is often associated with catheter obstruction due to mineral encrustation (*P. mirabilis*).

# Appropriate Microbiology Tests

- Existing, new, and approved diagnostic tests are summarised in Figure 4.5 and Table 4.2.

## Urine 'Dipstick' Testing

- *Nitrites:* Gram -ve bacteria reduce urinary nitrates to nitrites.
  - Nitrites react with aromatic amine reagent on dipstick and forms diazonium salt.
  - Diazonium salt interacts with hydroxybenzoquinolone.
  - It produces a *pink*-coloured azo dye (*Griess reaction*).
  - Causes of false +ve: contamination.
  - Causes of false -ve: non-nitrite converting

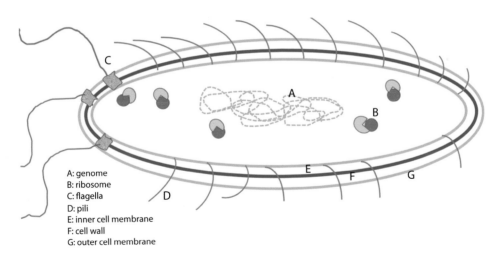

A: genome
B: ribosome
C: flagella
D: pili
E: inner cell membrane
F: cell wall
G: outer cell membrane

Figure 4.2 Gram-negative bacterial cell (e.g., *E. coli*). (A) Genome. (B) Ribosome. (C) Flagella. Each flagellum is powered by a 'motor' in the cell envelope – coordinated to allow bacteria to swim. not all gram-negative bacteria have flagella, gram-positive cocci rarely have them. (D) Pili. Dense layer on cell surface – scavenge ions, and function as attachment mechanisms to mammalian cells, and transmit DNA in bacterial sexual replication. (E) Inner cell membrane – same function as in gram-positive bacteria. (F) Cell wall. Gram-negative cell wall is much thinner than the gram-positive one. (G) Outer cell membrane: similar structure to the inner membrane. Has more functional proteins such as porins, that transport molecules into and out of the cell. Some gram-negative bacteria and a few gram-positive bacteria also produce a thick polysaccharide capsule (not shown in figure 2), that can protect them from phagocytosis, so it acts as a virulence factor.

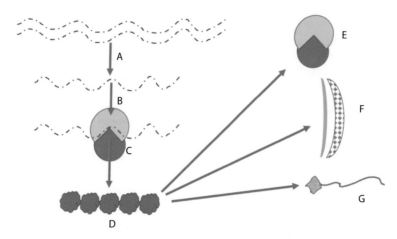

**Figure 4.3** The pathways from the bacterial genome (DNA) to synthesis of vital cell constituents. (A) Transcription of DNA to RNA. (B) The 'messenger' RNA (mRNA) attaches to specific receptors on the ribosome. (C) RNA is translated into peptides, that are assembled into proteins e.g., enzymes, toxins or structural components of the cell. (D), (E), (F) and (G). Enzymes and other peptides made in the ribosome are used to manufacture new cell constituents such as ribosomes (including modifications to existing ribosomes), new cell membrane and cell wall constituents, and new flagella and pili.

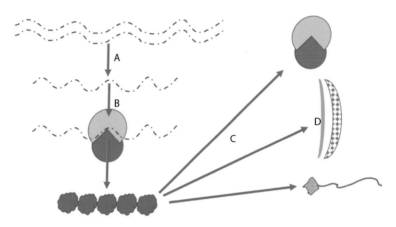

**Figure 4.4** Site of action of common antibiotics. (A) Trimethoprim inhibits new DNA synthesis, blocking successful cell replication Fluoroquinolones (e.g., ciprofloxacin) block the enzymes involved in translation of DNA to RNA. (B) Several antibiotics block attachment of RNA to ribosome, preventing further protein synthesis. Examples are gentamicin and tetracyclines. Some cause synthesis of faulty peptides that disrupt cell functions. Nitrofurantoin has an unusual mode of action, generating reactive substances that electrochemically inactivate or damage DNA, RNA, ribosomal proteins and enzymes. (C) Enzyme functional pathways are complex and can be inactivated by several antibiotics. Fosfomycin inactivates an enzyme near the inner cell membrane that is essential for cell wall synthesis, so the bacterial cell wall cannot be repaired or extended, as in bacterial replication. (D) Most antibiotics such as those that inhibit protein synthesis must be able to enter the cell. The beta-lactams – pivmecillinam, amoxycillin, cefalexin, exert their effect outside the inner cell membrane, at the point where the components of new cell wall are assembled, by binding to essential components. Bacteria replicate very rapidly (within an hour in ideal circumstances) and can generate alternative target sites for antibiotics very easily in many cases. Alterations to the ribosomal binding sites for mRNA can cause resistance to gentamicin. Production of altered enzymes can circumvent the action of many antibiotics, and production of alternative cell wall components can cause resistance to beta-lactams. Other resistance mechanisms include modification of cell membrane to prevent antibiotics from entering the cell or pumping them out again.

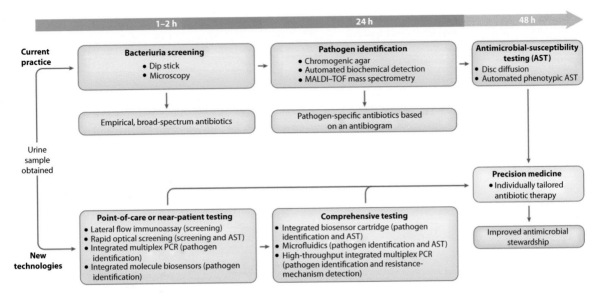

**Figure 4.5** Overview of the clinical workflow of existing and future diagnostic technologies for UTI. In *current practice*, once a urine sample is collected it is transferred to a clinical microbiology laboratory. In the laboratory, sample processing is initiated with a screening assay to assess for the presence of bacteria followed by pathogen identification, and, if positive, antimicrobial-susceptibility testing (AST). Information from each successive assay enables providers to prescribe specific antibiotic therapy. However, truly infection-specific antibiotic treatment cannot be prescribed until results from AST are available – at least 48 hours after sample submission. The *new technologies* in development have the potential to expedite this process and transform the clinical microbiology workflow. Urine samples collected in clinic can be analysed at the point of care. In this setting, integrated platforms can determine both pathogen identity and AST enabling precise, infection-specific treatment in a matter of hours from presentation. For complex samples or those collected from clinics without access to point-of-care testing, integrated platforms can provide similarly robust and efficient information in a clinical laboratory. MALDI-TOF, matrix-assisted laser desorption ionisation-time of flight. (Reprinted by permission from Springer Nature [5])

bacteria (e.g., *Pseudomonas* and gram +ve), ascorbic acid, urobilinogen, and dilute urine (low specific gravity).

- *Leucocytes:* neutrophils produce leucocyte esterase.
  - Leucocyte esterase hydrolyses dipstick indoxyl carbonic acid to indoxyl.
  - Indoxyl oxidises dipstick diazonium salt chromogen to produce a *purple* colour.
  - Causes of false +ve: contamination.
  - Causes of false -ve: dehydration, high urine specific gravity, ascorbic acid, glycosuria, urobilinogen present, and a non-fresh specimen (lysis of white blood cells).

- *Blood:* haemoglobin contains peroxidase.
  - Peroxidase oxidises dipstick orthotolidine.
  - Produces a *green* colour.
  - Causes of false +ve: exercise, dehydration, menstruation, povidone iodine, or hypochlorite solutions.
  - Causes of false -ve: – ascorbic acid (reducing agent).

- A positive result for nitrites or leucocyte esterase carries a sensitivity of ~75% and a specificity of ~80% for UTI.

## Urine Cultures

- Screen white blood cells, red blood cells, squamous epithelial cells, and other components (casts and crystals).
- Cellular components can be detected by microscopy or automated methods (urine analyser systems).
- Positive cellular components need further quantitative culture.
- Clinical details determine specifically which plates are needed for quantitative culture.
- A standard sample of urine is inoculated onto *blood agar*.
  - Cysteine-lactose -electrolyte-deficient (CLED) or chromogenic agar and incubated overnight at 37°C.
  - Cultures on chromogenic agar help identity bacteria and further tests might then be needed.

**Table 4.2** Approved Technologies for Pathogen Detection

| Technology | Commercial Assay | AST | Advantages | Disadvantages |
|---|---|---|---|---|
| Nitrite and leucocyte esterase | Dipstick (lateral flow assay) | No | Point of care | Poor specificity |
| Conventional culture | VITEK MicroScan | Yes | Standard of care, sensitive, and inexpensive | Time-consuming, not translatable to point-of-care applications |
| Urinalysis and microscopy | sediMAx | No | Fast, detects the presence of bacteria | No pathogen identification |
| | CLINITEK Atlas | | | |
| | Sysmex UF-1000i | | | |
| | Iris iQ200 | | | |
| MALDI-TOF mass spectrometry | VITEK MS | Under development | Fast, sensitive, specific, potential for simultaneous AST detection | Expensive for initial equipment |
| | Bruker MALDI-TOF | | | |
| FISH | AdvanDx | Under development | Rapid detection, high sensitivity and specificity | Requires multiple probes for all possible urinary pathogens |
| | QuickFISH | | | |
| Microfluidics | UTI Biosensor Assay (not FDA approved) | Under development | Integrated platform, rapid detection direct-from-patient samples, small footprint | System is not fully automated, poor data from low concentration of bacteria |
| PCR (clinical isolates) | GeneXpert SeptiFast | Resistance-gene probes available | Specific, sensitive, and rapid | Requires multiple probes for all possible urinary pathogens and extensive initial processing |
| | FilmArray | | | |
| Immunological-based assays | RapidBac | No | Rapid and inexpensive | Poor specificity and sensitivity |
| Forward light scattering | Uro-Quick BacterioScan | Under development | Inexpensive potential for AST | No species identification |

*Source:* Adapted from Springer Nature [5]
*Abbreviations:* AST, antimicrobial susceptibility testing; FISH, Fluorescent *in situ* hybridisation; MALDI-TOF, matrix-assisted laser desorption ionisation-time of flight; MS, mass spectrometry.

- Additional agar plates can be added based on microscopy or clinical details.
  - *Example:* if yeast cells are seen by microscopy, a *Sabouraud agar* plate can be added to detect Candida.
- Microorganism growth is assessed in terms of number of distinct species, and the total number of the predominating one.
- Expressed *in colony-forming units* (CFU)/mL (moving towards using CFU/L).
  - An assumption is made that each single bacteria cell in the original sample will give rise to one colony on the agar plate.
  - Does not consider that aggregates >1 bacteria cell still give rise to a single colony.
  - Hence, the use of CFU/mL rather than bacteria or yeast/mL.
- Cut-off count for UTI varies. Generally, $\geq 10^5$ CFU/mL ($10^8$ CFU/L) of a single predominating organism is indicative of it.
- $\geq 10^5$ CFU/mL may indicate ABU, but clinical interpretation is crucial.
- ABU should not be treated with antibiotics.
- Bacteria are tested further for susceptibility to a range of antibiotics suitable for treatment (sensitivities).

## Polymerase Chain Reaction (PCR)

- Amplification of DNA
- *Examples:* tuberculosis, chlamydia, gonorrhoea.

## Recommended Reading

1. Weiner LM, Webb AK, Limbago B, Dudeck MA, Patel J, Kallen AJ, et al. Antimicrobial-resistant pathogens associated with healthcare-associated infections: summary of data reported to the National Healthcare Safety Network at the Centers for Disease Control and Prevention, 2011–2014. Infect Control Hosp Epidemiol. 2016;37(11):1288–301.

2. National Institute for Health and Care Excellence. Urinary tract infection (lower): antimicrobial prescribing. NICE Guideline [NG109] Published date:31 October 2018.

3. Belfield K, Kalith S, Aimar K, Parkinson R, Bayston R. Microorganisms attached to the lumens and balloons of indwelling urinary catheters and correlation with symptoms, antibiotic use and catheter specimen of urine results. J Med Microbiol. 2019;68(4):549–54.

4. Nielubowicz GR, Mobley HLT. Host-pathogen interactions in urinary tract infection. Nat Rev Urol. 2010;7(8):43–41.

5. Davenport M, Mach KE, Shortliffe LMD. New and developing diagnostic technologies for urinary tract infection. Nat Rev Urol. 2017;14(5):296–310

# 5 Transplantation

*Jonathon Olsburgh and Rhana H. Zakri*

## Self Versus Non-Self: The Relevance to Clinical Transplantation

- The body detects 'self' from 'non-self' and reacts appropriately.
- Cell surface proteins (antigens, Ag) are recognised as self or non-self by immune cells.
  - Immune response occurs when non-self and foreign antigens are recognised, such as:
    - *Cancer* cells (altered expression of self-antigens by mutation)
    - *Foreign* or *'transplanted'* tissue → results in rejection
- An error within the immune system may result in recognising self-cells as foreign → auto-immune diseases can occur.

## Blood Groups

- There are four major red cell blood groups:
  - A, B, AB, and O
- Group A and group B Ag (or both) are expressed as oligosaccharides on the surface of red blood cells (RBC) → determines an individual's blood group.
- *In childhood*, dietary carbohydrates can mimic group A and group B Ag.
  - Children develop blood group antibodies (Ab) to these 'antigens'.
  - Blood group A: anti-blood group B Ab are produced.
  - Blood group B: anti-blood group A Ab.
  - Blood group O: anti-blood group A and B Ab.
  - Blood group AB: no anti-blood group Ab.
- Haemolytic reaction occurs if anti-group A or B Ab is mixed with group A or B Ag, respectively.
  - *Example:* blood group A patient (anti-B Ab) receives blood from group B (B Ag) → results in a haemolytic reaction
- *Blood group O:* ideal blood/solid-organ donor (no Ag)
- *Blood group AB:* ideal recipient (no Ab).
- ABO blood group compatibility is generally required for solid organ transplantation.
- As ABO blood groups are expressed on RBC, ABO blood group compatibility is not required for transplantation of cornea or heart valves.

## Major Histocompatibility Complex/Human Leucocyte Antigen

- The major histocompatibility complex (MHC) (Human Leucocyte Antigen (HLA) in humans) allows the differentiation of self vs non-self.
- HLA genes (alleles) are on chromosome 6p.
- There are *six antigens:*
  - *HLA-A, -B, -C, DR, DQ, and DP*
- *HLA-A, -B, -C antigens*
  - *Class I HLA*
  - Expressed on almost all nucleated cells.
- *HLA-DR, -DQ, and -DP antigens*
  - *Class II HLA*
  - Limited to antigen-presenting cells (APC)
    - B-cells, dendritic cells, and some endothelial cells.
- Each person has two alleles of HLA-A, -B, -C, DR, DQ, and DP:
  - One set inherited from each parent (each set is known as a haplotype).
  - Encodes two sets of HLA Ag corresponding to the HLA alleles- co-dominantly expressed. Some examples include:
    - Inheritance of HLA-A2 allele from both parents → homozygous at HLA-A, expressing only HLA-A2.
    - Inheritance HLA-A1 from father and HLA-A2 from mother → heterozygous at HLA-A, expressing both HLA-A1 and HLA-A2.
- The genes encoded within the HLA alleles are highly polygenic and polymorphic, which leads to an extensive range of expressed HLA Ag.
- The most important HLAs for matching are:
  - *HLA-A, HLA-B, and HLA-DR*
- HLA matching refers to the number of *HLA-A, -B, -DR* mismatches between donor and recipient.
- *Identical* HLA genes in donor and recipient = *0:0:0 mismatch.*
  - This gives the best outcomes with respect to graft survival.
- As there are two alleles for each gene,

- *Non-identical* HLA genes = *2:2:2 mismatch.*

## Syngeneic Versus Allogeneic

- *The Herrick twins* are genetically identical brothers.
  - The donor and recipient were genetically identical brothers – first successful living donor kidney transplant (23 December 1954)
  - Identical twins – *'syngeneic'* combination
- All other human transplantation is *'allogeneic'.*
  - Requires appropriate modulation to the immune system's response to differences in HLA and/or blood group.

## Clinical Transplantation (or Tissue-Typing) Laboratory

- The Clinical Transplantation (or tissue-typing) Laboratory (CTL) and blood-bank laboratories risk stratifies potential donor and recipient's compatibility and chooses appropriately compatible donor/recipient pairs.
- *Polymerase chain reaction* (PCR) using DNA extracts from blood specimens determines donor/recipient's HLA alleles.
- *Flow cytometry* technology determines any HLA Ab that a recipient may have developed following exposure to foreign cells.
  - i.e. from a blood transfusion, pregnancy, previous organ transplant, and previous episodes of organ rejection.
- Some Abs remain stable over time.
- HLA Abs (blood transfusion) are transitory.
  - Appear at ~day 10 post-blood transfusion.
  - Disappear after a month.
- HLA Ab that is no longer detectable may still have risks in triggering rejection through immunological memory.

## Kidney Donor Types

### Living Donation

- Donation of a single kidney by a *living* donor through donor nephrectomy.
- This is the preferred option because of better overall graft and patient survival.
- It helps with surgical planning, especially in complex recipients.
- *Direct* donation: specified recipient (e.g., relative or friend).
- *Non-directed* donation: non-specified; national waiting list (*altruistic* donation).
- *The national kidney sharing scheme* (NKSS) permits the matching of otherwise ABO and/or HLA non-compatible pairs of individuals.
  - This matches a few otherwise incompatible direct donation pairs but can also utilise a non-directed *'altruistic'* donor to initiate a chain of transplants.
- Direct donation can be performed between certain ABO/HLA incompatible pairs.
  - This requires the removal of the incompatible blood group/HLA Ab with strong immuno-suppression.

## Deceased Donation

There are two types of deceased donors:

1. Donation after brain death (DBD).
2. Donation after circulatory death (DCD).

### Donation after brain death

- Strict *neurological criteria*:
  - Brainstem testing set forth by the UK Code of Practice for the Diagnosis and Confirmation of Death.
- Applies to brain injury suspected to have caused an *irreversible loss of consciousness and capacity for respiration.*
  - Possible only for patients on mechanical ventilation.
  - Cessation is expected to lead to terminal apnoea, resulting in hypoxic cardiac arrest and circulatory standstill.

### Donation after circulatory death

- Where brainstem death criterion *cannot* be fulfilled.
- Where there is agreed 'futility' and occurs after an agreed period of cardiac arrest or circulatory standstill.
- DCD donation may be controlled or uncontrolled (Maastricht classification, Table 5.1).
- *Controlled DCD* has increased significantly in the UK, over the last 20 years.
  - ~39% of all UK deceased donation in 2018.
  - Variable in the rest of the world — may include legal, ethical, professional obstacles in countries where no DCD programmes exist.
- *Uncontrolled DCD* currently has no active organ retrieval programme in the UK.
- Mid- and long-term outcomes of DCD are equivalent to DBD kidney transplants.
  - The main difference is the duration of functional warm ischaemia at retrieval.
- *Functional warm ischaemia time* (f-WIT):
  - Commences when there is inadequate perfusion of organs defined by the following:
    - Systolic BP <50 mmHg, $O_2$ saturation <70%, or both until the initiation of cold perfusion.

**Table 5.1** The Maastricht Classification of Donation After Circulatory Death

| Category | Type | Circumstances | Typical Location |
|---|---|---|---|
| 1 | Uncontrolled | Death on arrival | Emergency Dept. |
| 2 | Uncontrolled | Unsuccessful resuscitation | Emergency Dept. |
| 3 | Controlled | Cardiac arrest follows planned withdrawal of life-sustaining treatments | Intensive care unit |
| 4 | Controlled | Cardiac arrest in a patient who is brain dead | Intensive care unit |

- *Organ retrieval and ischaemic time*
  - *DBD*
    - Donor is brain-dead.
    - The organs undergo cold perfusion just before retrieval starts, keeping WIT minimal.
  - *DCD* (Figure 5.1).
    - There is a time interval from withdrawal until asystole.
    - A further defined five minutes stand-off period and then the time until cannulation, during which organs are sub-optimally perfused and have yet to be cooled.
      - This leads to the accumulation of ischaemic metabolites, resulting in the potential for irreversible damage to the organs.
  - *First* WIT should be <20 min — once retrieved, organs are placed in slushed ice.
  - *Cold ischaemic time* (CIT)
    - Initial cold preservation until warm perfusion of the organ with the recipient's blood circulation during transplant surgery.
  - A *second* WIT takes place during surgical implantation of the kidney.
    - The time the organ is taken out of ice until the vascular clamps are removed, following vascular anastomoses, and the organ is perfused by the recipient circulation.

## Ischaemic Reperfusion Injury (IRI)

- Multi-factorial process
  - Paradoxical exacerbation of cellular dysfunction following reperfusion at the time of transplantation.
- Cold perfusion/storage slows down tissue metabolism → cannot prevent cellular injury completely
- Hypoxic environment and anaerobic metabolism:
  - Mitochondria increases the production of reactive oxygen species (ROS)
    - Superoxide anion ($O_2^-$), hydrogen peroxide ($H_2O_2$), hydroxyl radical ($OH^+$), and nitric oxide (NO)
  - Glycolysis supplies ATP to ischaemic cells → lactic acid and intracellular acidosis
  - Due to poor ATP production, failing Na/K ATPase pumps → imbalance between intracellular potassium and extracellular sodium → cell swelling → damage to cellular components → apoptosis
- The longer the CIT, the more likely that IRI will occur.
- Clinical manifestations can be early or late.
- Reperfusion of a kidney affected by IRI results in:
  - Inflammatory, microvascular, and oxidative damage to the transplanted organ.
  - Both endothelial cells and tubular epithelial cells are affected.
  - Loss of tubular epithelial cell integrity → sloughing of cells into tubules → tubular obstruction → acute renal tubular necrosis (ATN).
- *ATN manifests as:*
  - Delayed graft function (DGF)

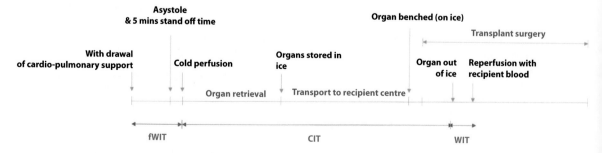

Figure 5.1 Timeline representing donation after circulatory death.

- Prolonged hospitalisation
- Ongoing dialysis post-transplantation
- Potential need for renal biopsies
- Loss of endothelial cell function causes impaired anticoagulant properties and potential intravascular thrombosis.
- *Strategies to minimise ischaemic cell death:*
  - Cooling to slow the metabolic rate.
  - Perfusing organs with cold preservation solution (reduces electrolyte imbalance, provides buffers against acidosis, and reduces osmotic swelling).
  - Machine perfusion.
- *A later complication* of IRI:
  - Cell- or antibody-mediated rejection (see below) by activation of pattern recognition receptors or activation of endothelial cells.
  - Prevention requires high dose steroids and T-cell depleting antibody at induction (see below).
- Donor/recipient factors that influence the incidence/severity of IRI include:
  - CIT
  - DCD donation
  - Donor age, male recipients, African-American race, obesity (BMI >30)
  - High sensitisation
- *Cold preservation fluid:*
  - University of Wisconsin (UoW) solution
    - Lactobionate, starch, raffinose limit swelling
    - Phosphate buffers H+ ions
    - Adenosine is a substrate for ATP synthesis
    - Glutathione is a free-radical scavenger
    - Allopurinol inhibits xanthine oxidase and frees radicals
    - Magnesium and dextromethorphan (DXM) stabilise membrane
    - Penicillin for antibiosis
    - Insulin

# Basic Immunology
## Antigen Presentation

- Occurs through antigen-presenting cells (APCs):
  - Macrophages and dendritic cells
  - Interact with the adaptive immune system (T cells and B cells)
- APCs are phagocytic and are recruited to areas of inflammation.
  - Ingest molecules → small fragments (peptides) bind to the antigen-binding groove of the HLA molecule (expressed on the APC surface) → antigen-peptide-HLA complex is recognised by the T-cell receptor (TCR) on the T-cell surface.
- There are three ways *'non-self'* donor HLA Ag is recognised as foreign Ag by the recipient:

1. *Direct*
   - Donor APCs have donor HLA molecule and donor peptide (from any cellular breakdown mechanism in the donor) all pre-assembled and visible on the donor *APC surface.*
   - Pre-assembled donor APC-HLA-Antigen complex is 'leaked' from donor cells into the recipient bloodstream.
   - *'Passenger'* donor APCs enter the recipient lymphatics and interact with recipient T-cells in lymph nodes.
   - Recipient TCR interacts with donor HLA-peptide complexes → immune response.
2. *Semi-direct*
   - Similar process to the direct mechanism.
   - Donor HLA molecule and donor peptide are assembled *in a donor-derived exosome* → shed from the graft into the recipient circulation.
   - *Recipient APCs* encounter the exosome → bound to the cell surface (*cross-dressing*).
   - *Cross-dressed APC* → recipient lymph nodes → presents intact donor HLA-peptide complex → recognised by TCR → initiates an immune response.
3. *Indirect*
   - Donor HLA molecules are shed from the donor kidney (naturally and in response to IRI) into the recipient circulation.
   - Molecules are engulfed by *recipient APCs* and presented to recipient T-cells.

# T-Cell Activation

- There are *three signal systems:*

## Signal 1

- Occurs in the early phase.
- TCR binds to its complementary HLA-2 Ag complex.

## Signal 2

- Complementary adhesion molecules on the T-cell surface (CD28) and the APC surface (B7) bind.
- Full activation (both signal 1 and 2) leads to signal transduction from the TCR via CD3 complex.
- Intracellular signalling pathways (IP3/diacylglycerol) → calcium mobilisation → activates the protein phosphatase *calcineurin.*
  - Calcineurin dephosphorylates NFAT (nuclear factor of activated T cells) → an active moiety translocates to the T-cell nucleus and binds to promoter regions of a variety of genes including cytokines (e.g., IL-2, IL-4, IL-5, IL-6, IFN-gamma) and regulatory genes.
  - Cytokines have paracrine stimulatory (helper) effects on cytotoxic T-cells and B-cells.

## Signal 3

- *IL*-2 expression leads to stimulation of T-cells via the IL-2 receptor (IL-2R).
- This leads to a signal transduction via the mammalian Target of Rapamycin (mTOR) pathway.
  - Important in the cell cycle, DNA synthesis, cell division, and replication that require purines as building blocks for DNA.

# Immunosuppression (IS)

- *Aims of IS strategies:*
  - Reduce the incidence of organ rejection.
  - Reduce short and long-term side-effects of IS and drug toxicity.
- Current approaches (Table 5.2):
  - Induction IS phase.
  - Post-transplant, less intense maintenance IS phase.
- Treatment for *rejection* is guided by features on transplant biopsy, such as:
  - T-cell- or B-cell-mediated rejection.
  - Evidence of donor-specific antibody (antibody-mediated rejection (AMR)).
  - Involvement of graft vasculature (vascular rejection).
- Combination IS strategies:
  - Target different key immune system interactions.
  - Achieve a synergistic IS with minimal toxicity.

## Steroids

- Prednisolone act on signal 1 and 2.

- *Regular doses* of glucocorticoid steroids act as agonists of steroid receptors.
  - Affect transcription through:
    - DNA-binding
    - Targeting transcription factors (e.g., activator protein 1 and nuclear factor kappa B).
- *Higher dose* steroids also have receptor-independent effects.
- *Side-effects* of steroids:
  - Infection, decreased wound healing, osteoporosis, diabetes, cardiovascular sequelae

# Calcineurin Inhibitors (CNI)

- Act on a downstream part of signal 2.
- *Examples:* Ciclosporin, Tacrolimus.
  - Both inhibit calcineurin phosphatase and T-cell activation.

- *Ciclosporin*
  - Isolated from Tolypocladium inflatum by Sandoz in 1970 in Basel, Switzerland.
  - J.F. Borel discovered its immunosuppressive activity in 1976.
  - First transplant use in humans by Sir Roy Calne in 1978.
  - Binds with cyclophilin — an intracellular protein of the immunophilin family.
  - Forms a complex that inhibits calcineurin.
- *Tacrolimus*
  - Derived from Streptomyces tsukubaensis (macrolide antibiotic).
  - Binds to a different immunophilin, FK506-binding protein 12 (FKBP12).

**Table 5.2** Immunosuppressive Drugs

| Class of IS | Drug Options | Main Use | Additional Use |
|---|---|---|---|
| Steroid | IV Methylprednisolone | Induction IS | Treat acute rejection |
| | Oral prednisolone | Maintenance IS in combination | |
| Nucleotide inhibitors | Azathioprine or MMF | Maintenance IS in combination | |
| Calcineurin inhibitors | Ciclosporin or Tacrolimus | Maintenance IS in combination | |
| mTOR inhibitors | Sirolimus or Everolimus | Maintenance IS in combination | |
| Depleting antibodies | ATG and Alemtuzumab | Induction IS | Treat severe acute rejection |
| Non-depleting protein drugs | Basiliximab | Induction IS | |
| | Belatacept | Maintenance IS (trials) | |

*Abbreviations:* mTOR, mammalian Target of Rapamycin; IV, intravenous; MMF, mycophenolate mofetil; ATG, anti-thymocyte immunoglobulin; IS, immunosuppression.

- Creates a complex that also inhibits calcineurin.
- Greater affinity than ciclosporin.
- CNIs *side-effects:* infection, diabetes tremor, and nephrotoxicity.

## Nucleotide Inhibitors

- Inhibit either purine or pyrimidine biosynthesis.
- Only inhibitors of *purine pathways* are used, and they target T- and B- cell proliferation.
- *Examples:* Azathioprine and Mycophenolic Acid.

- *Azathioprine*
  - Releases *6-mercaptopurine,* a metalloprotein-ase tissue inhibitor.
  - Causes thioguanine to be incorporated into nucleotides - interferes with DNA synthesis.
- *Mycophenolic acid (MPA)*
  - *Examples:* Mycophenolate Mofetil (MMF) and enteric-coated mycophenolate (Myfortic).
  - Discovered from Penicillium moulds.
  - Inhibits inosine monophosphate dehydro-genase (IMPDH).
  - Blocks purine synthesis.
- Nucleotide inhibitors *side-effects:* bone marrow suppression and infection.

## mTOR Inhibitors

- mTOR pathway is downstream of signal 3.
- Also have an anti-cancer effect (e.g., in Kaposi's sarcoma and renal cell carcinoma).
- *Examples:* Sirolimus (Rapamycin) and Everolimus.
- *Sirolimus*
  - Isolated from *Streptomyces hygroscopicus* found on Easter Island or Rapa Nui (hence, the name Rapamycin).
- mTORi *side-effects:* decreased wound healing, increased lymphocele, pneumonitis, and thrombo-cytopenia.

## Depleting Antibodies

- Destroy T cells, B cells, or both.
- *Examples:* anti-human thymocyte immunoglobulin (ATG), Alemtuzumab, Rituximab.
- Reduces early rejection, but increases the risks of infection and post-transplant cancers (e.g., lymphoma).
- *T-cell depletion*
  - Accompanied by cytokine release → severe systemic side-effects.
- *B-cell depletion*
  - Better tolerated than T-cell depletion.
  - Not usually accompanied by cytokine release.

- Recovery from immune depletion takes months to years.
- *Anti-human Thymocyte immunoglobulin*
  - Rabbit antibody.
  - Polyclonal drug which is given intravenously.
  - Used in some countries (e.g., USA) as part of the induction strategy.
  - Mainly used in the UK as treatment of severe rejection.
- *Alemtuzumab* (Campath-1H)
  - Humanised monoclonal antibody – sub-cutaneous injection.
  - Targets *CD-52* depleting both *T-cells* and *B-cells.*
  - Used as induction therapy for higher immunological risk kidney transplants.
- *Rituximab*
  - B-cell depleting monoclonal anti-CD20 antibody.
  - Used as part of protocols to help prevent rejection in ABO-incompatible kidney transplant programmes.
- *Basiliximab*
  - Humanised or chimeric monoclonal anti-CD25 antibody.
  - Interleukin-2 receptor inhibitor/antagonist.
  - Prevents T-cell activation and proliferation.
  - Administered intravenously.
  - Given at induction and on day 4 post-transplant.
- *Belatacept*
  - Soluble fusion protein.
  - Selectively inhibits CD28-mediated co-stimu-lation of T-cells.
  - Fusion protein with natural binding properties: CTLA-4-Ig (LEA29Y).
  - Limited to clinical trials – explore novel IS regimes to minimise CNI use/toxicity.

## Kidney Transplant Surgery

- Performed through an extraperitoneal approach into either iliac fossa.
- Rutherford Morrison incision.
- Careful planning about kidney transplant position is required prior to implant.
  - Ensure that the recipient vessels are not diseased.
  - Donor vessels and ureter are neither too long, too short, nor kinked.

## Vascular Anastomosis

- Donor kidney vessels may be implanted onto the external, internal, or common iliac.
- Usually end-to-side anastomoses.
- Aim for peak arterial systolic velocity (PSV) at <200 cm/sec (using Doppler USS).

- PSV >200 cm/sec is associated with poor graft function and hypertension.
  - Possibility of renal artery stenosis (RAS).
    - Confirmed with a CT/MR angiogram.
    - Treated with angioplasty where possible.
- The renal artery anastomosis is usually cephalad to the renal vein anastomosis.
- The *right* kidney donor renal vein is shorter.
  - With deceased donor kidneys, the right renal vein may require reconstruction with the IVC to provide additional length.

## Ureteric Anastomosis

- *Lich-Gregoir:* extravesical anastomosis onto the superolateral aspect of the bladder.
- *Necker* technique: donor ureter anastomosed onto the native ureter if native ureters are in situ and of reasonable calibre.
  - Useful if there is a short donor ureter.
- All anastomoses should be tension free, of good calibre, and well vascularised.
- A ureteric anastomosis is protected by a temporary JJ stent (removed at 2–6 weeks).
- Usually, the bladder catheter is removed 4–5 days post-operatively.

## Post-Operative

- Palpate peripheral leg pulses at the end of the operation to ensure that lower limb ischaemia has not occurred.
- Kidney transplant Doppler USS is performed in recovery/on the ward to assess immediate post-operative perfusion of the kidney and renal vascular blood flow.

## Complications

- Surgical, anaesthetic, medical/immunological consequences of renal failure and IS.
- Wound infection or dehiscence.
- Lymphocele.
- <1% arterial thrombosis.
- 2-5% venous thrombosis and can present with:
  - Sudden onset oligo-anuria.
  - Reversal of end-diastolic flow with absent venous flow.
- RAS (a more common complication):
  - Presents ~6 months after surgery.
  - Associated with hypertension and graft dysfunction.
- *Urine leak:* seen ~2 weeks post-surgery:
  - If the ureteric stent is still in situ, it is managed conservatively.
    - Reinsert urethral catheter and cystogram

14 days later prior to catheter and stent removal.
  - If a urine leak does not settle:
    - Place a percutaneous nephrostomy to divert the urine.
    - Revise the ureteric reimplantation surgery.
- *Ureteric stenosis:* commonly seen within three months of surgery.
  - Factors predisposing to ureteric ischaemia:
    - A stripped ureter during retrieval/bench work preparation.
    - Compromise of the lower pole blood supply.
    - Poor surgical technique.
    - Low blood pressures.
- *Ureteric obstruction:* can present early or late and may be due to:
  - Poor surgical technique.
  - Fibrosis secondary to rejection.
  - External compression from a lymphocele.
  - Ureteric ischaemia.
  - Management:
    - Percutaneous nephrostomy, nephrostogram, and insertion of a ureteric stent.
    - Ureteric reimplantation.
- Ureteric strictures may be managed with long-term stents or other endourological techniques.

## *Medical Complications*

- Acute and chronic rejection.
- Chronic allograft dysfunction.
- Recurrence of primary glomerular disease.
- *De novo* glomerulonephritis.
- New-onset diabetes after transplantation (NODAT).
- Cardiovascular disease.
- Post-transplant infection, especially opportunistic infections.
  - CMV, EBV, HSV, VZV, BK virus, candida, Aspergillus, PJP, TB.
- Post-transplant malignancy
  - The most common is a non-melanoma skin cancer.
  - The second most common is post-transplant lymphoproliferative disease (PTLD).
  - All other cancers are slightly more common in transplant recipients than in an age-matched general population.

## Rejection

- Rejection should be diagnosed on a kidney transplant biopsy.
- Can occur when:
  - The overall IS dosing is not adequate to prevent rejection.
    - Toxicity of the IS drugs prevents higher doses.

**Table 5.3** Type of Transplant Rejection

| Type of Rejection | Time Frame | Treatment Options |
|---|---|---|
| *Hyperacute* – (rare) pre-formed antibodies | Immediate – 24h | Nephrectomy |
| *Accelerated* – (rare) humoral or cell-mediated | Up to 10d post-transplant | Less common now with ATG induction |
| *Acute Antibody*-mediated | Usually early, occasionally late | Pulsed steroid |
| | | Plasma exchange and IV immunoglobulin |
| | | Optimise maintenance IS |
| *Acute T-cell*-mediated | Usually early, occasionally late | Pulsed steroid |
| | | Optimise maintenance IS |
| | | ATG for rejection affecting the vascular component |
| *Chronic Antibody*-mediated | Late | Optimise maintenance IS |
| | | Consider plasma exchange and IV immunoglobulin |

*Abbreviations:* ATG, anti-thymocyte immunoglobulin; IS, immunosuppression, IV, intravenous.

- Diseases such as infections require reduction in IS dose.
- Poor prescribing practices or drug unavailability.
- There is poor patient compliance with IS medication.
- *Types:* hyperacute (rare), accelerated (rare), acute or chronic (Table 5.3).

# Recommended Reading

1. Banff classification of Renal Allograft Pathology updated Banff '97 classification. Am J Transplant. 2008; 8: 753–60.
2. Gill J et al. Use and outcomes of kidneys from donation after circulatory death donors in the United States. J Am Soc Nephrol. 2017 Dec; 28(12): 3647–57.
3. Bohmig G et al. Strategies to overcome the ABO barrier in kidney transplantation. Nat Rev Nephrol. 2015; 11: 732–47.
4. Summers DM et al. Kidney donation after circulatory death (DCD): state of the art. Kidney Int. 2015; 88(2): 241–9.
5. Halloran PF et al. Immunosuppressive drugs for kidney transplantation. N Engl J Med. 2004; 351: 2715–29.
6. Hardinger KL et al. Selection of induction kidney transplantation. Transpl Int. 2013. 26(7): 662–72.
7. Nankivell BJ & Alexander SI. Rejection of the kidney allograft. N Engl J Med. 2010; 363: 1451–62.
8. Loupy A & Lefaucher C. Antibody-mediated rejection of solid organ allografts. N Engl J Med. 2018; 379: 1150–60.
9. Zhang Q & Reed E. The importance of non-HLA antibodies in transplantation. Nat Rev Nephrol. 2016; 12: 484–95.
10. Nieto T et al. Renal transplantation in adults. BMJ. 2016; 355: i6158.

# 6 Haemostasis and Thrombosis

*Karl H. Pang and Michael Laffan*

## Haemostasis

- *Haemostasis* is the mechanism that arrests bleeding.
- *Coagulation* is the generation of thrombin and the fibrin clot.
- Haemostasis comprises three steps: *vascular spasm, platelet plug formation, coagulation.*

1. **Vascular spasm (vasoconstriction) and the endothelium**
   - *Vasoconstriction*
     - A brief intense contraction of blood vessels.
     - Decreases blood flow to the area of injury.
   - *In response to vascular injury or inflammation,* the endothelium becomes prothrombotic.
     - It downregulates the expression of anti-thrombotic molecules.
     - It expresses procoagulant tissue factor (TF).
     - It expresses adhesion molecules which mediate platelet and leucocyte capture.
     - It releases the von Willebrand factor (VWF) which mediates platelet capture and aggregation.
     - It releases plasminogen activator inhibitor-1 (PAI-1: inhibits fibrinolysis).
   - *Vascular endothelium*:
     - A monolayer of endothelial cells (EC) lining all blood vessels – forms the intima with the basement membrane.
     - Produces the glycocalyx (sugar-protein) which coats the endothelium.
   - *In normal (resting) circumstances,* the endothelium has an *antithrombotic* function:
     - It secretes:
       - Prostacyclin (vasodilator and platelet inhibition)
       - Nitric oxide (vasodilator and platelet inhibition)
       - Tissue-plasminogen activator (tPA: activates fibrinolysis)
     - It expresses on its surface:
       - ADPase
       - Thrombomodulin (cofactor for activation of protein C)
       - Endothelial protein C receptor

- Heparan sulphate (potentiates antithrombin)
- Tissue factor pathway inhibitor (TFPI)

2. **Platelet plug formation (primary haemostasis)**
   - *Platelets:*
     - There are 150-400 billion platelets per litre of blood.
     - Produced by megakaryocytes in the bone marrow.
     - Life span of 8-12 days.
     - Recognises the disruption of EC and the exposed underlying extracellular matrix (primarily collagen).
   - *A haemostatic plug* is formed through *adhesion, activation, and aggregation.*
   - *Adhesion*
     - VWF binds to exposed collagen. Some VWF — released from the EC — is already bound to the extravascular collagen.
     - Platelets bind to the VWF under high shear via glycoprotein Ib (GPIb).
     - At low shear and after capture by the VWF, platelets bind to collagen via GPIaIIa and GPVI.
   - *Activation*
     - The binding of platelets to collagen and the VWF leads to their activation and thus:
       - The release of dense granule contents, most importantly adenosine 5'-diphosphate (ADP).
       - The synthesis of thromboxane A2 (TXA2) from membrane phospholipids.
       - ADP and TXA2 bind to platelet surface receptors, producing further activation (positive feedback).
       - The exposure of negatively charged phosphatidylserine on their surface supports the assembly of coagulation factor complexes.
       - Platelets also release platelet-derived growth factor (PDGF) and vascular endothelial growth factor (VEGF) to promote angiogenesis following injury.
   - *Aggregation*
     - The activation of platelets causes GPIIbIIIa

- to change into an active configuration which binds fibrinogen.
- Fibrinogen binding to IIbIIIa results in platelet aggregation and signalling, which further reinforces activation.
- Other adhesion molecules — including VWF and fibronectin — also bind to IIbIIIa and contribute to aggregation.
- Platelets change configuration to mediate clot retraction which strengthens the clot.

3. **Coagulation** (Figure 6.1)
- Results in the generation of thrombin which converts soluble fibrinogen to insoluble fibrin strands so that they precipitate into a mesh that strengthens and stabilises the primary platelet plug (secondary haemostasis).
- The fibrin molecules are covalently cross-linked by the action of Factor XIII, which is also activated by thrombin.
- Most procoagulants and anticoagulants are produced by the liver — except factors VWF and Factor VIII which are produced by the endothelium.
- The enzymes of the cascade II, VII, IX, and X require Vitamin K for their synthesis in the liver (as do the anticoagulant proteins C and S).
- Standard coagulation tests activate thrombin generation by the pathways shown in Fig X. These are of practical use but differ from the pathways *in vivo*, which is of some practical significance.

- The pathways in Figure 6.1 are divided into three components: *extrinsic, intrinsic, common.*
  - *Extrinsic*:
    - Initiated by the TF.
    - A TF-VIIa complex is formed which activates factor X to factor Xa, and begins coagulation and joins the common pathway.
    - This is the physiological pathway which follows the exposure of extravascular TF to the blood.
  - *Intrinsic*:
    - This is initiated by the exposure of blood to negatively charged molecules (contact activation).
    - The negatively charged surface activates FXII and activation proceeds via the intrinsic and common pathways.
    - Contact activation is not necessary for normal haemostasis (patients with complete FXII deficiency do not bleed). However, FXI, FVIII, and FIX *are* all required. The explanation for this paradox is that *in vivo* TF-VIIa also activates FIX and thrombin will back activate FXI and FVIII (as well as FV).
  - *Common*:
    - Factor Xa combines with FVa to form the prothrombinase complex which converts prothrombin to thrombin.

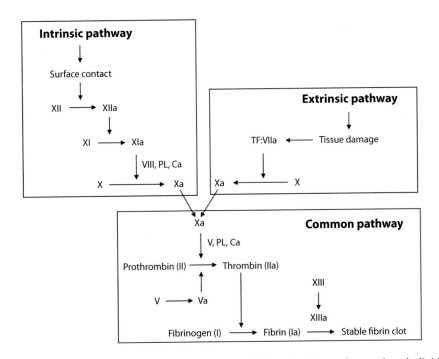

Figure 6.1 The coagulation cascade. TF, tissue factor; a, activated; PL, platelet membrane phospholipid; Ca, calcium.

- Thrombin also activates FXIII which cross-links fibrin and stabilises the clot.

# Anticoagulant Mechanisms

- The procoagulant mechanisms are continually active at a low level as evidenced by the presence of d-dimer and thrombin activation peptide (F1.2) in the blood of healthy individuals.
- This activity is held in check by a corresponding set of anticoagulant or inhibitory factors in the blood and endothelium.
- This prevents inappropriate coagulation events which would result in thrombosis.
- Thrombosis is the formation of a blood clot inside an intact vessel (as opposed to haemostatic clot formation).
- The anticoagulant systems also limit the extent of haemostatic events so that after injury, the haemostatic mechanisms arrest blood flow but do not propagate into undamaged vessels.
- *Anticoagulant factors:*
  - Tissue factor pathway inhibitor (TFPI)
    - Present in plasma and released by platelets, but the majority is on the surface of EC. It binds FXa and then TF-FVIIa and thus acts to dampen any procoagulant stimulus.
  - Antithrombin
    - Binds and inhibits the coagulation proteases, particularly thrombin (FIIa) and FXa. Its action is greatly potentiated by the heparans on the surface of EC and by heparin administered therapeutically.
  - Protein C-Protein S
    - Thrombin escaping from the haemostatic event is captured by thrombomodulin on the surface or normal endothelium. This drastically changes its specificity so that it now activates protein C (APC). APC in concert with Protein S degrades FVa and FVIIIa, thus limiting further thrombin generation.

# Fibrinolysis

- When the fibrin clot forms, it exposes binding sites (lysine residues) for plasminogen and tPA.
- The binding of plasminogen and tPA to fibrin promotes the cleavage of plasminogen to plasmin — its active form.
- Plasmin then degrades the cross-linked fibrin, releasing d-dimers and other fibrin degradation products.
- Plasmin is inhibited by antiplasmin in plasma.
- Tranexamic acid is a lysine analogue which binds to plasminogen, blocks its binding to fibrin, and so prevents its activation.

- tPA (and other agents) can be given therapeutically to promote plasmin generation and break down thrombi, but there is a significant risk of bleeding.
- The fibrinolytic system is also important in wound healing and extravascular repair and fibrosis. This involves interactions with the urokinase system and matrix proteases.

# The Balance of Haemostasis

- Principle. From the above description, it can be seen that the blood and vessels contain a complex mix of opposing factors that tend to form and prevent clot formation. It is useful to think of this system as normally existing in an equilibrium, or balance retains blood in liquid form, so that pathological states can be thought of as an imbalance.
  - *Haemorrhagic disorders may arise from*:
    - A deficiency of procoagulant factors (e.g., haemophilia)
    - An excess of anticoagulant factors (usually therapeutic)
  - *Thrombotic disorders may arise from*:
    - A deficiency of anticoagulant factors (e.g., antithrombin)
    - An excess of procoagulant factors (e.g., FVIII)
- The alterations in balance may be hereditary or acquired and involve single or multiple factors.
- The same principle applies to therapy. For example, warfarin reduces the risk of thrombosis by reducing the levels of procoagulant factors.

# Laboratory Measurement

- Samples for coagulation tests are taken into citrate anticoagulant. Unlike most other samples, this anticoagulant has a significant volume. Thus, the volume of blood in the tube must be correct to avoid dilution: always fill to the indicated line.
- Similarly, very high haematocrits can cause a similar problem due to the smaller volume of plasma.
- Coagulation in the tests is initiated by a trigger in combination with recalcification.
- The normal ranges are reagent dependent and so vary between laboratories.

1. *Prothrombin time (PT)*
   - PT = the time it takes for plasma to clot after adding TF, phospholipid, and Ca++.
   - *Normal range:* c11-13.5 sec
   - Evaluates *extrinsic* and *common* coagulation pathway (II, VII, X, V).
   - Requires clotting factors I (fibrinogen), II, V, VII, X

- *Prolonged by:*
  - Congenital deficiency of any of these factors
  - Warfarin and Vitamin K deficiency
  - Direct anticoagulants and high levels of heparin
  - Liver damage
  - Consumption, dilution
  - Acquired inhibitors (relatively unusual)

2. *International normalized ratio (INR)*
   - The ratio of a patient's PT to a normal (control) sample corrected for the reagent (thromboplastin) used.
   - Used to monitor warfarin (or other vitamin K antagonist) anticoagulant therapy.
   - *Normal range: 0.8-1.1*

3. *Activated partial thromboplastin time (APTT)*
   - Evaluates *intrinsic* and *common* coagulation pathway (all factors except factor VII).
   - *Normal range: 30-40 sec*
   - Prolonged by:
     - Congenital deficiency of any factor except FVII
     - Warfarin and Vitamin K deficiency (less marked than PT)
     - Direct anticoagulants and heparin
     - Inhibitors – including lupus anticoagulant and acquired anti-FVIII antibodies (acquired haemophilia)

4. *Anti-Xa assays*
   - These are used to measure heparins and direct FXa inhibitors. It is important to specify what is being measured because they are all calibrated and reported differently.

5. *Thromboelastography (TEG) or thromboelastometry (ROTEM)*

- Viscoelastic haemostatic assay – usually performed on un-anticoagulated whole blood.
- Performed as a point of care test for rapid assessment of coagulation status and to guide replacement therapy.
- Approved by NICE for cardiac surgery but is widely used outside this indication. https://www.nice.org.uk/guidance/DG13/chapter/1-Recommendations
- Measures the global viscoelastic properties of whole blood clot formation under low shear stress.
- TEG shows the interaction of platelets with the coagulation cascade.
  - Thromboelastogram gives details regarding (Figure 6.2).
  - *R:* reaction time (sec) – time to initiate fibrin formation.
  - *K:* kinetic (sec) – time to achieve a certain level of clot strength.
  - *alpha:* angle-rate of clot strengthening through polymerisation of available fibrinogen.
  - *TMA:* time to maximum amplitude (sec).
  - *MA:* maximum amplitude (mm) – includes platelet contribution (number, function) to clot strength through interaction with fibrinogen/fibrin.
  - *A30 (LY30):* amplitude at 30 min
  - *CLT:* Clot lysis time (sec) – fibrinolytic activity derived from percentage decrease in clot strength 30 min after MA is reached.
- The corresponding ROTEM terms are:
  - CT (clot time)
  - CFT (clot formation time)
  - Alpha angle (the same)
  - MCF (maximum clot firmness)
  - CLI 30 (clot lysis index at 30 minutes)

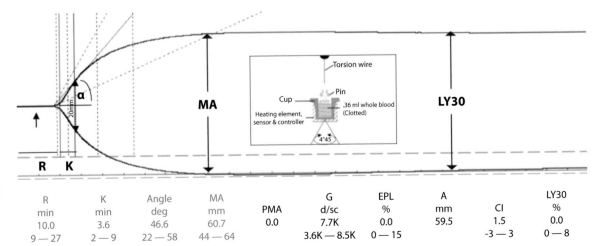

| R min | K min | Angle deg | MA mm | PMA | G d/sc | EPL % | A mm | CI | LY30 % |
|---|---|---|---|---|---|---|---|---|---|
| 10.0 | 3.6 | 46.6 | 60.7 | 0.0 | 7.7K | 0.0 | 59.5 | 1.5 | 0.0 |
| 9 — 27 | 2 — 9 | 22 — 58 | 44 — 64 | | 3.6K — 8.5K | 0 — 15 | | -3 — 3 | 0 — 8 |

**Figure 6.2** Normal human thromboelastogram (citrated native blood). The ROTEM produces a similar tracing but with slightly different nomenclature. (Reprinted by permission from Springer Nature [3])

| **Table 6.1** Risk Factors for Thrombosis (Virchow's Triad) | | |
|---|---|---|
| **Blood flow stasis** | **Endothelial dysfunction** | **Hypercoagulability** |
| Long surgical procedures | Hypertension | Malignancy |
| Prolonged immobility | Diabetes | Factor V Leiden mutation |
| Atrial fibrillation | Atherosclerosis | Antithrombin III deficiency |
| Left ventricular dysfunction | | Protein C or S deficiency |
| | | Venous insufficiency/obstruction |
| | | Obesity |
| | | Cigarette smoking |
| | | Hormonal contraceptives |
| | | Pregnancy |

# Thrombosis

- Haemostasis is the normal physiological process in response to vascular injury.
- A pathological thrombus forms in intact vessels when there is an imbalance in the coagulation system.
- *Type of thrombus:*
  - Venous (deep vein thrombosis, pulmonary embolism, superficial thrombophlebitis)
  - Arterial (cerebral vascular accident, myocardial infarction, bowel ischaemia, limb ischaemia)
- *Virchow's triad* – the risk of thrombosis depends on three factors:
  - *The blood* – hypercoagulability, hyperviscosity
  - *The endothelium* – injury and inflammation
  - *The blood flow* – stasis/turbulence (Table 6.1)
- Thrombosis arises from an imbalance in the pro and anticoagulant mechanisms (see above).

# Specific Pathological States

1. **Disseminated intravascular coagulation (DIC)**
   - Also called 'consumptive coagulopathy'.
   - Usually triggered by the intravascular expression of TF which causes widespread coagulation activation.
   - This results in:
     - Thrombin generation and fibrin formation which is deposited in critical organs leading to organ failure.
     - Consumption and deficiency of coagulation factors (including platelets) leading to haemorrhage.
     - Excess generation of plasmin causing degradation of fibrinogen and leading to haemorrhage.
   - Intravascular TF expression on leucocytes and EC is stimulated by inflammation (e.g., sepsis, shock, malignancy).

- Coagulation tests: In established DIC, all coagulation tests are prolonged, platelets and fibrin are reduced, and D-dimers are elevated. In the initial stages, the platelet count falls first, followed by prolongation of clotting tests. Defibrination is a relatively late feature.

2. **Sickle cell disease (SCD)**
   - Most commonly seen in patients with ancestry in malarial areas: sub-Saharan Africa, the Mediterranean Basin, the Middle East, and India.
   - Multisystem disorder caused by a single gene mutation.
   - Characterised by the presence of abnormal erythrocytes (sickle or crescent shape) damaged by polymerisation of sickle haemoglobin (HbS).
   - SC anaemia is defined as homozygosity for the HbS gene- mutation on the beta-globin gene (*HBB*).
   - Many other forms of varying severity arise from compound heterozygosity with another Hb variant. For example, HbSC disease and HbS-beta thalassaemia.
   - Inherited in an autosomal recessive pattern.
   - Vaso-occlusion and haemolytic anaemia are central to the pathophysiology of SCD and precipitate a cascade of pathological events:
     - Vascular-endothelial dysfunction
     - Functional nitric oxide deficiency
     - Inflammation
     - Oxidative stress and reperfusion injury
     - Hypercoagulability
     - Increased neutrophil adhesion
     - Platelet activation
   - Signs and symptoms of SCD usually begin in early childhood and is a result of the above pathological mechanisms:
     - The typical event is vaso-occlusion. In children, this may present as dactylitis; in

older patients, a painful occlusive crisis may involve the limbs, abdomen, or the chest (chest syndrome).

- Vessel vasculopathy results in cerebrovascular disease and stroke at a young age, pulmonary hypertension, priapism, leg ulcers, and retinopathy.
- Progressive ischaemic organ damage: hyposplenism, renal failure, bone disease, and liver damage.
- General: anaemia, infections, jaundice, pain (acute chest syndrome).

- Association with priapism (See Chapter 21)
  - The prevalence of priapism in SCD is up to 48%.
  - >95% ischaemic type priapism.
  - Altered vascular homeostatic actions in the penis and deficient erection control mechanisms.
  - Possible molecular mechanisms:
    - Aberrant signalling of the endothelium-derived nitric oxide and PDE5 signal transduction pathway in the penis.
    - Dysfunctional signal transduction systems involving adenosine and RhoA/Rho-kinase.
    - Opiorphins also demonstrate a role in regulating corporal smooth muscle tone and, thereby, dysregulation of erection physiology in priapism.

- Management of acute priapism (see Chapter 21):
  - SCD: aspiration, corporal irrigation, +/- shunting
  - Intravenous fluids, alkalinisation, and exchange transfusion
  - Limited evidence for a medical prophylaxis role for hydroxyurea, etilefrine, pseudoephedrine, leuprolide, sildenafil, and other agents.
- Long term consequences:
  - Stuttering priapism
  - Erectile dysfunction

# Recommended Reading

1. van der Meijden PEJ and Heemskerk JWM. Platelet biology and functions: new concepts and clinical perspectives. Nat Rev Cardiol. 2019;16(3)166–179.
2. Saito H, Matsushita T, Kojima T. Historical perspective and future direction of coagulation research. J Thomb Haemost. 2011;9 Suppl 1:352–363.
3. Othman M and Kaur H. Thromboelastogram (TEG). Methods Mol Biol. 2017;1646:533–543.
4. Gando S, Levi M, Toh CH. Disseminated intravascular coagulation. Nat Rev Dis Primers. 2016;2:16037.
5. Piel FB, Steinberg MH, Rees DC. Sickle cell disease. NEJM. 2017;376(16):1561–1573.
6. Kato GJ. Priapism in sickle-cell disease: a hematologist's perspective. J Sex Med. 2012;9(1):70–78.
7. Hoffbrand AV, Higgs, DR, Keeling DM, Mehta AB. Postgraduate Haematology, 7th Edition. Wiley-Blackwell.

# Systemic Response to Surgery and Shock

*Nadir I. Osman*

## Systemic Response to Surgery

- Interlinked/overlapping physiological changes occur.
- Mix of immune, endocrine, metabolic, and haemodynamic responses (Figure 7.1).
- Classically described as biphasic *'ebb'* and *'flow'* process.
  - *Ebb phase:* reduced metabolic activity (2–3 days).
  - *Flow phase:* prolonged catabolic and hypermetabolic phase lasting over a week.
- In reality, the two phases are less clearly defined.

## Activations of Stress Response

- Tissue injury → afferent signals from the site of injury → dorsal root ganglion → hypothalamus.
- *Cytokines:* mediate and maintain inflammatory response. Initial release from activated macrophages and monocytes in damaged tissue (IL1 and TNF-a) → simulates mass release of IL6.
- *Acute phase response:* series of changes stimulated by IL6. This includes production of acute phase proteins in the liver which act as inflammatory mediators (e.g., CRP, fibrinogen, antiproteinases).

## Elements of Stress Response

- *Sympatho-adrenal:* release of epinephrine and norepinephrine from adrenal medulla → increase in heart rate and blood pressure.
- *Sympatho-renal:* release of renin from juxtaglomerular cells of kidneys → activation of renin–angiotensin–aldosterone axis → $Na^+$ absorption from distal convoluted tubule and increase of peripheral resistance → increase in blood pressure.
- *Hypothalamic–pituitary–adrenal axis:* ACTH (anterior pituitary) → cortisol (adrenal medulla) → increase in blood glucose (via gluconeogenesis, lipolysis) and anti-inflammatory effect.
- *Growth hormone* from anterior pituitary: increased glycogenolysis → increases blood glucose.
- *ADH* from posterior pituitary: upregulation of aquaporin channels in collecting ducts → reabsorption of free water.

- *Sympatho-pancreas:*
  - Reduced insulin secretion → reduced inhibition of protein catabolism and lipolysis.
  - Increased glucagon → stimulates lipolysis, gluconeogenesis, and glycogenolysis → increases blood glucose.

## Metabolic Sequalae of Stress Response

- Net effect = secretions of catabolic hormones and release of substrate from catabolism of carbohydrate, protein, and fat.
- *Carbohydrate* metabolism: due to the decreased insulin production and increased resistance → blood glucose levels are related to intensity of surgical insult.
- *Protein* metabolism: stimulated by cortisol, protein breakdown mainly in the skeletal muscle.
- *Fat metabolism:* stimulated by cortisol, catecholamines, and growth hormone.
- *Water and electrolyte* metabolism: ADH and renin result in net water and sodium retention.

## Unregulated Stress Response

- Potentially harmful and may result in:
  - Systemic inflammatory response syndrome (SIRS)
  - Acute respiratory distress syndrome (ARDS)
  - Multiorgan failure

## Strategies to Mitigate Stress Response

- Minimally invasive surgery → reduction of tissue injury
- Reduction of operative time
- Regional anaesthesia → neural blockade
- Enhanced recovery after surgery (ERAS) protocols

## Enhanced Recovery After Surgery

- ERAS protocols aim to reduce stress and improve response to stress.
- Mainly for abdominal-pelvic surgery, such as radical cystectomy/cystoprostatectomy.
- Maintains homoeostasis and prevents catabolic

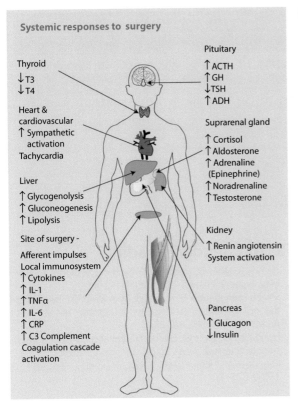

**Systemic responses to surgery**

**Thyroid**
↓T3
↓T4

**Heart & cardiovascular**
↑ Sympathetic activation
Tachycardia

**Liver**
↑ Glycogenolysis
↑ Gluconeogenesis
↑ Lipolysis

**Site of surgery -**
Afferent impulses
Local immunosystem
↑ Cytokines
↑ IL-1
↑ TNFα
↑ IL-6
↑ CRP
↑ C3 Complement
Coagulation cascade activation

**Pituitary**
↑ ACTH
↑ GH
↓TSH
↑ ADH

**Suprarenal gland**
↑ Cortisol
↑ Aldosterone
↑ Adrenaline (Epinephrine)
↑ Noradrenaline
↑ Testosterone

**Kidney**
↑ Renin angiotensin System activation

**Pancreas**
↑ Glucagon
↓ Insulin

**Figure 7.1** Summary of changes in hormones and effects of the stress response to surgery. ACTH, adrenocorticotrophic hormone; ADH, antidiuretic hormone; CRP, C-reactive protein; GH, growth hormone; IL, interleukin; TNF, tumour necrosis factor; TSH, thyroid-stimulating hormone. (Reprinted with permission from Elsevier [1])

responses that cause loss of protein/muscle strength and cellular dysfunction.

- Pre-operative nutrition and carbohydrate loading aim to minimise post-operative insulin resistance.
- Epidural/spinal anaesthesia reduces the endocrine stress response.
- Anti-inflammatories reduce inflammation.
- Early feeding avoids insulin resistance.
- Maintains euvolemia, cardiac output, and delivery of oxygen and nutrients which supports cellular function after surgery.

## Shock

- Life-threatening circulatory disorder which causes inadequate organ perfusion and tissue hypoxia.
- *Three types:*
  - Cardiogenic
  - Hypovolaemic
  - Distributive shock

## Cardiogenic Shock

- Definition: systolic blood pressure (BP) of <90 mmHg, urine output of <20 mL/hour, and normal or elevated filling pressure.
- *Pathophysiology:* reduced contractility → decreased cardiac output
- *Aetiology:*
  - *Non-obstructive:* myocardial infarction, arrhythmias, heart failure
  - *Obstructive:* tension pneumothorax, cardiac tamponade, pulmonary embolism

## Hypovolaemic Shock

- *Pathophysiology:* loss of >20% intravascular volume. The faster the rate, the less likely for compensation.
- *Aetiology:*
  - *Haemorrhagic* (trauma, surgical)
  - *Non-haemorrhagic* (gastrointestinal loss, third space, post-obstructive diuresis)
- *Classification* (see Table 7.1)

## Distributive Shock

- *Septic:* see Chapter 16.
- *Neurogenic:* loss of sympathetic vascular tone → peripheral vasodilation → reduction in blood pressure
  - *Causes:* spinal cord injury, severe pain, cerebral haemorrhage
- *Anaphylactic:* Type 1 hypersensitivity reaction → mast cell degranulation → histamine release → systemic vasodilation → capillary leak → drop in blood pressure and tissue oedema

## Compensatory Mechanisms

- *Baroreceptor* reflex: drop in BP sensed → increases heart rate, contractility, and peripheral resistance
- *Chemoreceptor* reflexes: acidosis sensed → further sympathetic stimulation
- *Humoral* mechanism: renin-angiotensin–aldosterone pathway → further catecholamine release and ADH release

## Decompensatory Mechanisms

- Result after failure of compensatory mechanisms:
- *Cardiogenic shock:* impaired coronary blood flow → cardiac ischaemia
- *Sympathetic escape:* accumulation of metabolic vasodilators in tissues impairs sympathetic mediated vasoconstriction
- *Cerebral ischaemia:* loss of sympathetic outflow from medulla

**Table 7.1** Classification of Haemorrhagic Shock

| Class | I | II | III | IV |
|---|---|---|---|---|
| Blood loss | <15% (750 mL) | 15–30% (750-1500 mL) | 30–40% (1500-2000 mL) | >40% (>2000 mL) |
| Heart rate | <100 | 100–120 | 120–140 | >140 |
| Systolic blood pressure | Normal | Normal | ↓ | ↓ |
| Pulse pressure | Normal or ↑ | ↓ | ↓ | ↓ |
| Respiratory rate per min | 14–20 | 20–30 | 30–40 | >35 |
| Urine output mL/h | >30 | 20–30 | 5–15 | Absent |
| Mental status | Anxious | Mildly anxious | Anxious, confused | Confused, lethargic |

- *Metabolic acidosis:* depresses cardiac contractility and reduces smooth muscle tone
- *Systemic inflammatory response:* endotoxins from ischaemic bowel lead to cytokine production → $NO_2$ and oxygen-free radical → cardiac depression and vasodilation
- *Rheological factors:* stasis in microcirculation → increases viscosity and plugging of microcirculation by white blood cells and platelets → intravascular coagulation

# Recommended Reading

1. de Bois J, Moor D, Aggarwal G. Systemic response to surgery. Surgery (Oxford). 2020; 38(3): 172–6.
2. Manou-Stathopoulou V, Korbonits M, Ackland GL. Redefining the perioperative stress response: a narrative review. Br J Anaesth. 2019; 123(5): 570–83.
3. Ljungqvist O, Scott M, Fearon KC. Enhanced recovery after surgery: a review. JAMA Surg. 2017; 152(3): 292–8.
4. Cannon JW. Hemorrhagic shock. N Engl J Med. 2018; 378(4): 370–9.

# Section II

## EMBRYOLOGY, ANATOMY, AND PHYSIOLOGY

# 8 Embryology, Anatomy, and Physiology of the Kidneys and Ureters

*Paul Sturch, Sanjeev Madaan, and Seshadri Sriprasad*

## Embryology of the Kidney and Ureters

- 4th week of gestation – development of the urogenital system begins.
- Involves three structures (Figure 8.1):
  - *Pronephros* (week 4)
  - *Mesonephros (weeks 5–8)*
  - *Metanephros* (week 5 onwards)
- The pronephros and mesonephros regress.
- The metanephros persists to become the mature kidney.
- The intermediate mesoderm forms a urogenital ridge on either side of the aorta.
  - The *pronephros* is the first structure to develop.
  - It acts as a blueprint for the subsequent formation of the renal tract.
- 5th week – pronephros degenerates as the mesonephros forms.
  - Starts cranially and progresses caudally.
- 8th–9th week – mesonephros stops working as a functional unit and the metanephros takes over.
  - *Males* – mesonephros becomes the epididymis, vas, and seminal vesicles.
  - *Females* – without the action of anti-müllerian hormone (AMH), the mesonephros regresses.
- *Metanephros* forms from the intermediate mesoderm caudal to the mesonephros.
  - Does not regress – forms the mature functioning kidney.
  - The ureteric bud develops from the metanephros.
- The surrounding tissue of the metanephric mesenchyme forms:
  - The glomeruli, the proximal convoluted tubule (PCT), the Loop of Henle (LOH), and the distal convoluted tubule (DCT).

## The Collecting System

- 5th week onwards – metanephros penetrates the surrounding tissue as the ureteric bud.
- This *ureteric bud* forms:
  - The collecting system (collecting duct, CD), renal pelvis, and ureter.
  - This process is known as renal induction.
- The metanephric mesenchyme becomes the rest of the kidney.
- Ureteric bud bifurcates ~4 days after it forms and penetrates the mesenchyme.
  - Each end of the bifurcating duct dilates into an ampulla—becoming the renal pelvis.
  - Further sequential branching of each part of the duct forms the major calyces.
- Branching continues up to week 32 → results in 1–3 million collecting tubules.
- 4th–5th weeks – the lumen of the ureter becomes patent starting from its centre point, progressing both cranially and caudally.
- As the bladder continues to develop, the mesonephric (Wolffian) duct and the ureter are incorporated into the bladder base.
- *Chwalla's membrane* forms at the point at which the ureter enters the urogenital sinus (UGS).
  - Normally ruptures, allowing the passage of urine.
  - Failure of normal perforation leads to a *ureterocoele* (Figure 8.2).
- 9th week – metanephros starts producing urine and drains down the ureter maintaining its patency.
- Smooth muscle develops in the ureteric wall.
  - Failure of normal muscular development results in an *aperistaltic segment, dilatation*, and *megaureter*.

## The Development of the Nephron

- As the collecting system forms, the bifurcating ureteric bud secretes growth factors.
  - Induces the adjacent metanephric mesenchyme to differentiate into:
    - The *renal vesicle*
      - Forms the PCT, LOH, and DCT
    - The *s-shaped tubule*
      - One end acquires capillaries and forms the glomerulus and Bowman's capsule.
      - The other end fuses with the ureteric duct.

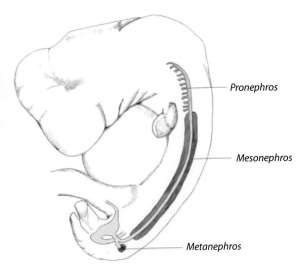

Figure 8.1 Location of the pre-, meso- and metanephros. (Reuse with permission from John Wiley and Sons [1])

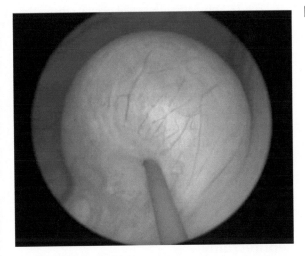

Figure 8.2 Cystoscopic view of a left ureterocoele. A ureterocoele Results from failure of the Chwalla's membrane to rupture.

- Formation of the nephron continues until birth.
- The loss of function of any of the inductive factors involved in this process can lead to *hypoplasia or agenesis.*

## Disorders of Renal Development

- *Renal agenesis* – failure of the ureteric bud to arise from the mesonephric duct.
- If the ureteric bud arises more medially and closer to the UGS:
  - Renal dysplasia may occur and the ureteric orifice will lie laterally and superiorly to its normal position as the mesonephric duct and ureter rotate during the development of the bladder.
  - This can lead to a short intravesical portion of the ureter, resulting in loss of anti-reflux mechanism and reflux of urine.
- If the *ureteric bud* arises further away from the UGS:
  - A dysplastic kidney may occur with an ectopic ureter opening medially and inferiorly (*Weigert-Meyer*).
  - The ectopic ureter may open at the bladder neck, urethra, vagina, or vas.
- *Duplication* → results in duplex ureters, with or without ectopia or ureterocoele (Figure 8.3)
- *Abnormal ascent* → results in pelvic kidney
- *Fusion* → results in a horseshoe kidney

# Anatomy of the Kidney and Ureters

## Kidneys

- Paired organs, ~11 cm in length, weighing 130–150 g.
- Receive ~25% of the cardiac output (~1300 mL/min).
- Mobile within the retroperitoneum.
- Position varies with respiration and body position.
- *The right kidney* is slightly lower (1–2 cm), shorter, and wider than the left due to compression by the liver.
- Lie on the psoas and quadratus lumborum muscles of the posterior abdominal wall.
- Longitudinal axis lies obliquely along the line of the psoas.
- Renal hila face anteromedially by ~30°–50°.
- The upper pole is larger and positioned more medial and posterior than the smaller lower pole.
- The kidneys are enclosed:
  - in a fibrous capsule surrounded in perirenal fat.
  - then Gerota's fascia, surrounded in pararenal fat.

## Gerota's Fascia

- Consists of an anterior and posterior layer.
- The anterior fascia is thinner and adherent to the peritoneum.
- *Superiorly* – fuses with the infra-diaphragmatic fascia above the adrenal glands.
- *Laterally* – fuses behind the colon.
- *Medially* – fuses with the fascia of paraspinal muscles and connective tissue of the great vessels.

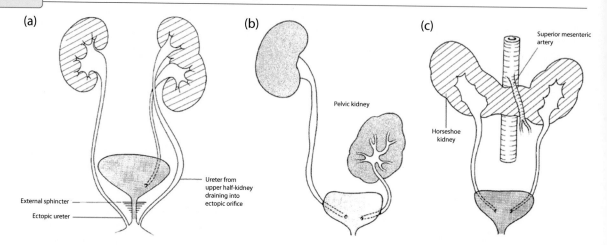

**Figure 8.3** Abnormal renal and ureteric development. (a) Duplex system: the ureter draining the upper moiety opens inferio-medially and may drain ectopically into the vagina or urethral sphincter; (b) Pelvic kidney: remains rotated; (c) Horseshoe kidney: ascent is halted by the inferior mesenteric artery. (Reuse with permission from John Wiley and Sons [1])

- *Inferiorly* – fascia is open, acting as a potential space allowing perinephric collections to track into the pelvis.

## Anatomical Relations

- *Right* kidney:
  - *Superior* – liver, separated by peritoneum.
    - Parietal peritoneum runs as the hepatorenal ligament to the liver.
    - Excessive downward traction on the kidney can lead to a capsular tear.
  - *Medial* – duodenum, can potentially be injured during laparoscopic nephrectomy.
  - *Hepatic flexure* – anterior to the right lower pole.

- *Left* kidney:
  - *Superior* – spleen and stomach.
  - *Superio-medially* – left adrenal gland.
  - *Inferior* – jejunum and splenic flexure.
  - *Medial* – tail of the pancreas and splenic vessels.
  - The parietal peritoneum runs as the splenorenal ligament between the upper pole of the left kidney and spleen.
  - Splenic flexure – anterior to the left lower pole.

## Percutaneous Access

- The lungs and diaphragm are closely related to the kidneys.
- Diaphragm covers posterior part of the upper third of both kidneys.

- The 12th rib, with its invested pleura, crosses the kidneys just inferior to the diaphragm.
  - Supra-costal punctures and many punctures below the 12th rib may pass through the diaphragm.
- Lungs lie just superior to the 11th rib.
  - Punctures in the 10th intercostal space involve risks of lung injury.
- Intercostal punctures should be made in the *lower half* of the intercostal space — *on top of the rib* below — to avoid damage to the intercostal vessels.
- Punctures through the fornix of a calyx carry much lower risk of vascular injury compared to the infundibulum.

## Nephrectomy

- *Transabdominal approach*:
  - Colon must be mobilised along the white *line of Toldt*.
    - *Toldt* – a lateral reflection of the posterior parietal peritoneum over the ascending and descending colon.
  - *Kocher's manoeuvre* – mobilisation of the second part of the duodenum. Often required to access the *right* renal hilum.

## Sectional Anatomy

- The kidney consists of (Figure 8.4):
  - The outer cortex and inner medulla.
  - A collecting system of calyces and renal pelvis draining into the ureter.
  - Renal medulla – made up of conically shaped 'pyramids'.

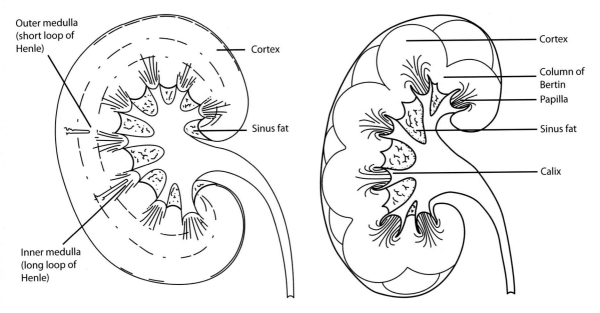

**Figure 8.4** Section through the kidney. (Reuse with permission from John Wiley and Sons [1])

- Pyramid bases point laterally.
- The pyramid apex points to the renal papilla as it enters its individual minor calyx.
- The cortex covers the pyramids peripherally and extends between each pyramid as the *Columns of Bertin*.

## Vascular Anatomy

- The kidneys develop in the true pelvis.
- The vascular pedicle is derived sequentially from different sources along its ascent to the adult para-aortic position.
  - Failure of renal ascent results in a pelvic kidney.
  - Therefore, blood vessels may be derived from anomalous sources (Figure 8.5).
- Renal arteries arise from the aorta at the level of the intervertebral disk between the L1 and L2 lumbar vertebrae.
- The right renal artery passes behind the inferior vena cava (IVC).
- The right renal artery is longer than the left.
- Each renal artery gives branches to the following:
  - The adrenal gland, renal pelvis, and upper ureter.
  - The artery divides into anterior and posterior divisions after entering the hilum.
  - The anterior division supplies the anterior two-thirds of the kidney through five segmental branches.

- The posterior division supplies the posterior third of the kidney.
- Variations in renal anatomy may occur in 25–40% of the population.
- Multiple renal arteries may arise from the

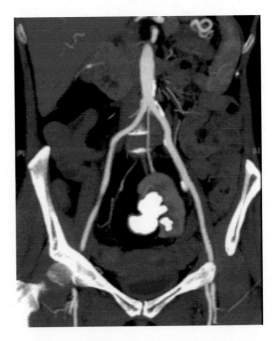

**Figure 8.5** CT (coronal section) showing a pelvic Kidney with a staghorn stone and blood supply from the iliacs at the aortic bifurcation.

aorta/iliac vessels in horseshoe or pelvic kidneys.

- ~5% of the main right renal artery passes anteriorly to the IVC.

## Key Points

- The renal artery divides into five segmental branches (Figure 8.6).
  - Segmental branches are end arteries and do not significantly anastomose.
  - Injury to one branch will cause an infarction to the segment of kidney supplied by that vessel.
- The *line of Brodel* is a relatively avascular plane just posterior to the lateral convex border of the kidney.
  - Preferred point of access for percutaneous puncture of posterior calyces, and was of

importance when an atrophic nephrolithotomy was practised due to reduced bleeding.

- *Horseshoe kidney*
  - Most common renal fusion abnormality (1:400).
  - The inferior mesenteric artery can arrest ascent of the midline isthmus.
  - Associated with abnormal vascular supply depending on the final position of the kidneys.

## Venous Drainage

- The venous drainage closely follows the arterial supply.
- Extensive communication between venous collaterals around calyceal infundibulae, subcapsular plexus, and perirenal veins.
- 3–5 segmental veins join to form the renal vein.
- Renal vein lies anterior to the artery.

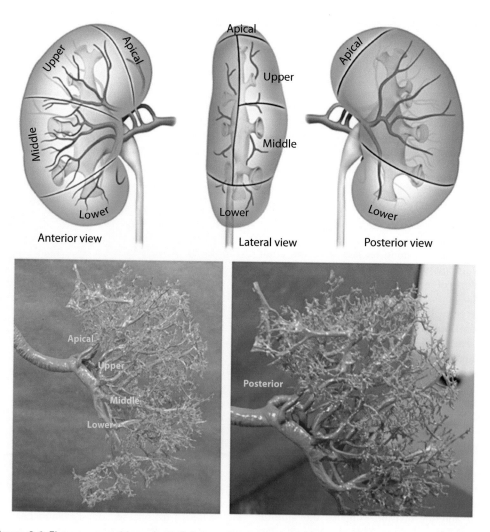

**Figure 8.6** Five segmental branches of the renal artery. (Reprinted with permission from Elsevier [7])

- Occlusion of a segmental venous branch has little impact on venous drainage.
- Both renal veins drain into the IVC.
- The left renal vein is longer than the right.
  - Receives the left gonadal and adrenal veins (right gonadal vein drains into IVC)
  - May also receive a lumbar vein.
  - May travel through a narrow angle between the superior mesenteric artery anteriorly and the aorta posteriorly.
    - Compression of the vein may cause 'nutcracker syndrome' (pain, haematuria, or varicoceles from venous congestion).

## Lymphatics

- Closely related to renal vessels.
- Lymph vessels running *anterior* to the respective renal vein drain into:
  - paracaval, precaval, retrocaval, and inter-aortocaval nodes.
- Lymphatics travelling *posterior* to the vein drain into:
  - paracaval, retrocaval, and inter-aortocaval nodes.
- Retrocaval nodes connect with the thoracic duct.
- The thoracic duct drains into the junction of the left subclavian and internal jugular vein.
- On the left side, lymph vessels may pass through the left crus of the diaphragm and connect with the thoracic duct directly, without draining into any lymph nodes.
- Variations in lymphatic drainage are common and make lymphatic spread in renal cell carcinoma unpredictable.

## Key Points

- *Renal hilum*
  - Renal vein anterior
  - Renal artery behind
  - Ureter most posterior
- *Renal pedicle* – single paired renal artery and vein enters the hilum and extends into the kidney via the renal sinus.
- The renal arterial blood supply, venous, and lymphatic drainage follow a similar segmental pattern → travel between the renal hilum to the peripheral tissue through renal sinuses.

## Nerve Supply

- Th kidneys have a rich nerve supply from the autonomic nervous system.
- *Sympathetic innervation*
  - Preganglionic sympathetic nerves originate from the T8-L1 segments.
    - Contributions from the coeliac and greater splanchnic, intermesenteric, and superior hypogastric plexuses.
  - Postganglionic sympathetic fibres from the autonomic plexus surrounding the renal artery follow the paths of the arterial supply through the cortex and outer medulla.
  - Controls renal blood flow through vasoconstriction.
  - Thought to transmit pain sensation.
- *Parasympathetic* fibres
  - Originate from the Vagus nerve (cranial X).
  - Travel with sympathetic fibres to the autonomic plexus.
  - Their role is unknown.

## The Ureters

- Muscular tubes – continuation of the renal pelvis.
- Run along the retroperitoneum.
  - The abdominal portion run along the anterior surface of the psoas crossing anteriorly to the tips of the L3-5 transverse processes.
  - Pass over the bifurcation of the common iliac artery as they enter the pelvis.
  - Run a lateral course (along with internal iliac artery) before passing medially to enter the urinary bladder.
  - Ureters cross the obturator vessels and nerve at the lateral wall of the pelvis.
  - At the level of the ischial spine, the ureters pass medially through the endopelvic fascia along with the hypogastric nerves.
- Both ureters are crossed anteriorly by the gonadal and are close to the pelvis.
- The left ureter is crossed by the colic vessels and sigmoid colon.
- *Males* – vas swings medially, crossing in front of the ureter.
- *Females* – ureter passes through the base of the broad ligament, under the uterine vessels (water under the bridge).
- *Distal* ureter – enveloped in a muscle layer (*Waldeyer sheath*) before it enters the bladder in an oblique line.
  - Waldeyer muscle fibres fuse with the detrusor muscle, preventing reflux during bladder contraction.
- *Blood supply* is segmental from:
  - The renal artery, gonadal, and vesical arteries.
  - Smaller branches from the aorta, common iliac, and vaginal arteries.

## Key Points

- Total length – 22–30 cm
- The ureter consists of *three layers:*

- *Inner* mucosa – transitional epithelium on a layer of lamina propria, which the vessels and nerves supplying the ureter run in.
- Muscular *middle* layer – layers either side of a layer of circular fibres in between.
  - Extends into the minor calyces where the ureters peristaltic pacemaker is situated.
  - *Outer* adventitia – collagen and elastic fibres with blood vessels and nerves.
- The ureter is divided into abdominal and pelvic segments — or into three, according to its position relative to the sacrum.
  - *Upper* – above the sacrum.
  - *Mid* – over the sacrum.
  - *Lower* – below the sacrum.
- *Three narrowing points* – potential for ureteric stones to obstruct.
  - Pelviureteric junction (PUJ).
  - As it crosses the iliac vessels.
  - Vesicoureteric junction (VUJ).

## Ureteric Function

- Baseline ureteric pressure: 0–5 cm $H_2O$
- Pressure during contraction: 20–80 cm $H_2O$
- Resting potential: –30 to –70 mV
- Urine production is continuous.
- Minor calyces have pacemakers—atypical smooth muscle cells.
- Urine is propagated into the upper ureter from the renal pelvis.
- The PUJ acts as a gate.
- Urine peristalses happens once there is sufficient volume for a bolus.
- Peristaltic waves occur 2–6 times per minute.
- Peristaltic contractions can occur in the ureter even when denervated.
  - Can occur from stimulation at any point along its length.
- VUJ: telescoping and lengthening, allows urine to pass into the bladder (not relaxation).

## Ureteric Duplication

- Duplex ureters may be partial or complete.
- *Partial duplication*:
  - Premature division of a single ureteric bud before it fuses with the mesenchyme.
  - Ureter fuses and enter the bladder as a single tube.
- *Complete duplication*:
  - This is less common.
  - Two ureteric buds forming two complete and separate ureters.
  - The *Weigert-Meyer* Rule:
    - The ureter draining the upper pole moiety crosses and enters the bladder inferio-medially to the lower pole moiety ureter.

- The ectopic duplex ureter may be associated with:
  - Ureterocoele, causing obstruction and dilatation of the upper pole ureter.
  - Reflux of the lower pole ureter.
  - Urinary incontinence if it opens distal to the urinary sphincter.
- *'Drooping lily sign'*
  - The inferolateral displacement of the opacified lower pole moiety due to an obstructed (and unopacified) upper pole moiety in duplicated collecting system.

# Physiology of the Kidney
## Functions of the Kidney

- Excretion of metabolic waste products, drugs and toxins.
- Regulation of water and electrolyte balance.
- Regulation of arterial pressure.
- Regulation of acid–base balance.
- Erythropoiesis.
- Hormone regulation.

- Water and solutes are filtered out of the blood, leaving only red cells and large proteins.
  - Free filtration of neutral and small molecules.
  - Some filtrations of neutral and positively-charged particles up to 60 Å.
  - No filtration of larger molecule or highly negatively-charged molecules (e.g., albumin).
    - Proteinuria may be due to the abnormal 'leak' of molecules and may be indicative of glomerular disease.

- Oncotic pressure is constant at ~25 mmHg.
- Urine is formed through reabsorption of water and salts and the secretion of waste products.
  - Blood passes into the glomerulus (an extension of the renal capillaries) and into the Bowman's capsule.
  - The high permeability of the glomerulus is achieved through:
    - Fenestration of the negatively-charged capillary endothelial layer.
    - Filtration slits in the glomerulus.
  - Passive ultrafiltration of plasma across the semipermeable membrane into the proximal tubule creates urine.
  - Fine-tuning of urine occurs in the LOH, distal tubule, CD, and renal pelvis.

- *The nephron* (~1 million per kidney) consists of:
  - Glomerulus (filtration)
  - Proximal tubule (reabsorption)
  - Loop of Henle (concentration)
  - Distal tubule (reabsorption and secretion)
  - Collecting duct (reabsorption and secretion)

- *Renal clearance* – amount of plasma where a substance is completely removed from the body (mL/min).
- The *glomerular filtration rate* (GFR) is determined by:
  - Glomerular permeability
  - Glomerular surface area
  - Hydrostatic pressure gradient
  - Oncotic pressure gradient (maintained at a constant 25 mmHg)
- *Glomerular filtration* is maintained over a range of blood pressures through several mechanisms:
  - *Myogenic autoregulation*
    - With increasing arterial pressure, the walls of the afferent arterioles stretch and then contract to regulate flow.
    - Glomerular blood pressure at ~50–60 mmHg.
  - *Osmotic autoregulation*
    - The macula densa cells in DCT monitor flow.
    - With increased pressure and flow, granular cells of the juxtaglomerular apparatus release substances (endothelin, TXA2, AT2) → afferent arteriole constriction.
  - *Central regulation*
    - Sympathetic innervation of the afferent arteriole cause:
      - Constriction in response to blood loss.
      - Dilatation in response to hypertension.

## Assessment of Glomerular Filtration

- Glomerular filtration cannot be directly measured.
  - Estimation is based on the clearance of plasma creatinine or other markers.
- The ideal substance to estimate GFR through clearance includes the following:
  - It should achieve a steady state on the plasma.
  - Be solely and freely filtered by the kidney without metabolism, secretion or reabsorption in the tubule.
  - Inulin is ideal but impractical.

- *Others:* diethylene triamine pentaacetic acid (DTPA).
- Typically, *creatinine clearance* is used.
  - Creatinine is produced at a constant rate.
  - Varies depending on age, gender, race, and muscle mass.
  - Creatinine clearance overestimates GFR because ~10% is secreted by the proximal tubules.
  - Overestimation increases with deteriorating renal function due to an increase in the proportion of secreted creatinine.

1. The *Cockcroft & Gault* equation calculates creatinine clearance in individuals with normal renal function:

$$C_{cr} = \frac{(140 - age) \times weight}{72 \times Scr} \times 0.85 \text{ (if } female)$$

Ccr, creatinine clearance (mL/minute); age (year's); weight (kg); SCr, serum creatinine (mg/dL).

2. The clearance of a substance in the plasma is another way of estimating GFR:

$$Cl = \frac{U \times V}{P}$$

Cl denotes clearance; U as urine concentration of substance; V as volume of urine; and P as plasma concentration of substance.

3. The Modification of Diet in Renal Disease (MDRD) formula for calculating estimated GFR is:
   eGFR = 186 × (*Cr* / 88.4) –1.154 × (*Age*) –0.203 × (0.742 *if female*) × (1.210 *if black*)

# Tubular Function

## Proximal Convoluted Tubule

- Electrolyte and glucose reabsorption.
- Secretion of drugs and toxins.
- Reabsorption (Table 8.1):
  - 15% $Mg^{2+}$

**Table 8.1** Solute and Water Reabsorption

| Solute | PCT | LOH | DCT/CD |
|---|---|---|---|
| Sodium | 65% | 25% | 10% |
| Potassium | Majority | | Intercalated cells |
| Water | 65% | 15% | 15% |
| Magnesium | 15% | 60% | 10% |
| Phosphate | 90% | | |
| Calcium | 60% passive | 20% | 10% active |
| Bicarbonate, glucose, amino acids | Majority | | |

*Abbreviations:* PCT, proximal convoluted tubule; LoH, Loop of Henle; DCT, distal convoluted tubule; CD, collecting duct.

- 65% $Na^+$, $K^+$, $Ca^{2+}$
- 80% water, phosphate, bicarbonate ($HCO_3^-$)
- 100% glucose and amino acids
- Sodium is *actively* pumped back into the blood in exchange for potassium.
- Sodium is the only solute *actively* reabsorbed.
- Water and chloride ions follow sodium from the tubular lumen *passively* down the concentration gradient.
- Glucose and amino acids follow sodium through a *co-transport* system.
- 75% of filtrate has been reabsorbed by the time the urine has reached the LOH.

## Loop of Henle

- Situated in the medulla of the kidney.
- Generates a *counter-current mechanism* and *osmotic gradient* for variable water reabsorption.
- Acts as the site for additional sodium chloride reabsorption.
- Divided into three *distinct parts:*
  - *Descending limb*
    - Passive reabsorption of water occurs through highly water permeable aquaporin 1 channels.
    - Very little movement of salt with low permeability to salt and no active transport, which creates an osmotic gradient.
  - *Thin ascending limb*
    - Highly permeable to sodium chloride with very low permeability to water.
    - No active salt transport.
    - Sodium chloride and urea diffuse down a concentration gradient.
  - *Thick ascending limb*
    - Very low permeability to water.
    - Sodium, potassium, and chloride passively diffuse into the cells and are actively transported out of the basolateral surface using ATP.

## Distal Convoluted Tubule and Collecting Tubule

- Distal tubules fine-tunes salt reabsorption.
- *Principle cells* (CD) secrete potassium and absorb sodium under the influence of aldosterone.
- *Intercalated cells* (CD) absorb sodium.
  - *Sodium*
    - Sodium is absorbed passively via sodium–potassium–chloride co-transport, and pumped out actively of the basolateral surface of the cells.
  - This co-transporter mechanism is inhibited

by thiazide (DCT) and diuretics (CD), which reduces the concentration gradient and causes net loss of sodium.
- Anti-diuretic hormone (ADH)
  - Secreted by the posterior pituitary gland.
  - Increases collecting duct permeability to water.
  - Increases LOH and collecting duct reabsorption of sodium chloride.
- *Calcium*
  - Reabsorbed by passive diffusion independent on sodium transport.
  - Pumped out of cells by sodium-calcium exchange pump.
- Rate of potassium secretion is dependent on the amount of sodium and the rate of urine production.

## Renin–Angiotensin–Aldosterone System

- *Renin*: released by granular cells of the juxtaglomerular apparatus in response to:
  - Reduced renal blood pressure.
  - Reduced sodium delivery to macula densa.
  - Sympathetic stimulation.
- Renin converts angiotensinogen (produced by the liver) to angiotensin I.
- Angiotensin I is converted into angiotensin II by angiotensin converting enzymes (ACE – lung enzyme).
- *Angiotensin II*
  - At low levels, constricts afferent arterioles, raising glomerular filtrations.
  - At higher levels, constricts efferent arterioles, reducing glomerular filtration.
  - Increases reabsorption of sodium and water in DCT.
  - Causes the release of aldosterone from the adrenal cortex and vasopressin from the pituitary.
  - Increases thirst.
- Renin is the rate-limiting step of this axis.
- Factors that influence renal blood flow:
  - Angiotensin II constricts afferent and efferent arterioles → reduces flow.
  - ADH, adenosine triphosphate (ATP), platelet-activating factor (PAF), and endothelin → vasoconstriction → reduce flow and GFR.
  - Nitric oxide (NO), prostaglandin → vasodilatation → increases blood flow.
  - Atrial natriuretic peptide (ANP) → afferent arteriole dilatation → increases flow and GFR.

## Acid–Base Balance

- pH 7.35–7.45 (Figure 8.7)

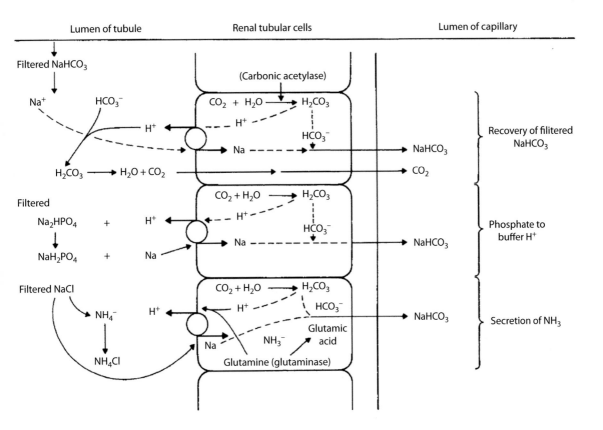

Figure 8.7 The regulation of acid–base balance. Reuse with permission from John Wiley and Sons [1].

- Buffers: bicarbonate ($HCO_3^-$), phosphate ($HPO_4^-$), proteins
  - *Carbonic anhydrase* catalyses: $H_2O + CO_2 \leftrightarrow H_2CO_3 \leftrightarrow HCO_3^- + H^+$
  - Occurs in tubular cell, tubular lumen, and blood.
- Kidneys alter pH through:
  - Glomerular filtration of hydrogen ($H^+$) and bicarbonate.
  - Excretion of hydrogen ions in the DCT ($H^+/Na^+$ pump).
    - $H^+ + HPO_4^- \rightarrow H_2PO_4^-$ (excreted)
  - Reabsorption of 85% of bicarbonate in the PCT.
- PCT – glutamine converted into ammonia ($NH4^+$) and bicarbonate.
  - Glutamine $\rightarrow NH4^+ + HCO_3^-$
  - Ammonia is excreted and bicarbonate is reabsorbed.

## Erythropoiesis

- *Erythropoietin* (EPO) is produced by interstitial cells in response to falling concentrations of red blood cells and low oxygen tension.
- *Hypoxia-inducible factor* -1a and -2a (HIF-1a and HIF-2a) are stabilised in hypoxic conditions to assemble apparatus for promoting transcription of EPO.
- *EPO:*
  - Increased in some cancers (e.g., renal cell carcinoma) through a mutation on the von Hippel-Lindau (VHL, 3p25) tumour suppressor gene and increased expression of HIF-1a.
  - Reduced in the presence of inflammation.
- Chronic renal failure leads to anaemia through the loss of EPO-producing cells.

## Calcium Regulation

- Calcium homoeostasis is maintained by parathyroid hormone (PTH) and vitamin D.

## Vitamin D

- Vitamin D is a fat-soluble vitamin found in very few foods.
- Increases absorption of calcium and phosphate in the intestine.
- Increases calcium resorption in bones.
- Increases renal reabsorption of calcium in the distal tubules.
- Cholecalciferol (vitamin D3) is synthesised in the skin from cholesterol in reaction to sunlight.

- Liver 25-hydroxylase converts Vitamin D3 to 25-hydroxycholecalciferol (calcidiol).
- Calcidiol is transported to the kidneys and bound to vitamin D-binding protein, where a second hydroxylation occurs within the renal tubular cells.
- 1α-hydroxylase converts calcidiol to 1,25-dihydroxycholecalciferol (calcitriol).
- 24α-hydroxylase converts calcidiol to 24,25-dihydroxycholecalciferol (inactive).
- Unregulated calcitriol synthesis can occur in macrophages in granulomatous conditions and in prostate cancer cells.

## Parathyroid Hormone

- *Hypocalcaemia* causes:
  - Increased synthesis and release of PTH.
  - Decreased degradation of PTH.
- The opposite occurs in hypercalcaemia.
- Calcitriol suppresses PTH synthesis.
- High phosphate stimulates PTH secretion.
- *In kidneys*:
  - PTH increases active calcium reabsorption in the distal tubule.
  - Decreases phosphate reabsorption in the proximal tubule.
  - Increases 1α-hydroxylase levels and calcitriol production.
- *In bones*: increases bone resorption, increasing serum calcium, and phosphate.
- Fibroblast growth factor 23 maintains phosphate levels by:

- Increasing renal excretion and suppressing 1α-hydroxylase activity.
- Acting on parathyroid glands to reduce calcitriol and PTH activity.

## Recommended Reading

1. Omar M. Aboumarzouk. Blandy's Urology, 3rd Edition. John Wiley and Sons; 2019.
2. Hamdy FC, Eardley I. Oxford Textbook of Urological Surgery. Oxford University Press; 2017.
3. El-Galley R, Keane T. Embryology, anatomy, and surgical applications of the kidney and ureter. Surg Clin North Am. 2000;80(1): 381–401.
4. Wein A, Campbell M, Walsh P. Campbell-Walsh Urology. Philadelphia, PA: Elsevier Saunders; 2012.
5. Standring S, Gray H. Anatomy. Gray's anatomy. Edinburgh: Churchill Livingstone; 2015.
6. Sampaio F. Renal anatomy. Urol Clin North Am. 2000;27(4): 585–607.
7. Klatte T, Ficarra V, Gratzke C et al. A literature review of renal surgical anatomy and surgical strategies for partial nephrectomy. Eur Urol. 2015;68(6):980–992
8. Karmali RJ, Suami H, Wood CG, Karam JA. Lymphatic drainage in RCC. Bju int. 2014;114:806–817.
9. Hutch JA. Anatomy and physiology of the bladder, trigone and urethra. London, New York: Butterworths Appleton-Century-Crofts; 1972.
10. Callahan M. The drooping Lily sign. Radiology. 2001;219(1): 226–228.
11. Cockcroft DW, Gault MH. Prediction of creatinine clearance from serum creatinine. Nephron. 1976;16(1): 31–41.
12. Lote C. Principles of Renal Physiology. Springer; 2019.

# 9 Embryology, Anatomy, and Physiology of the Adrenal Glands

*Karl H. Pang and Fausto Palazzo*

## Embryology and Anatomy

- The foetal adrenal gland is evident from weeks 6–8.
- *Two layers:*
  - The *outer cortex* is derived from mesenchymal cells.
    - The inner zone later regresses.
    - The outer zone forms the adult cortex.
  - The *inner medulla* is derived from ectodermal neural crest cells.
    - Formed by week 20.
- Paired retroperitoneal structures.
- Antero-superior and medial to the kidney.
  - *Left:* behind the pancreas and splenic artery.
  - *Right:* postero-lateral to the inferior vena cava.
- Pyramidal in shape and measures ~5 × 2 × 1 cm and weighs ~5 g.
- Rich blood supply estimated at ~6–7 mL/g per minute.
  - Superior adrenal artery arises from the inferior phrenic artery.
  - Middle artery arises from the aorta.
  - Inferior artery arises from the renal artery.
  - Right adrenal vein drains into the IVC.
  - Left vein drains into the left renal vein.

- Innervated by the coeliac plexus and greater splanchnic nerves.
- *Adrenal cortex* – three layers (Figure 9.1).
  - Outermost – *zona glomerulosa* (ZG).
  - Middle – *zona fasciculata* (ZF).
  - Innermost – *zona reticularis* (ZR).
- *Adrenal medulla*
  - A large sympathetic nerve terminal (T10-L1).
  - Chromaffin cells.

## Physiology

- *Zona glomerulosa* (ZG)
  - Secretes the mineralocorticoid aldosterone and increases sodium reabsorption and potassium excretion.
  - Expresses aldosterone synthase.
- *Zona fasciculata* (ZF)
  - Constitutes up to 75% of the cortex.
  - Secretes mainly cortisol glucocorticoid and some androgen precursors.
  - Cortisol increases in response to stress.
    - Maintains blood pressure (increases the effect of vasoconstrictors).
    - Suppresses the immune system.
    - Increases gluconeogenesis and decreases peripheral glucose uptake.

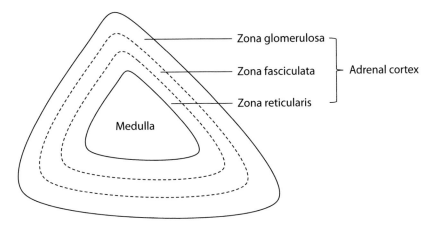

Figure 9.1 Zonal anatomy of the adrenal gland.

- Activates lipolysis.
- Bone resorption.
- Skin thinning.
- *Zona reticularis* (ZR)
  - Secretes androgens, dehydroepiandrosterone (DHEA), androstenedione, and cortisol (Figure 9.2).
  - Adrenal androgens are important in puberty.
- Pituitary adrenocorticotrophic hormone (ACTH) regulates the ZF/ZR secretion of cortisol and sex steroid precursors.
- Aldosterone (ZG) production is controlled by the RAA system and circulating electrolyte concentration.
- *Adrenal medulla*
  - Secretes catecholamines noradrenaline and adrenaline in response to neuro-humeral activation by the autonomic nervous system and other endocrine mediators → bind adrenergic receptors → executes the 'fight-or-flight' response.
- In the absence of 'stressors', the integrity of physiological systems is maintained in a dynamic fashion over 24 hours by an internal *'circadian clock'* (Figure 9.3).

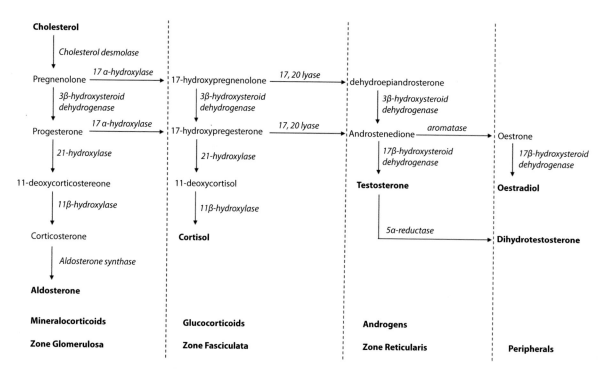

Figure 9.2 Metabolic pathways generating glucocorticoids, mineralocorticoids and androgens. Disruption in the control and components of metabolic pathways can result in diseases (e.g., 21-hydroxylase deficiency is the most common cause of congenital adrenal hyperplasia). Some drugs also act on these pathways (e.g., abiraterone inhibits 17α-hydroxylase and finasteride inhibits 5α reductase).

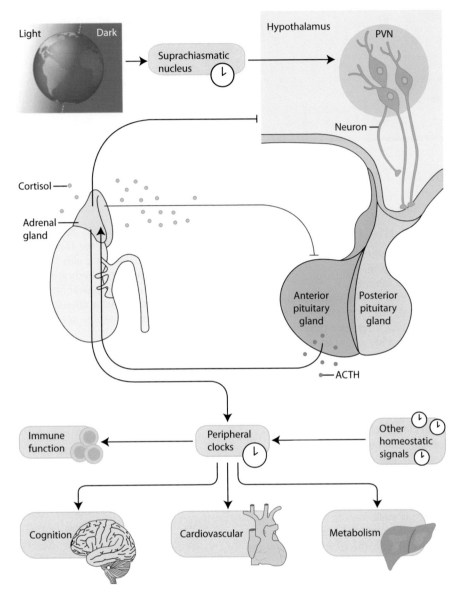

**Figure 9.3** Coordination of central and peripheral clocks by glucocorticoids. The suprachiasmatic nucleus central clock receives light-dark signals that, in turn, influence hypothalamic -pituitary -adrenal and sympatho -adreno-medullary activity leading to circadian cortisol production. Cortisol activates glucocorticoid receptors in peripheral tissues, which synchronises peripheral clocks and downstream metabolic, cardiovascular, neuronal and immune pathways. Other zeitgebers such as food, temperature and social cues can also entrain or influence the entrainment of clocks and can alter the output of these downstream pathways. ACTH, adrenocorticotropic hormone; PVN, paraventricular nucleus. (Reprinted by permission from Springer Nature [3])

## Recommended Reading

1. Omar M. Aboumarzouk. Blandy's Urology, 3rd Edition. UK: John Wiley and Sons, 2019.

2. Hamdy FC, Eardley I. Oxford Textbook of Urological Surgery. UK: Oxford University Press. 2017.

3. Russell G, Lightman S. The human stress response. Nat Rev Endocrinol. 2019;15(9):525–534.

# 10 Embryology, Anatomy, and Physiology of the Bladder

*Allan Johnston, Tarik Amer, Omar Aboumarzouk, and Hashim Hashim*

## Embryology of the Bladder

- The urogenital system develops from the intermediate mesoderm.
- During embryonic folding:
  - The mesoderm is carried ventrally and forms a longitudinal ridge on either side of the dorsal aorta—the *urogenital ridge*.
  - The urogenital ridge gives rise to:
    - The *nephrogenic cord* → urinary system
    - *The gonadal ridge* → genital system
- The key stages in bladder development and ureteric insertion are highlighted in Table 10.1.
- The *Cloaca* forms from yolk sac dilatation.
- The common cloacal channel divides into:
  - Anterior urogenital sinus
  - Posterior anorectal canal
- The *Allantois* develops at ~day 16 as a small diverticulum (Figure 10.1).
  - It extends from the yolk sac caudal wall into the connecting stalk.
  - It is involved in early blood formation.
  - It is associated with the development of the urinary bladder.
- The bladder enlarges and the allantois becomes the *urachus* - represented by the *median umbilical ligament* in neonatal life.
- The *cloaca* is the terminal portion of the embryonic hindgut:
  - Lined with endoderm.
  - Forms a pit in contact with the embryonic surface ectoderm (proctodeum/anal pit).
  - Receives the allantois ventrally.
  - Divided into a dorsal and ventral part by the *urorectal septum* (Figure 10.1).
- The *urogenital sinus (UGS)* (Figure 10.1) arises from the division of the cloaca during the 5th and 6th week.
  - Consists of three parts (cranial, middle, caudal):
    - The *cranial* vesical part forms the majority of the urinary bladder. It is continuous with the allantois.
  - The *middle* UGS forms the pelvic part:
    - Urethra in the bladder neck
    - Prostate in males
    - Complete urethra in females
  - The *caudal* (phallic part) is the precursor to the penis or clitoris.
- There are two theories to explain the separation process:
  1. *Rathke and Tourneux* (the traditional theory)
     - An upper fold (Tourneux) develops caudally.
     - Two lateral (Rathke) folds fuse at the cloacal wall midline forming the *urorectal septum*.
     - Completed when the urorectal septum fuses with the cloacal membrane by 5–6 weeks' gestation.
  2. *Kluth and van der Putte*
     - Both suggested that there is neither a descending septum nor a lateral walls fusion. These studies aimed at determining the cause of congenital anorectal malformations.

- *Wolffian duct (mesonephric duct)* (Figure 10.2):
  - Fuses with the cloaca during embryonic folding.
  - Follows the development of the UGS.
  - The common excretory ducts are the portion of the Wolffian duct:
    - Lie distal to the developing ureteric bud.
    - Ducts dilate by ~day 33 and insert into the UGS.
    - Duct orifices move caudally and away from the ureteral orifices.
  - Apoptosis allows the ureters to disconnect from the Wolffian duct.
  - Ureters are incorporated into the bladder at the trigone.
    - Migrate cranially and laterally within the floor of the bladder.

## Bladder Histology

- By week 10: a single layer of cuboidal cells is surrounded by loose connective tissue.

**Table 10.1** Timelines of the Developing Urinary Bladder

| Gestation | Development |
|---|---|
| 3rd Week | Cloaca exists as a bilaminar flat structure with an endoderm and ectoderm surface. |
| 4th Week | Embryonic folding. |
| | Distal yolk sac dilates and becomes the cloaca. |
| | Cloaca membrane is forced ventrally. |
| | The Wolffian duct fuses with the cloacal membrane by day 24. |
| 5th and 6th Week | Formation of the anterior urogenital sinus. |
| | The common excretory duct dilates and fuses with the urogenital sinus by day 33. |
| | By day 37, the ureteral orifices have evaginated into the urinary bladder. |
| 7–12th Week | The bladder is lined by a single layer of cuboidal cells. |
| | The apex is continuous with the urachus. |
| | During this time, the connective tissue surrounding the bladder condenses and smooth muscle appears. |
| 12th Week | The urachus becomes a fibrous cord—the median umbilical ligament in the human. |
| 13–17th Week | Cuboidal cells change morphologically to become mature urothelial cells. |
| | By week 15, striated muscles develop at the bladder neck and development of the urethral sphincter. |
| 21st Week | The bladder continues to develop. |
| | It is now made up of 4–5 layers. |
| 21–38th Week | Increasing bladder compliance. |
| | Increasing thickness of the bladder muscle wall. |

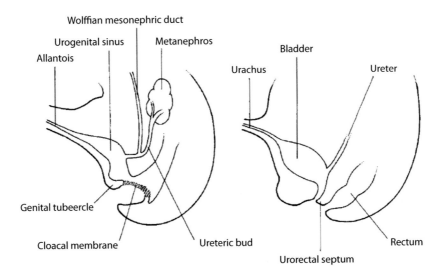

**Figure 10.1** Wolffian (mesonephric duct). The urogenital sinus arises from the division of the cloacal and forms the bladder. The cloacal membrane is divided by the urorectal septum. (Reuse with permission from John Wiley and Sons [3])

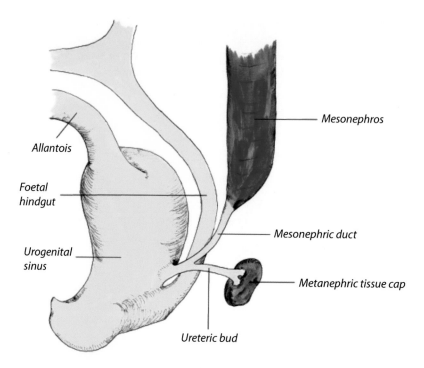

**Figure 10.2** Wolffian (mesonephric) duct and ureteric bud. The Wolffian duct follows the development of the UGS. The ureteric bud develops as an outgrowth of the Wolffian duct (5th week). (Reuse with permission from John Wiley and Sons [3])

- Week 12: increased layers of cuboidal cells.
- Week 13–17: cells undergo morphological changes.
- Week 21: mature urothelial cells develop.
- Loose connective tissue condenses and is replaced by smooth muscles, migrating from the bladder dome to the bladder base.

## Sphincter

- Development begins after cloaca division into an anterior and posterior chamber.
- Mesenchymal cells migrate and condense around the inferior aspect of the UGS.
- Week 15: striated muscle fibres first appear.

## Bladder Trigone

- There are two theories described regarding trigone development:
1. *Weiss et al.*
   - The lateral common excretory ducts fuse in the midline after attaching to the UGS - forms the primitive trigone which is structurally different from the bladder and urethra.
2. *Viana et al.*

- The trigone develops from the bladder smooth muscle, with minor contributions from the ureters.

## The Developing Bladder in Neonatal Life and Infancy

1. *Voiding during sleep*
   - *Neonates:* voiding reflex develops some cortical connections
   - Function remains immature until later years.
2. *Bladder capacity*
   - First increase in capacity: 4-fold increase around birth.
   - Second increase: age of toilet training (~3 years)
     - Stimulant due to the ability of the child to remain dry overnight, resulting in higher bladder volumes.
3. *Urine production and number of voids*
   - Urine rate (mL/kg/hour) decreases with age, but the total volume every 24 hours increases - small, frequent voids
   - The number of voids and volume is critical in the development of increased bladder capacity.

4.  *Residual urine*
   - Neonates and children up to the age of two years do not completely empty.
   - During 3rd year, voiding control increases → bladder is completely emptied.

# Congenital Anomalies of the Urinary Bladder and its Outlet

## Urachal Anomalies

- Urachal cyst, sinus, or fistula

## Exstrophy of the Bladder

- ~1 in 10,000–40,000 births
- More common in males
- Failure of the mesenchymal cells to migrate between the ectoderm of the abdomen and cloaca during the 4th week.
  - Lack of muscle and connective tissue in the anterior abdominal wall.
  - Exposure and protrusion of the posterior urinary bladder wall.
  - The trigone and ureteric orifices are external.
- Epispadias is associated with this anomaly.

## Posterior Urethral Valves

- ~1 in 5,000 births per year.
- Hugh Hampton Young (1919) described three lesions.

- Type 1 is most common, where bicuspid valves/leaflet arise from the verumontanum. They run anteriorly and fuse with the midline.
- Type 2: Hypertrophied band of tissue. Now known not to be associated with posterior urethral valves.
- Type 3: Sheet membrane with central aperture - possibly a variation of Type 1. arise from the verumontanum.
- Now termed congenitally obstructing posterior urethral membrane (COPUM) - iris-shaped deformity that is converted to a 'Type 1' deformity following the passage of a urethral catheter/feeding tube.
- Long-term implications:
  - Bladder hypertrophy and dysfunction
  - Urinary reflux and hydronephrosis

# Anatomy of the Urinary Bladder

- Lies in the lesser pelvis when empty.
- Has anterior/posterior/lateral walls, dome, trigone, and ureteric orifices (Figure 10.3).
- Distends antero-superiorly to the abdominal cavity when filling.
- *Male:* rectum is separated postero-superiorly by the rectovesical pouch (Figure 10.4a).
  - Posterior inferior are the seminal vesicles and vas deferens.
- *Female:* anterior vaginal wall lies posteriorly. (Figure 10.4b).

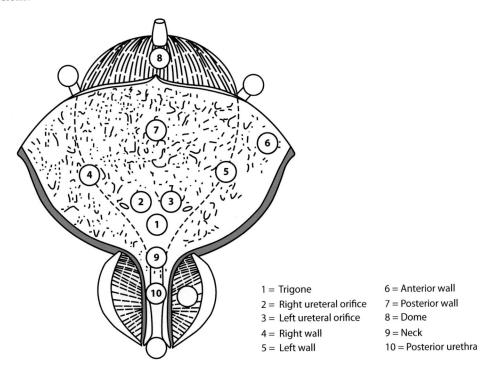

| | |
|---|---|
| 1 = Trigone | 6 = Anterior wall |
| 2 = Right ureteral orifice | 7 = Posterior wall |
| 3 = Left ureteral orifice | 8 = Dome |
| 4 = Right wall | 9 = Neck |
| 5 = Left wall | 10 = Posterior urethra |

Figure 10.3 Bladder diagram. (Reproduced with permission of the EAU guidelines office [8])

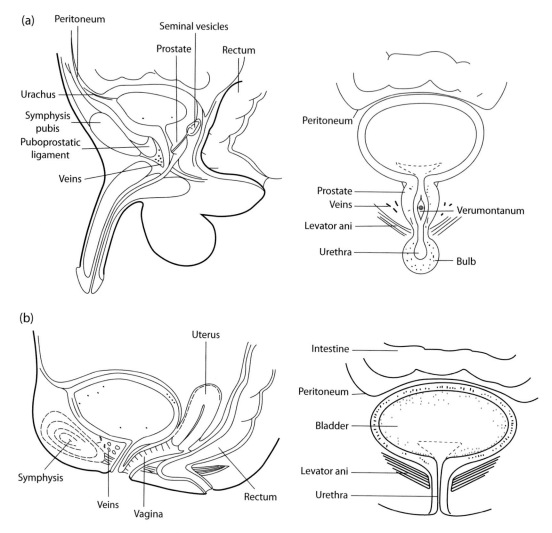

**Figure 10.4** Sagittal and coronal section through the pelvis. (a) Male; (b) Female. (Reuse with permission from John Wiley and Sons [3])

- The *bladder apex* is attached to the medial umbilical ligament and ascends to the umbilicus.
- The *space of Retzius* separates the bladder from the transversalis fascia anteriorly.
- The normal histology of the bladder is described in Table 10.2.

## Internal Structure of the Bladder

- Mucosa
- *The trigone*:
  - Posterior-lateral: ureteric orifices/openings (UOs)
    - Beyond the UOs, it extends as ureteric folds (terminal portion of the ureters as they enter the bladder).
  - *Anterior apex*: internal urethral opening
  - *Posterior*: inter-ureteric bar

- There are *two layers of muscle*:
  - *Deep* – continuous with the rest of the bladder.
  - *Superficial* – continuous with the fibres of the intramural ureters posteriorly and the smooth muscle of the proximal urethra.

## Blood Supply

- Branches of the anterior trunk of the internal iliac artery (Figure 10.5):
  - Superior and inferior vesical arteries
  - Obturator artery
  - Inferior gluteal artery
- *Superior vesical artery*
  - First large anterior branch of the internal iliac artery
  - Runs inferior to the pelvic brim

**Table 10.2** Histology of the Bladder

1. **Urothelium**
   a. Multi-layered, approximately seven layers thick.
   b. Apical/umbrella cells in contact with urine—largest cells.
      i. Hexagonal
      ii. Barrier function
      iii. Involved in signalling pathway to higher centres
   c. Produce uroplankins which form plaques—important in barrier function.
2. **Lamina Propria**
   a. 'Functional Centre' for local control of the bladder.
   b. Coordinates urothelium and detrusor muscle.
      i. Filled with unmyelinated nerve fibres.
      ii. Also includes microvasculature.
   c. Myofibroblasts that regulate interaction of the detrusor muscle and urothelium.
3. **Stroma**
   a. Collagen and elastin matrix composed of prostaglandins.
   b. Fibroblasts
   c. Involved in passive mechanical properties of the bladder.
4. **Smooth muscle**
   a. Myofibrils arranged in bundles in random directions.
   b. Motor innervation post-ganglionic parasympathetic nerve fibres.
   c. Gap junctions allow nerve signalling pathways to be transferred throughout the bladder smooth muscle.

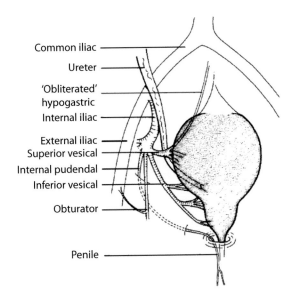

Common iliac
Ureter
'Obliterated' hypogastric
Internal iliac
External iliac
Superior vesical
Internal pudendal
Inferior vesical
Obturator
Penile

**Figure 10.5** Artery ssupply of the bladder. (Reuse with permission from John Wiley and Sons [3])

- Traverses the pelvis from its sidewall medially towards the upper portion of the bladder.
- *Supplies:*
  - Distal ureter, bladder, the proximal end of the vas deferens, seminal vesicles.
  - Gives rise to the umbilical artery in the foetus (medial umbilical ligament in adults).
- *Inferior vesical artery*

- Often replaced by the middle rectal/vaginal artery in females.
- Passes medially along the floor of the pelvis to the fundus of the bladder.
- *Supplies:*
  - Bladder and trigone, seminal glands, prostate, vas deferens.
- *Obturator artery*
  - Passes immediately from the lateral pelvic wall to the upper aspect of the obturator foramen.
  - Leaves the true pelvis via the obturator foramen.
  - Crossed on its most medial aspect by the ureter (and the vas deferens in the male).
  - Provides a vesical branch to the bladder.

## Lymphatics

- Important when performing lymph node dissection in bladder cancer (Chapter 24).
- Majority of the three collecting vessels end in the external iliac nodes.
- *Lymph nodes:*
  - External iliac
  - Obturator
  - Internal iliac (hypogastric)
  - Common iliac
  - Presacral
  - Abdominal (paracaval, interaortocaval, para-aortic)

# Physiology of the Urinary Bladder

- *Function:* to store and expel urine.
- Multiple reflex pathways – spinal reflexes involving higher centres.
- *Storage phase:*
  - Reflexes prevent contraction of the urinary bladder.
    - Sympathetic reflex for receptive relaxation.
  - Ensures contraction of the urinary sphincter.
    - *Guarding* reflex increases the sphincteric tone of the rhabdosphincter.
- Afferent sensory feedback relays fullness to spinal reflexes and sacral micturition centre, which in turn relays to higher centres.
- *Micturition:*
  - Contraction of the bladder.
  - Relaxation of the urethral sphincter.
- The innervation of the bladder is summarised in Table 10.3 and Figure 10.6.

- *Sensory* feedback from the *bladder:*
  - Conveyed by the pelvic, hypogastric, and pudendal nerves.
- *Fullness:*
  - Spinal cord – pelvic and hypogastric nerves.
- *Sensory* feedback from the *bladder neck and sphincter* (hypogastric and pudendal nerve).
- The differing fibres are shown in Table 10.4.

- The *bladder urothelium* is also important in sensory feedback.
  - Expresses nicotinic, muscarinic, tachykinin, adrenergic, bradykinin, and transient receptor vanilloid receptors.

- Releases chemical mediators (e.g., ATP, ACh, and nitric oxide).

## Control of the Micturition and Storage Cycle

- The pontine micturition centre (PMC, Barrington's nucleus)
- Periaqueductal grey matter
- Pre-optic hypothalamus
- Neurons of the cerebral cortex

## Bladder Filling and the Guarding Reflex

- Detrusor muscle is relaxed (sympathetic – *hypogastric nerves*).
- Urethral sphincter smooth muscle is contracted (sympathetic).
- Urethral external (striated muscle) sphincter is contracted (*pudendal nerve*).
  - Promotes filling and inhibits bladder emptying — *guarding reflex* (Figure 10.7a).
- Parasympathetic efferents are turned off.
- Critical level of bladder distension:
  - Tension receptors switch afferent pathways to maximal activity.
  - Maintain continence due to *voluntary control:*
    - Registration of bladder filling.
    - Regulation/manipulation of the voiding reflex.
- *Periaqueductal grey matter:*

---

**Table 10.3** Neural Control of the Urinary Bladder

1. **Parasympathetic, S2-4** (p for 'pee')
   a. Urine expulsion – bladder contraction, M3 receptor>M2 receptor
   b. Outflow at sacral level – pelvic nerves
   c. Lateral part of sacral grey matter (Sacral Parasympathetic Nucleus)
   d. *Acetylcholine* neurotransmitter (excitation)
   e. Non-adrenergic non-cholinergic transmitters (ATP, P2X – detrusor excitation; nitric oxide – urethral relaxation)
   f. Post-ganglionic neurons in detrusor muscle wall
2. **Sympathetic, T11-2** (s for 'stores')
   a. Urine storage
   b. Outflow from lumbar spinal cord
   c. *Noradrenergic* neurotransmitter
   d. Excitatory to sphincter (alpha1 receptor)
   e. Inhibits bladder wall (beta3 receptor)
3. **Somatic**
   a. Urine storage
   b. Pudendal Nerve (guarding reflex)
   c. *Acetylcholine* neurotransmitter (excitation)
   d. Onuf's Nucleus (S2-4)
   e. Motor neurons form the ventral horn to the external urinary sphincter.

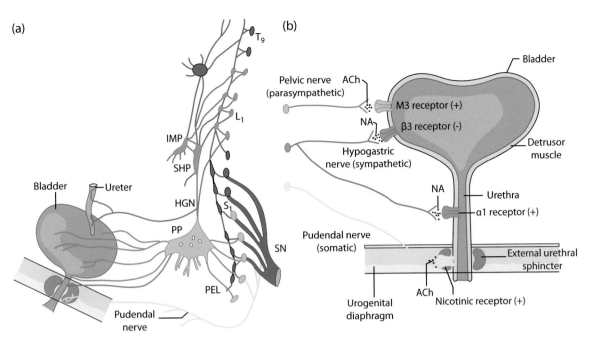

Figure 10.6 Efferent pathways of the lower urinary tract. (a) Innervation of the bladder; (b) Efferent pathways. IMP, inferior mesenteric plexus; SHP, superior hypogastric plexus; HGN, hypogastric nerve; PP, pelvic plexus; PEL, pelvic nerves; SN, sciatic nerve; ACh, acetylcholine; NA, noradrenaline. (Reprinted by permission from Springer Nature [7])

**Table 10.4** Fibres Supplying the Bladder

| Fibre | Myelination | Innervation | Function |
| --- | --- | --- | --- |
| A-Delta | Myelinated | Smooth muscle | Bladder fullness |
| C | Unmyelinated | Mucosa | Stretch and volume |
| C | Unmyelinated | Mucosal muscle | Nociception to increasing distension |

- Receives and communicates ascending signals to higher centres.
- Receives signals from the higher centres and the PMC.
- Many other neuronal circuits are relayed to the:
  - *Insula* – desire to void
  - *Thalamus* and *cerebral cortex* – noxious stimuli
  - *Anterior cingulate cortex* – conscious attention of filling and how to react to them
- *Frontal lobe:* has a role in the behavioural mechanism in bladder control.

## Bladder Voiding

- Mediated by a spino-bulbospinal pathway that passes through the PMC.

- PMC activates descending pathways (Figure 10.7b):
  - Urethral relaxation
  - Sacral parasympathetic outflow (*pelvic nerve*)
    - Bladder contraction
    - Increase in intravesical pressure
- A disruption in the control mechanism causes a *'neurogenic bladder'*:
  - Overactive/underactive bladder
  - Detrusor-sphincter-dyssynergia (DSD)

## Bladder Compliance

- Change in volume/Change in detrusor pressure:

$$\text{Compliance (mL/cmH}_2\text{0)} = \Delta V \text{ (mL)}/\Delta Pdet \text{ (cmH}_2\text{0)}$$

- Compliance is high in normal adult (<10 cmH$_2$0 rise during filling).

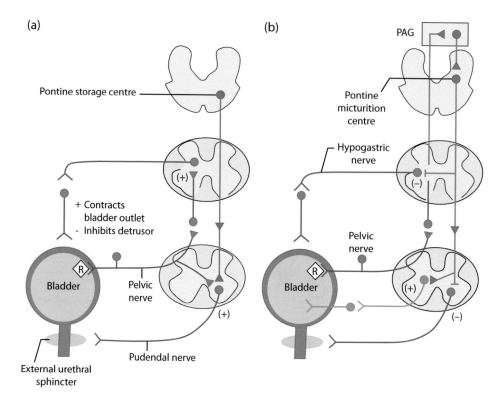

**Figure 10.7** The efferent pathways of the lower urinary tract. (a) Urine storage reflexes: sympathetic and pudendal outflow causes bladder relaxation and urethral sphincter contraction (red). The pontine storage centre increases striated urethral sphincter activity (grey); (b) Voiding reflexes: spino-bulbospinal reflexes activated (blue). Parasympathetic outflow causes bladder contraction (green) and inhibition of sympathetic and pudendal outflow (red). PAG, periaqueductal grey; R, afferent nerve receptors. (Reprinted by permission from Springer Nature [7])

- *Mechanisms:*
  - *Early* filling – elastic bladder wall (smooth muscle, elastin, collagen)
  - *Late* filling – inhibition of parasympathetic tone
- The causes of poor compliance include:
  - *Mucosa:* infective/interstitial/radiation cystitis
  - *Detrusor:* hypertrophy, neurogenic

## Acknowledgement

Professor Alice Roberts, Professor of Public Engagement in Science, School of Biosciences, University of Birmingham, B15 2TT.

## Recommended Reading

1. Sadler TW. Langman's Medical Embryology 10th Edition. USA:Lippincott Williams and Wilkins. 2006 Chapter 15 Urogenital System.
2. Wein AJ, Kavoussi LR, Partin AW, Peters CA. Campbell-Walsh Urology 11th Edition. Philadelphia: Elsevier. 2016 Volume 4 Chapter 15 Embryology of the Genitourinary Tract.
3. Aboumarzouk O. Blandy's Urology 3rd Edition. UK: John Wiley and Sons, 2019. Chapter 3 Embryology for the Urologist.
4. Tourneax F. Fur le premiers developpements du cloaque du tubercle genitale et de l'anus chez Fembryon moutons, avec quelques remarques concemant le developpement des glandes prostatiques. J Anat Physiol (1888);24:503–17.
5. Sillen U. Bladder function in healthy neonates and its development during infancy. J Urol. (2001);166:2376–81.
6. Standring S. Gray's Anatomy: The Anatomical Basis of Clinical Practice 40th Edition. Edinburgh: Churchill Livingstone. 2008 Chapter 75 Bladder, Prostate and Urethra.
7. Fowler CJ, Griffiths D, De Groat WC. The neural control of micturition. Nat Rev Neurosci (2008);9:453–66.
8. EAU Guidelines on Non-muscle Invasive Bladder Cancer, 2020 (Figure 5.1, p. 13). ISBN 978-94-92671-04-2.

# 11 Embryology, Anatomy, and Physiology of the Prostate

*Joseph Tam and Hashim Ahmed*

## Embryology of the Prostate

- Prostate development begins at ~week 10.
- Driven by dihydrotestosterone (DHT) – produced from the reduction of testosterone by 5α reductase.
- Five paired epithelial buds form on the posterior side of the urogenital sinus.
  - *Top* pair arise from the mesoderm and forms the *periurethral/transitional* zones.
  - *Lower* pair arises from the endoderm and forms the *peripheral* zone.
- The *central* zone arise from the Wolffian duct.
- Development continues in concentric rings with the urethra in the centre.
- Forms acini and collecting ducts by arborisation into the urethra.
- Sertoli cells release Müllerian inhibiting substance.
  - Causes virilization of the male characteristics.
  - Regression of the Müllerian duct (Hydatid de Morgagni).
- At maturation, the fully formed prostate has different growth levels depending on the area.
  - Glandular tissue nearest to the ducts is mostly secretory.
  - Glandular tissue in the peripheries of the ducts has a higher mitotic index and contribute less to secretions.

## Anatomy of the Prostate
### Surfaces and Relations

- The prostate is one of four sex accessory glands; the other three structures include (Figure 11.1):
  - Seminal vesicles
  - Cowper's glands (bulbourethral)
  - Glands of Littre (urethral/peri-urethral)
- The prostate is
  - 70% glandular tissue, 30% fibromuscular tissue.
  - Surrounds the prostatic urethra.
  - Important in ensuring anterograde ejaculation.
  - Surrounded by Denonvillier's fascia, which separates the rectum.

- *Anterior prostate*
  - Mostly consists of thick fibromuscular layers.
  - Narrow and convex.
  - 2 cm behind the pubic symphysis and is attached to the pubis by puboprostatic ligaments at its superior aspect.
  - A retroperitoneal fat layer (Cave of Retzius) and the dorsal vascular complex (Santorini's plexus) are between the prostate and pubic symphysis.
- *Lateral*
  - Separated from levator ani by the Denonvillier's fascia.
  - The prostatic venous plexus and neurovascular bundle lie between the inner and outer lamina.
  - Should always be divided laterally to avoid damage to the neurovascular bundle during prostatectomy.
- *Inferior/apex*
  - Smooth muscle fibres are continuous with the external urethral sphincter.
  - The isthmus connects the left and right lobes anteriorly from the external urethral sphincter to the bladder neck.
- *Superior/base*
  - Continuous with the bladder base.
- *Posterior*
  - Muscle fibres fuse with Denonvillier's fascia.
  - Highest density of prostate capsule.

## Prostate Lobes

- Consists of an anterior lobe (isthmus), middle lobe, left and right lateral lobes, and a posterior lobe.
- *Landmarks*
  - Ejaculatory ducts lie in a depression on the posterior surface, which separates the small middle lobe superiorly and lateral lobes inferiorly.
  - Shallow longitudinal central furrow separates lateral lobes posteriorly.
  - The *isthmus*—a band of fibromuscular tissue—connects the lateral lobes anteriorly.

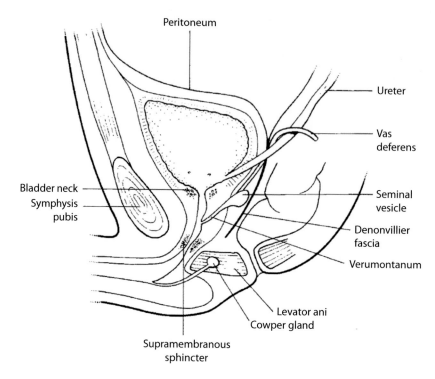

Peritoneum

Ureter

Vas deferens

Bladder neck

Symphysis pubis

Seminal vesicle

Denonvillier fascia

Verumontanum

Levator ani
Cowper gland

Supramembranous sphincter

Figure 11.1 Sagittal view of prostate. (Reuse with permission from John Wiley and Sons [9])

## Arrangement and Zones

- Concentrically arranged inward:
  1. *Fibrous capsule*
     - Thin anteriorly and dense posteriorly.
     - Fuses with fibromuscular fibres at the base and apex, making histological margins difficult to determine at that point.
     - *Two layers*
       - *Inner* lamina – tightly adherent to prostate

- *Outer* lamina – continuous with Denonvillier's fascia
- In benign prostatic hyperplasia (BPH), a 'false' capsule can develop when hypertrophic tissue compresses the peripheral zone.
  2. Layer of *smooth muscle* with branching septa into the stroma.
  3. *Supporting stroma* containing (Figure 11.2) the following:
     - *Peripheral* zone – 75% of all glandular

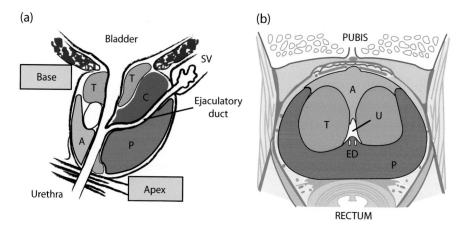

(a)

Bladder

SV

Base

T

T

C

Ejaculatory duct

A

P

Urethra

Apex

(b)

PUBIS

A

T

U

ED

P

RECTUM

Figure 11.2 Zonal anatomy of the prostate. (a) Sagittal section; (b) Axial section. A, anterior; T, transitional; C, central; P, posterior; SV, seminal vesicle; ED, ejaculatory duct; U, urethra. (Reuse with permission from John Wiley and Sons [9])

tissue in the prostate, where 75% of prostate cancer arises.

- *Central* zone – encloses the urethra and contains ~25% of all glandular tissue.
- *Peri-urethral* zone – gives rise to the median lobe in BPH.
- *Transitional* zone – peri-urethral glandular area contains 2% of all the glandular tissue and gives rise to lateral lobes in BPH.
- Differentiation of peripheral and central zones is difficult histologically, which can be seen on MRI T2 diffusion-weighted imaging.

## Arterial Supply

- Supplied by branches of the *internal iliac artery* (Figure 11.3):
  - Inferior vesical
  - Internal pudendal
  - Middle rectal arteries
- *Anterior:* 1 and 11 o'clock (Flock's artery).
- *Posterior:* 5 and 7 o'clock (*Badenock's* artery) positions.
- Inferior vesical artery branches into urethral and capsular vessels.
- Urethral arterial branches enter the prostate at the prostatovesical junction.
- Capsular arterial branches run posteriorly, laterally, and inferiorly alongside the neurovascular bundles-enter the prostate at the prostatourethral junction at the apex.

## Venous Supply

- The peri-prostatic venous plexus envelopes the prostate anteriorly and laterally.

- It is anterior to the bladder and posterior to the arcuate pubic ligament and lower part of the pubic symphysis.
- Main tributary – deep dorsal vein of the penis
  - Drains into the vesical plexus and internal pudendal vein, which drains into the vesical and internal iliac veins.

## Lymphatic Drainage

- Internal iliac, sacral, and obturator nodes.

## Nerve Supply

- Supplied by the inferior hypogastric (pelvic) plexus and peri-prostatic nerve plexus.
- Somatic pudendal nerve supplies the external urethral sphincter, entering at the five and seven o'clock positions.

## Internal Structures of the Urethra

- *Urethra:* peri-prostatic, prostatic, and membranous parts (Figure 11.4).
- *Crista phallica*
  - Longitudinal muscular fold at the posterior midline, where glandular fluid drains into the prostatic sinuses.
  - Extends from the uvula of the bladder through the prostatic urethra, ending at the external urethral sphincter.
  - At the midpoint, the urethra angles anteriorly (~35°, varies between 0° and 90°) and divides the prostatic urethra into proximal (peri-prostatic) and distal (prostatic) parts.

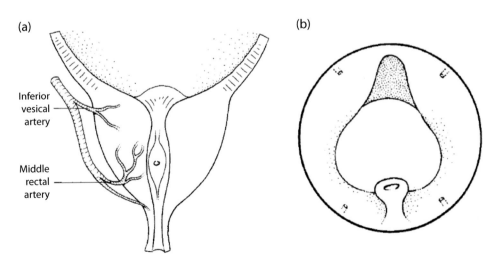

(a)

Inferior vesical artery

Middle rectal artery

(b)

**Figure 11.3** Arterial supply of the prostate. (a) Main arterial supply: inferior vesical and middle rectal; (b) Position of arteries seen in transurethral resection of the prostate: 5 and 7 o'clock (Badenock's artery), 1 and 11 o'clock (Flock's artery). (Reuse with permission from John Wiley and Sons [9])

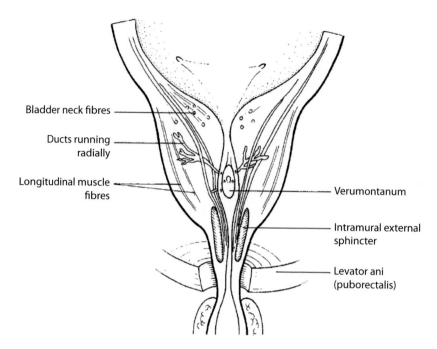

Bladder neck fibres

Ducts running radially

Longitudinal muscle fibres

Verumontanum

Intramural external sphincter

Levator ani (puborectalis)

Figure 11.4 Coronal section of the prostate and sphincter. (Reuse with permission from John Wiley and Sons [9])

- Peri-prostatic urethra contains the *involuntary internal urethral sphincter.*
- Prostatic urethra collects major glandular secretions.
- Widens at the posterior wall and continues to become the seminalis (verumontanum).
- *Verumontanum*
  - Prostate utricle (6 mm blind Müllerian remnant) – a small orifice that opens at the upper border of the verumontanum.
  - Ejaculatory ducts lie either side of the verumontanum.

## Urethral Sphincters

- *Internal sphincter*
  - Located at the bladder neck.
  - Continuation of the detrusor muscle.
  - Autonomic control of micturition:
    - *Sympathetic* fibres
      - Innervated by lumbar splanchnic nerves (L1-2).
      - Causes contraction and closure of the bladder neck.
      - Norepinephrine stimulation of $\beta2/\beta3$ adrenergic receptors results in bladder relaxation.
      - Norepinephrine stimulation of $\alpha1A$ adrenergic receptor results in urethral contraction.
    - *Parasympathetic* fibres
      - Innervated by inferior hypogastric plexus (S2-4).

- Results in relaxation and opening of the bladder neck.
- Mediated by acetylcholine and adenosine triphosphate, which stimulate M2/M3 muscarinic receptors and P2X1 receptors, respectively, causing detrusor contraction.
- Nitric oxide causes urethral relaxation via cyclic guanosine monophosphate pathways.
- *External sphincter*
  - Innervated by the perineal nerve—a branch of *pudendal* nerve (S2-4).
- *Male* – surrounds the membranous urethra.
- *Female*
  - Distal end of the bladder neck.
  - *Three parts:* sphincter urethrae, urethrovaginal muscle, and compressor urethrae.
  - Contraction causes vaginal contraction simultaneously.

## Histology of the Prostate

- *Glandular tissue*
  - Consists of follicles with internal papillae.
    - Opens into canals and joins to form 12–20 ducts.
  - Supported by muscular stroma.
  - *Epithelium:* predominantly columnar and can be single-layered or pseudostratified.
- *Prostatic ducts*

- Bi-layered epithelial layer with basement membrane.
- *Secretory cells*
  - Located along lumen near the apex of columnar cells.
  - *Positive stains:* prostatic acid phosphatase (PAP), prostate-specific antigen (PSA), keratin.
  - Characterised by small colloid amyloid bodies known as corpora amylacea.
- *Columnar cells*
  - Tall and lined in a row.
  - Apex microvilli projecting into the lumen, with the base attached to the basement membrane.
  - Golgi apparatus separates the nucleus from the cytoplasm.
- *Neuroendocrine cells*
  - Sparsely and irregularly populated between columnar and cuboidal cells.
  - *Type I* – open and contains microvilli.
  - *Type II* – closed with long dendrite-like processes extending to nearby epithelial cells and basal cells close to nerves.
  - There are three types of $\alpha$-1 adrenergic receptor ($\alpha_{1A}$, $\alpha_{1B}$ and $\alpha_{1D}$). The $\alpha_{1A}$ receptors are linked to smooth muscle contraction.
- *Transit-amplifying cells*
  - Intermediate cells between the basal layer and undifferentiated stem cells.
- *Basal/Stem cells*
  - *Type I* – small and flattened with little cytoplasm and condensed chromatin.
  - *Type II* – large cuboidal cells with less condensed chromatin.
  - Growth is not influenced by testosterone levels as basal cells lack androgen receptors (AR).
    - Androgen deprivation therapy will eliminate secretory cells in the luminal compartment and *not* the basal layer.
- *Tissue matrix* – cells anchored in a tissue matrix via direct attachments of the nuclear matrix, cytomatrix, basement membrane, extracellular matrix, and stroma.

# Physiology of the Prostate

## Endocrinology

- Majority of steroid and androgens are bound to protein dependent on *two factors:*
  - The affinity of the steroid to the protein.
  - The capacity of the binding protein.
- Common *binding proteins* include:
  - Serum albumin
  - Testosterone–oestrogen-binding globulin
  - Corticosteroid binding globulin
  - Progesterone binding globulin
  - $\alpha$-acid glycoprotein
- Increasing levels of oestrogen will increase levels of circulating binding proteins resulting in more protein-bound testosterone and less free testosterone
- *Prolactin*
  - Secreted from the anterior pituitary gland.
  - Involved in regulating zinc levels in the prostate.
- *Testosterone*
  - Secreted by Leydig cells from the testes (but some also from adrenals)
  - Adrenal steroid hormones which are converted to testosterone include:
    1. Dehydroepiandrosterone (DHEA)
       - The rate of conversion to testosterone is slow via prostate sulfatase hydrolysis.
       - Levels are not sufficient to replace testosterone levels in castrate studies.
       - Dehydroepiandrosterone sulfate is the conjugate form of DHEA.
    2. Androstenedione cannot be directly converted to DHT.
    3. Adrenal sources of testosterone do not contribute sufficiently to support the growth of the prostate.
  - Insoluble in water and are mostly bound in plasma to sex hormone-binding globulin (~60%) and albumin (~38%).
  - Secretion is controlled by the hypothalamic–pituitary–gonadal axis in a negative feedback loop:
    - Hypothalamus secretes gonadotrophin-releasing hormone (GnRH), which stimulates the anterior pituitary gland;
    - The anterior pituitary secretes luteinizing hormone, which stimulates Leydig cells; and
    - Leydig cells in the testes secrete testosterone.
    - Testosterone negatively inhibits further production of GnRH.
  - The secretion of testosterone from the adrenals is controlled by the same axis—the anterior pituitary secretes adrenocorticotrophic hormone (ACTH) and prolactin, which stimulates the adrenals.
  - Testosterone is irreversibly reduced in the prostate by 5$\alpha$ reductase to DHT. It can be irreversibly converted to estradiol by aromatase.
- *Dihydrotestosterone (DHT)*
  - Product of reduction from testosterone.
  - High affinity to AR and induces higher levels of AR activity.

- Plasma DHT is 99.12% bound to plasma proteins and synthesised in the skin and liver by 5α reductase type I.
- *5α reductase*
  - *Type I* – found in the skin and prostate, responsible for plasma DHT.
  - *Type II* – expressed in the prostate.
  - 5α reductase is involved in BPH – inhibitors are used in its treatment.
  - *Finasteride* – 5α reductase type II isozyme inhibitor.
  - *Dutasteride* – 5α reductase type I and II isozyme inhibitor.
  - *5α reductase type II deficiency* (autosomal recessive, chromosome 2p):
    - Incomplete/insufficient differentiation and development of male characteristics.
    - Ambiguous genitalia, micropenis, hypospadias. Do not develop BPH.
- *Oestrogen*
  - 10–25% secreted by testes
- *Growth factors, suppressors, and signalling*
  - EGF (epidermal growth factor), TGF-α (transforming growth factor alpha), and bFGF (basic fibroblast growth factor) – *stimulatory* growth factors involved in upregulating gene expression.
  - TGF-β (transforming growth factor beta) – *inhibitory*.
  - IGF (insulin-like growth factor) – required in prostate proliferation, but levels do not drive it.
- *Androgen receptor (AR)*
  - Critical in normal function and development.
  - Dysregulation is involved in prostate cancer.
  - Found in the cytoplasm in a complex with multiple heat shock proteins.
  - AR signalling is induced when an androgen (DHT) binds to it:
    - Phosphorylation causes the release of AR from its cytoplasmic complex.
    - AR undergoes a second phosphorylation to allow ligand binding of the androgen to its ligand-binding domain.
    - Induces a conformation change to form a homodimer, which translocates to the nucleus and induces transcription of associated AR genes.
  - AR can be transactivated in the absence/low concentration of DHT (e.g., castrate-resistant prostate cancer) via pathways including small GTPase (Ras) and tyrosine kinase (JAK1).
    - Extracellular peptides: insulin-like growth factor, epidermal growth factor, and interleukin-6 can induce transactivation of AR.
  - Epithelial and stromal cells contain AR.
    - AR is found at much lower expression in basal cells compared to secretory cells, and within the epithelial layer compared to the stroma.
  - Growth and secretion of the epithelial layer is dependent on AR and transcription within the stroma—which is integral in the development of BPH.
  - Androgen deprivation therapy is used in managing prostate cancer to target AR and its downstream regulation.
- *Prostate-specific antigen (PSA)*
  - Serine protease enzyme
  - Also known as human Kallikrein-3
  - PSA exists in five isoforms
  - The predominant isoform is 237 amino acid.
    - Quantified by mass spectrometry at ~28.4 kDa
    - Protein electrophoresis by SDS–PAGE: molecular weight ~32–33 kDa
    - Literature quote: 30–34 kDa
  - *PSA gene:* chromosome 19 long arm (19q13.2-q13.4)
  - Shares significant similarities with the Kallikrein family:
    - 63% similarity to pancreatic-renal kallikrein
    - 80% similarity to glandular kallikrein 2
  - Synthesised as pre-pro-PSA → pro-PSA → PSA
  - *Three forms of serum PSA:*
    - Free (active)/unbound with a half-life of ~2–3 hours.
    - Bound to α1-antichymotrypsin (ACT) with a half-life of ~4–5 days.
    - Bound to α2-macroglobulin (AMG) with a half-life of ~4–5 days.
  - Monoclonal PSA antibody assays detect free PSA, complexed PSA, or any cross-reactivity with glandular kallikrein.
    - Total PSA = free PSA + complexed PSA
    - AMG is not detected by immunoassays.
    - Complexed PSA is largely ACT-bound.
  - *PSA kinetics:*
    - *PSA velocity* (PSAV): rise in PSA per year (ng/mL/year)
    - PSAV >0.75 ng/mL/year: increased risk of prostate cancer
    - *PSA doubling time:* time for PSA to double
    - *PSA density* (PSAD): PSA per mL prostate tissue (volume)
      - Vol = height × width × length × 0.52
      - PSAD >0.15 ng/mL/mL: increased risk of prostate cancer
    - Free/total PSA: % free PSA compared to total.
      - When total PSA is 4.0–10.0 ng/mL, <25% fPSA is associated with increased risk of prostate cancer.
  - PSA is not specific to prostate cancer, it can be elevated by:
    - Age, prostate size/BPH

- Digital rectal examinations, ejaculation, or cycling
- Acute prostatitis, urinary tract infection, or urinary retention
- Prostate biopsy and transurethral procedures
- Neuroblastomas produce PSA.
- PSA liquefies semen.

## Continence

- Plays no active role in continence despite its location.

## Ejaculation

- Antegrade if bladder neck mechanism is competent.
- *Steps:*
  1. Tightening of the bladder neck (alpha receptors).
  2. Transportation of spermatozoa from the ampullae of vasa into the prostatic urethra (emission).
  3. Contraction of prostatic smooth muscle, including pre-prostatic sphincter.
  4. 5–6 contractions of prostatic muscle (ejaculation).

## Prostatic Secretions

- 2 mL secreted by the seminal vesicles (alkaline).
- 0.5 mL secreted by the prostate.
- 0.1 mL secreted by the Cowper's glands and glands of Littre.
- Minimal contribution of volume from sperm cells.
- *Glands of Littre* – produce lubrication for the urethra and for penetration (although penetration may have occurred before secretion).

- Fertilising promote peptide acts to increase the fertility of sperm.
- Glycerylphosphocholine is produced by the seminal vesicles and is split by acid phosphatase into glyceryl-phosphate—which has protective effects for sperms.
- Secretions contain high concentrations of zinc and citrate.

## Recommended Reading

1. McNeal JE. Regional morphology and pathology of the prostate. Am J Clin Pathol. 1968,49(3):347–357.
2. McNeal JE. Normal histology of the prostate. Am J Surg Pathol. 1988;12(8):619–633.
3. Standring S (ed.) et al. Gray's Anatomy, 41st Edition, London, United Kingdom: Elsevier Limited; 2016.
4. Moore KL, Dalley AF, Agur AMR. International Edition: Moore Clinically Oriented Anatomy. 7th Edition, Baltimore: United States of America (printed in China), Lippincott Williams & Wilkins; 2014.
5. Stevens A, Lowe JS. Human Histology, 3rd Edition, Philadelphia: United States of America (printed in Spain): Elsevier Mosby; 2005.
6. Feneley M, Mundy AR, Emberton M. The Prostate and Benign Prostatic Hyperplasia, The Scientific Basis of Urology, 3rd Edition, London, United Kingdom: Informa Healthcare; 2010.
7. Wein AJ (ed.) et al. Campbell Walsh Urology, 10th Edition, Volume 1, Philadelphia: (printed in the United States of America): Elsevier Saunders, 2012.
8. Wein AJ (ed.) et al. Campbell Walsh Urology, 9th Edition, Volume 3, Philadelphia: (printed in China), Elsevier Saunders; 2007.
9. Omar M. Aboumarzouk. Blandy's Urology, 3rd Edition. UK: John Wiley and Sons; 2019.
10. Lonergan PE, Tindal DJ. Androgen receptor signalling in prostate cancer development and progression. J Carcinog. 2011;10:20, doi:10.4103/1477-3163:83937.

# 12 Embryology, Anatomy, and Physiology of the Male Reproductive System

*Maria Satchi and Asif Muneer*

## Introduction

- *Mesonephric (Wolffian) ducts* are the embryological origin of the male reproductive system.
  - They form the epididymis, vas deferens, seminal vesicles, and the central zone of the prostate.
- The *paramesonephric (Müllerian) duct* forms the genital system in females.
  - Regresses in males, but remnants can persist.
- The urogenital system develops from the intermediate mesoderm.
  - Sexual differentiation occurs between the 7th–17th week of gestation.
- The initial stages of development are similar in both sexes up to the 7th week.

## Embryology of the Testis

### Testis Development

- The primitive gonads initially form as a pair (gonadal ridges).
- By the *3rd week,* the primordial germ cells are found in the yolk sac wall (endoderm).
- During the *5th week,* migration happens along the dorsal mesentery to reach the primitive gonads.
- By the *6th week,* germ cells appear in the genital ridges and the epithelium proliferates to form gonocytes.
  - Failure of migration to the gonadal ridge results in gonadal development failure.
  - Epithelial cells of the genital ridge penetrate the mesenchyme, forming primitive sex cords.
- *Male:* the Y chromosome short arm (Yp11) carries the *sex-determining region Y* gene (SRY, also known as testis determining factor).
  - Signals differentiation of primitive sex cords to form the testis/medullary cords.
  - The SRY and SOX9 genes are responsible for testes differentiation.

- *Sertoli cells* develop in the testis cord.
  - Support development of Leydig cells and primordial germ cells.
  - *Leydig cells* are derived from the mesenchyme of gonadal ridge.
  - Sertoli produces *anti-Müllerian hormone* (AMH).
    - It is also known as *Müllerian inhibitory substance* (MIS).
  - SOX9 activates AMH.
    - In males, AMH causes the regression of paramesonephric ducts and may leave a remnant (testis appendix – hydatid of Morgagni).
- By the *8th week,* Leydig cells produce testosterone.
  - In target cells, testosterone is converted to dihydrotestosterone (DHT) by the 5-alpha reductase enzyme.
  - DHT stimulates the development of the male external genitalia, penis, scrotum, and prostate.
  - Testosterone induces mesonephric (Wolffian) duct development into the vas deferens, seminal vesicles, efferent ductules, and epididymis.
- By the *4th month,* testis cords are made of primitive germ cells and Sertoli cells.
- During puberty, seminiferous tubules form from the canalisation of the cords.

## Testicular Descent

- Occurs in *two stages* (Figure 12.1).
- Failure results in an undescended testis (UDT).
  - The testis can be intraabdominal, in the inguinal canal, or high in the scrotum.
- The caudal genital ligament and gubernaculum extend from the testis caudal pole to the inguinal region to guide descent.

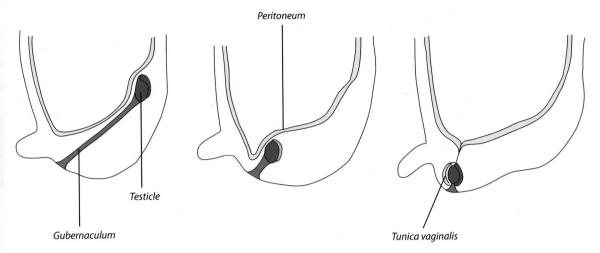

Peritoneum

Testicle

Gubernaculum

Tunica vaginalis

**Figure 12.1** Testicular descent. Testicular descent is guided by the gubernaculum and acquires a layer of peritoneum, which forms the tunica vaginalis. (Reuse with permission from John Wiley and Sons [8])

## Transabdominal Stage: Weeks 8–15

- Mediated by *insulin-like 3 hormone* (Leydig cells).
- AMH may have a role, but there is no clear evidence.
- The testis descends along the posterior abdominal wall to the inguinal region.
- The gubernaculum extends from the inguinal region to the scrotum.

## Inguinoscrotal Stage: Weeks 24–35

- Androgen-dependent.
- The testis passes through the inguinal canal (week 24–28), drawn caudally into the scrotum (week 28–35) by the gubernaculum.
- The abdominal cavity peritoneum forms a reflected fold — processus vaginalis (PV).
  - PV descends along with the testis and gubernaculum to the scrotum.
  - Pulls with it the layers of the abdominal wall muscles and fascia to form the inguinal canal.
  - The PV is obliterated at/soon after birth.
  - Failure to obliterate may result in an infant hernia or hydrocele.
- The *spermatic fascia* (three layers) surrounds the spermatic cord.
  - *External spermatic fascia* is derived from the external oblique.
  - *Cremasteric fascia* from the internal oblique.
  - *Internal spermatic fascia* from the transversalis fascia.
  - Contents of the spermatic cord are detailed in Table 12.1.

## Scrotal Development

- Develops from the inferio-medial migration and midline fusion of the genital folds which forms the midline raphe.
  - Failure of fusion leads to the separation of the labioscrotal folds without a median raphe - Appears as a bifid scrotum, often seen with proximal hypospadias.
- Ectopic scrotum or hemiscrotum may occur in the supra/infrainguinal or perineal regions.
  - Associated with UDT, inguinal hernia, and bladder exstrophy.

## Embryology of the Penis

- Androgens cause the *genital tubercle* to lengthen.
  - The *mesoderm* gives rise to the corpus cavernosa and glans.
  - The *ectoderm* gives rise to the shaft skin and prepuce.
- An increase in testosterone (Leydig cells) and loss of inhibitory effect of maternal oestrogens on the foetal pituitary leads to an increase in penile length.
- Table 12.2 summarises the hormones and genes associated with the development of the male reproductive system.

## Anatomy of the Male Genitalia

- The male perineum is diamond-shaped – bordered by:
  - The pubis anteriorly;
  - The coccyx posteriorly; and
  - The ischial tuberosities laterally.

**Table 12.1 Contents of the Spermatic Cord**

| Structure | Origin | Drainage |
|---|---|---|
| Testicular artery | Aorta | |
| Deferential artery | Superior vesical artery (off internal iliac) | |
| Cremasteric artery | Inferior epigastric artery (off external iliac) | |
| Pampiniform plexus of testicular veins | | Testicular vein (into left renal vein and IVC on the right) |
| Lymphatics | | Para-aortic nodes |
| Genital branch of genitofemoral nerve | Lumbar plexus | |
| Vas deferens | | |
| Processus vaginalis | Abdominal wall peritoneum | |

*Abbreviation:* IVC, inferior vena cava.

**Table 12.2 Summary of the Hormones and Genes that Play a Role in the Embryology of the Male Reproductive System**

| Hormone/Gene | Origin | Action |
|---|---|---|
| Testosterone | Leydig cells | The development of internal genitalia from mesonephric duct: seminal vesicles, epididymis, vas deferens. Testis descent during inguinoscrotal stage. |
| Dihydrotestosterone (DHT) | Testosterone converted by 5α reductase in target tissue | Development of external genitalia: prostate, penis, scrotum. |
| Anti-Müllerian hormone (AMH)/ Müllerian inhibiting substance (MIS) | Sertoli cells | Regression of paramesonephric duct. |
| Insulin-like 3 hormone | Leydig cells | Testis descent during the transabdominal stage. |
| SRY gene | Short arm Y chm Yp11 | Testis differentiation. |
| SOX9 | Long arm chm 17 | Activates AMH. |

- A line between the two ischial tuberosities divides the perineum into:
  - The smaller anterior urogenital triangle.
  - The larger posterior anal triangle.
- The superficial *Scarpa's fascia* of the anterior abdominal wall is continuous with the fascial layers of the perineum.
- *Colle's fascia* – superficial layer at the root of the penis.
  - Attached posteriorly to the perineal membrane and to the inferior ischiopubic rami.
- The Scarpa's fascia is continuous with the superficial dartos fascia of the scrotum and penis.
- Deep to the Scarpa's is the deep penile fascia - *Buck's* fascia of the penis.
  - Continuous with Gallaudet's fascia proximally.
    - Covers the bulbospongiosus, ischiocavernosus, and superficial transverse perineal muscles that cover the root of the penis.
- The *superficial pouch* is the space between the perineal membrane and attachments of Colle's fascia → houses the root of the penis and its attachments.

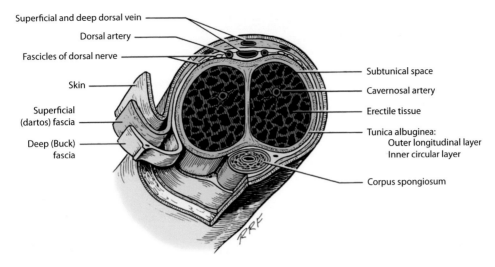

Superficial and deep dorsal vein
Dorsal artery
Fascicles of dorsal nerve
Skin
Superficial (dartos) fascia
Deep (Buck) fascia

Subtunical space
Cavernosal artery
Erectile tissue
Tunica albuginea:
    Outer longitudinal layer
    Inner circular layer
Corpus spongiosum

**Figure 12.2** Transverse section of the penis. (Reprinted with permission from Elsevier [3])

# Penis

- The male sexual organ consists of the root, shaft, and glans (Figure 12.2).
  - The root has *two crura*.
  - Each is attached to the ipsilateral ischiopubic ramus, perineal membrane, and urethral bulb, which is attached to the perineal membrane alone.
- The paired *ischiocavernosal muscles* cover the two crura.
  - The crura converge to form the *corpora cavernosa*.
  - The corpus cavernosa (erectile tissue) consists of lacunar spaces with smooth muscle and endothelium — filled with arterial blood during an erection.
- The *Bulbospongiosus muscle* covers the penis bulb.
  - The bulb continues as the *corpus spongiosum*.
  - Lies ventrally between the two dorsal corpora cavernosa, forming the penile shaft.
  - The corpus spongiosum continues distally, expands to form the glans, and covers the corporal tips.
- The bulbar and penile urethra traverse the length of the bulb and corpus spongiosum, respectively.
- The *glanular* part is composed of the fossa navicularis and the urethral meatus.
- *Tunica albuginea:*
  - Thick fibrous sheath – type I and type III collagen interlaced with elastin fibres.
  - Has an outer longitudinal layer and an inner circular layer.

- Contains emissary veins that are compressed during an erection.
- Surrounds the corpora cavernosa and fuses medially to form the median septum – has fenestrations to allow communication between the two corpora.
- Fuses ventrally, so longitudinal fibres are absent in the ventral groove.
- The tunica albuginea of the corpus spongiosum is a single layer of circular fibres.
  - Thinner than those around the corpora cavernosa.
  - The corpus spongiosum fills to a lower pressure during tumescence and allows the urethra to remain patent.
- *Buck's fascia* fuses with the tunica albuginea to surround corporal bodies.
  - Splits ventrally to surround the spongiosum.
  - The superficial dartos fascia which is highly elastic is superficial to Buck's.
    - Confers mobility to the penile skin.
- The foreskin extends above the glans.
  - Folds over to attach below the corona of the glans.
- The penis is supported by the *suspensory ligament* of the penis.
  - Formed by the attachment of the fibrous Buck's fascia to the pubic symphysis.
  - The fundiform ligament lies superficial to the suspensory ligament.
    - This is an extension of the linea alba of the abdominal wall Scarpa's fascia.
    - Slings around the penis to support it.
    - Continues inferiorly to form the scrotal septum.

| Table 12.3 The Neurovascular Supply to the Penis (3–4) | | |
|---|---|---|
| **Arterial Supply** | **Origin** | **Supply** |
| Bulbourethral artery | Internal pudendal artery | Corpus spongiosum, glans, antegrade supply to urethra |
| Dorsal artery | Internal pudendal artery | Penile skin, fascial layers, retrograde supply to urethra |
| Cavernosal artery | Internal pudendal artery | Erectile tissue of the crura and corpus cavernosa |
| Superficial dorsal artery | External pudendal artery | Penile skin |
| **Venous drainage** | **To** | **From** |
| Deep dorsal vein | Periprostatic venous plexus of Santorini | Erectile tissue and deep fascial layers |
| Superficial dorsal vein | Superficial external pudendal veins | Penile skin and subcutaneous tissue |
| **Lymph drainage** | | **From** |
| Superficial inguinal nodes | | Penile skin, glans, corpora |
| Deep inguinal nodes | | Corpus cavernosum and spongiosum |
| External/iliac nodes | | Any penile structure and urethra |
| **Nerve supply** | **Origin** | **Supply** |
| Dorsal nerves (sensory) | Pudendal nerve | Dorsal penile skin, glans, glanular urethra |
| Posterior sacral nerves (sensory) | Perineal nerve | Ventral penile skin |
| Perineal nerve (motor) | Perineal nerve | Bulbospongiosus muscle, ischiocavernosus muscle |
| Parasympathetic nerves | S2, S3, S4 | Erectile tissue |
| Sympathetic nerves | T11-L2 | Erectile tissue |

## Neurovascular Supply to the Penis (Table 12.3)

- Internal iliac artery → internal pudendal artery → common penile artery
- The common penile artery divides into *three branches* (Figure 12.3):
  - *Bulbourethral, dorsal,* and *cavernosal* artery.
  - The cavernosal artery gives off helicine arteries which supply cavernous sinuses and vasodilate during penile tumescence.
- The *neurovascular bundle* is found within Buck's fascia.
  - Consists of deep dorsal vein, dorsal arteries, and dorsal nerves.

## Urethra

- *Male:* ~18–20 cm long
  - The *posterior* urethra is proximal to the perineal membrane.

- Comprised of the *prostatic* and *membranous* urethra.
- The *anterior* urethra is distal to the perineal membrane.
  - Contained within the corpus spongiosum.
  - Comprised of the *bulbar* and *penile* urethra.
- *Prostatic urethra*
  - Continuous with the bladder transitional epithelium.
  - Surrounded by inner longitudinal and outer circular smooth muscle.
- *Ejaculatory ducts:* ~2 cm long
  - Begin at the junction of the seminal vesicles and vas deferens.
  - Open into the prostatic urethra at the verumontanum at an acute angle to prevent urinary reflux into the ducts.
- *Membranous urethra,* ~2 cm
  - Suspended from the pubis by connective tissue and inserts into the puboprostatic and suspensory ligaments.

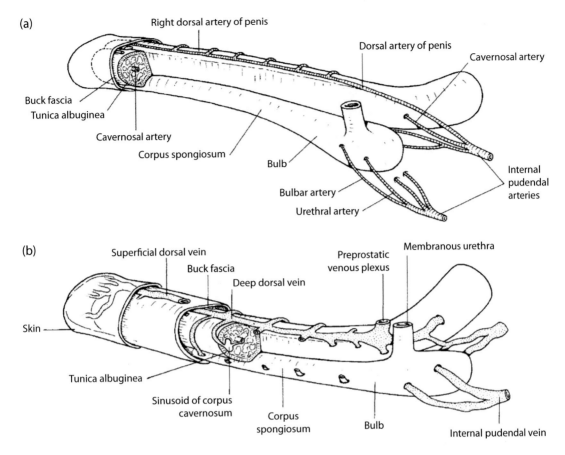

**Figure 12.3** Arterial (a) and Venous (b) Supply of the penis. (Reuse with permission from John Wiley and Sons [8])

- Surrounded by signet-shaped striated *external urethral sphincter*.
- The sphincter inserts into the perineal body posteriorly.
- During sphincter contraction, the urethra pulls posteriorly towards the perineal body.
- *Anterior urethra*
  - Lined by stratified and pseudostratified columnar epithelium proximally.
  - Lined by stratified squamous epithelium near the fossa navicularis and urethral meatus.
- Mucous secreting *Littre's glands* are found in the mucosa along its course.

## Scrotum and Testis

- Originates from the anterior urogenital triangle.
- The scrotum is made up of an outer layer of skin, dartos muscle, and spermatic cord fascia which surrounds the spermatic cord.
- *The testis* is enveloped by:
  - *Tunica vaginalis* (outermost layer)
  - The *tunica albuginea* (intermediate layer) is a dense adherent layer to the testis.
- Gives rise to fibrous tissue at the posterior aspect (mediastinum), where testicular artery and veins supply the testis.
- The *tunica vasculosa* (innermost layer) consists of blood vessels and connective tissue.
- *Adult male testis:* ~14–22 mL in volume, 3.6–5.5 cm in longitudinal axis.
- Testis parenchyma is composed of coiled seminiferous tubules.
  - Contains developing germ cells and interstitial tissue.
    - Made up of Leydig cells, nerves, blood, and lymph vessels.
  - Sertoli cells are found in the basement membrane.
    - Support and provide nutrition to developing germ cells.
- The testis is divided into lobes by septa (Figure 12.4).
  - Seminiferous tubules within each septum terminate in the rete testis → gives rise to efferent ductules (15–20) → open into the convoluted duct of the epididymis.

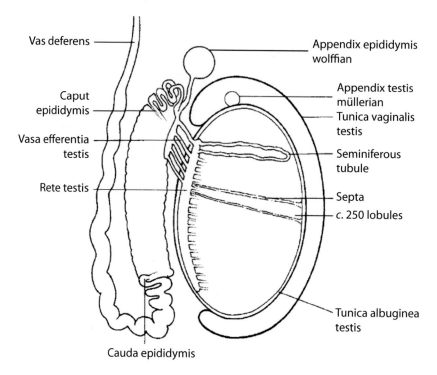

**Figure 12.4** Anatomy of the testis. (Reuse with permission from John Wiley and Sons [8])

- *Epididymis* – a tightly coiled and compressed tube.
  - Divided into caput (head), corpora (body), and cauda (tail).
  - Main site of mature sperm storage.
  - Continues as the vas deferens.
- *Vas deferens* – a fibromuscular tube ~45 cm long.
  - Transports sperm to the ipsilateral ejaculatory duct during ejaculation.
  - Commences as the convoluted part.
  - Continues as the straight part from the scrotum and into the spermatic cord (contents summarised in Table 12.1).
  - Enters the inguinal canal through the superficial ring.
  - Continues through the deep inguinal ring and emerges lateral to inferior epigastric vessels.
  - Routes medially to reach the posterior base of the prostate.
    - The dilated ampulla is the terminal end which stores sperm.
- *Seminal vesicle:* ~4 cm and is the lateral outpouching of the vas deferens.
  - Located at the posterior base of the prostate.
  - A tubular structure which does not store sperm.
  - Contributes a majority of secretions to the ejaculate.
- The seminal vesicle and vas deferens are supplied by the deferential artery.

- They form ejaculatory ducts and open into the prostatic urethra.

## Physiology of the Testis

- The hypothalamic pituitary gonadal (HPG) axis maintains the male reproductive physiology.
- The testes are the male reproductive organs which produce sperm and male androgens.
- Foetal testosterone production is initially independent of gonadotropin stimulation.
  - At ~14th week, the maternal human chorionic gonadotropin (hCG) stimulates a peak.
  - It becomes responsive to foetal luteinising hormone (LH) thereafter.
- After birth, gonadotropin levels start to rise.
- At ~3 months, a peak in LH is reached in boys.
  - UDT at birth may be expected to descend to coincide with the LH surge.
- By 6–9 months, gonadotropin and testosterone levels start to drop and remain low until puberty.
- At puberty, the HPG axis is activated and the hypothalamus produces pulsatile gonadotrophin-releasing hormone (GnRH).
  - Regulation of the HPG axis is through negative feedback (Figure 12.5).
  - GnRH is released from the hypothalamus (plasma half-life ~5–7 minutes).
    - Release is *circadian*.

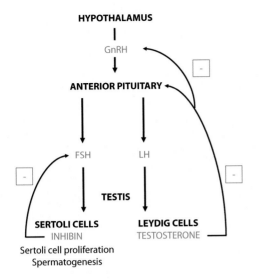

**Figure 12.5** The hypothalamic pituitary gonadal axis.

- Stimulates peak testosterone levels in the morning.
- Pulsatile approximately every 90–120 minutes.
- Acts on the anterior pituitary and stimulates the release of gonadotropins, LH, and follicle-stimulating hormones (FSH) to adult levels.
- FSH stimulates Sertoli cell proliferation and spermatogenesis.
  - Stimulates the release of inhibin from the Sertoli cells.
  - Inhibin affects the release of FSH from the pituitary gland through negative feedback.
- LH stimulates testosterone release from the Leydig cells.
- Testosterone is a steroid hormone.
  - Supports spermatogenesis by binding the androgen receptor of Sertoli cells.
  - Responsible for the development of male secondary sexual characteristics.
  - In an adult male: normal levels >12 nmol/L, equivocal 8–12 nmol/L, low <8 nmol/L.
  - ~60% bound to sex hormone-binding globulin (SHBG)
    - ~38% bound to albumin (bioavailable)
    - ~2% free (bioavailable)
- SHBG levels *increased* (lowers bioavailable free testosterone) by:
  - Ageing
  - Hepatic disease
  - Hyperthyroidism
  - Drugs: anticonvulsants, oestrogens
  - Smoking
  - HIV infection

- SHBG levels *decreased* by:
  - Drugs: glucocorticoids, testosterone, anabolic steroid
  - Obesity
  - Hypothyroidism
  - Cushing disease, acromegaly
  - Nephrotic syndrome
  - Insulin resistance
- *Prolactin* is released from the anterior pituitary.
  - Its role is less well understood
  - Thought to increase LH receptors on Leydig cells, maintaining normal/high intratesticular testosterone levels.
  - Plays a role in maintaining libido.
  - Hyperprolactinaemia can inhibit GnRH release and lower gonadotropin levels.

## Spermatogenesis

- At 2–3 months, LH surge causes testosterone levels to rise.
- From 6-9 months, gonadotropins and testosterone levels remain low.
- By ~12 years (puberty), the HPG axis is reactivated and the hypothalamus generates pulsatile GnRH.
  - Increased levels of gonadotropins reach adult levels.
  - Elevated testosterone levels stimulate androgen-dependent development of male sexual function, characteristics, and growth.
  - FSH initiates and regulates spermatogenesis.
  - Testosterone levels increase and reach a further peak in the 2nd–3rd decade of life, then plateau until a slow decline during the ageing process.
- Spermatogenesis occurs within the seminiferous tubules.
  - Sertoli cells support germ cells and provide nutrition during the maturation process.
  - Within tubules, germ cells are layered from the basement membrane to the lumen in order of differentiation.
- The full cycle of *spermatogenesis* takes ~74 days (but varies among individuals).
- Consists of three phases (Figure 12.6).

1. Proliferative phase
   - Spermatogonial stem cells (diploid, 2n) located near the basement membrane divide by mitosis to form type A and type B spermatogonia.
   - Type A replenish the spermatogonial stem cells.
   - Type B spermatogonia form primary spermatocytes.

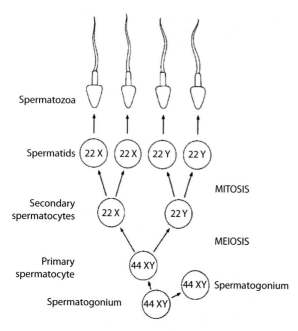

**Figure 12.6** Spermatogenesis. 44 XY, 2n Diploid; 22 X or Y, n Haploid. (Reuse with permission from John Wiley and Sons [8])

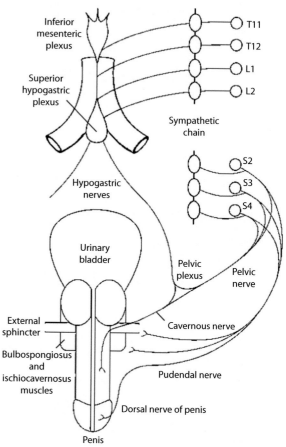

2. Meiotic phase
   • Primary spermatocytes (diploid, 2n) undergo the 1st meiotic phase.
   • Give rise to two secondary spermatocytes.
   • Secondary spermatocyte (haploid, n) divides in the 2nd meiotic phase.
   • Each give rise to two spermatids (haploid, n).
3. Spermiogenesis phase
   • Spermatid undergoes structural changes in the nucleus and cytoplasm to form mature spermatozoa.
      • The round spermatid loses its cytoplasm and acquires an asymmetrical nucleus.
      • The nucleus contains chromatin which is condensed and compacted.
      • Acrosome and flagellum are formed.
      • Mitochondria reorganise in the midpiece of the tail.

• A mature spermatozoon has a head, a connecting neck, and a tail.
   • The head contains the nucleus and acrosome — which contains enzymes for fertilisation.
   • The tail contains mitochondria for energy and sperm flagellar movement.
• Formed spermatozoa are pushed through seminiferous tubules.
   • Migrate through the epididymis and acquire motility.
   • Become fully motile when they reach the cauda for storage.

**Figure 12.7** Innervation of the penis. Sympathetic pathways from the T10-L2 segments of the spinal cord pass via the sympathetic chain ganglia to the prevertebral ganglia in the inferior mesenteric and superior hypogastric plexuses. From there, fibres descend to the pelvic plexus via the hypogastric nerves. In the sacral area, postganglionic fibres from the sympathetic chain ganglia pass to the sacral nerves and then to the pelvic or pudendal nerves. Parasympathetic preganglionic axons arising in the S2 to S4 segments of the spinal cord pass via the pelvic nerve to the pelvic plexus. Ganglion cells in the pelvic plexus send axons into the cavernous nerve, which innervates the penis. The pudendal nerve originates in the S2 to S4 segments of the spinal cord and innervates the external sphincter, the bulbospongiosus muscle and the ischiocavernosus muscle. The pudendal nerve also provides sensory fibres to the dorsal nerve of the penis. (Reprinted by permission from Springer Nature [9])

• Mature sperm can fertilise the egg.
   • Unlike non-motile sperm within the testis, which may require intracytoplasmic sperm injection, in the case of asthenospermia, to faciliate fertilisation.

# Physiology of Ejaculation and Erection

## Neurophysiology (Figure 12.7)

- *Sympathetic fibres* (T11-L2) → sympathetic chain ganglia → hypogastric nerves → pelvic plexus → cavernous nerves
- *Parasympathetic* nerves (S2-4) → pelvic nerve → pelvic plexus → cavernous nerves
- Cavernous nerves carry sympathetic and parasympathetic fibres to innervate the penis
- *Sympathetic* – detumescence and ejaculation
- *Parasympathetic* – erections and activation of the veno-occlusive mechanism
- Sensory receptors of the penis are located in the skin, glans, and urethra.
  - Sensory information is sent via the dorsal penile and pudendal nerves which enter the spinal cord at S2-S4 to relay information to the thalamus and sensory cortex.
- *Somatomotor centre* (S2-4) Onuf's nucleus: efferent innervation (*pudendal* nerve) to the ischiocavernosus and bulbocavernosus muscle.
- Medial preoptic area (MPOA), paraventricular nucleus (PVN) and periaqueductal grey – central coordination of afferent sensory information.
  - Responsible for sexual function and attaining and maintaining an erection.

## Ejaculation

- Ejaculate – secretions from seminal vesicles and prostate.
  - Seminal vesicles contribute to ~65–75% of the volume.
    - *Alkaline* secretion – fructose (energy substrate for spermatozoa) and semenogelin (coagulates sperm).
  - Prostate contributes to ~25–30% of the seminal fluid volume.
    - *Acidic* – serine proteases (PSA) that liquefy the coagulated ejaculate.
    - ~5–10% are spermatozoa from the vas deferens.
    - ~1% are from bulbourethral glands (Cowper's gland) secretions.
- *Ejaculation* is described in two phases – *emission* and *expulsion*.
  - Mediated by the autonomic nervous system, predominantly the sympathetic nervous system
  - Sympathetic nerves release noradrenaline (NA) to stimulate smooth muscle contraction and epithelial secretion.
  - Dopamine is excitatory; serotonin is inhibitory.
  - Spermatozoa and seminal fluid are propelled through the epididymis → vas deferens → ejaculatory ducts → prostatic urethra.
- *Emission* is stimulated by:
  - Tactile stimulation of the glans penis when sensory information is transmitted to the lumbar sympathetic nuclei.
  - Following visual or physical stimulation under cerebral control.
- *Expulsion* happens when seminal fluid and spermatozoa exit the urethral meatus.
  - Contraction of the internal urethral sphincter with relaxation of the external urethral sphincter (rhabdosphincter) prevent retrograde ejaculation and promote antegrade ejaculation.
  - Propulsion of seminal fluid by rhythmic contraction of bulbocavernosus (under somatic nerve control).
  - Somatosensory information via dorsal penile and pudendal nerves to S2-S4.
  - Somatomotor information sent from Onuf's nucleus in S2-S4 to stimulate muscle contraction.

## Erection

- Dependent on cavernosal smooth muscle and arterial smooth muscle.
- *Five Phases* of erection:
  - 0 – Flaccid
  - 1 – Latent
  - 2 – Tumescence
  - 3 – Full erection
  - 4 – Rigid erection
  - 5 – Detumescence
- *Flaccid* state – the smooth muscle is tonically contracted and sinusoids are empty.
- Psychological, tactile, or audiovisual stimulation can initiate an erection.
- Mediated by the autonomic nervous system (Figure 12.8).
  - Cavernous nerves innervate the helicine arteries and cavernosal smooth muscle.
  - *Two types* of cavernous nerves: *cholinergic* and *non-noradrenergic non-cholinergic* (NANC).
- Parasympathetic nerves release nitric oxide (NO) from NANC cavernous nerve terminals via neuronal NO synthase (nNOS).
- Smaller amount of NO is released from the endothelium via endothelial NOS (eNOS).
  - L-citrulline + $O_2$ → NO
- NO half-life is ~5 seconds.
- NO activates guanylyl cyclase to convert guanosine triphosphate (GTP) to cyclic guanosine monophosphate (cGMP).
  - Activates protein kinase G, which opens calcium channels through phosphorylation.
  - Reduction in intracytosolic calcium.

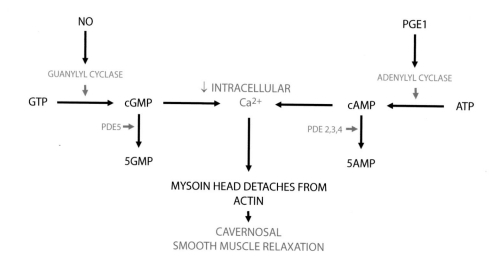

TUMESCENCE

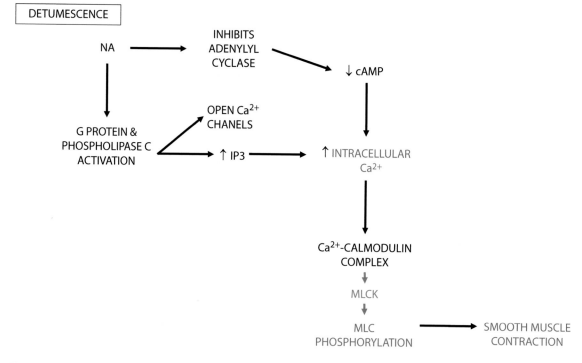

DETUMESCENCE

Figure 12.8 The physiological pathways involved in tumescence and detumescence. NO, nitric oxide; PDE, phosphodiesterase; GTP, guanosine triphosphate; cGMP, cyclic guanosine monophosphate; ATP, adenosine triphosphate; cAMP, cyclic adenosine monophosphate; $Ca^{2+}$, calcium; PG, prostaglandin; NA, noradrenaline; IP3, inositol triphosphate; MLCK, myosin-light chain kinase.

- Dissociation of calcium from calmodulin deactivates myosin-light chain kinase (MLCK).
- Reduced phosphorylation of myosin-light chain (MLC) causes dissociation of myosin heads from actin.

- Causes smooth muscle relaxation and *tumescence.*
- Prostaglandin E1 (target of alprostadil) activates adenyl cyclase to convert adenosine triphosphate (ATP) to cyclic adenosine monophosphate (cAMP).

- Reduce intracellular calcium → smooth muscle relaxation and increase in arterial inflow into sinusoidal spaces through arterial and arteriolar dilatation.
- Intracavernosal pressure rises during tumescent phase to the rigid erection phase.
  - Sinusoidal spaces expand against the tunica albuginea → tunica stretches to capacity and subtunical plexus and emissary veins are compressed between layers of the tunica albuginea → venous outflow decreased → penis raised from the dependent position to erect state – *full erection*
  - Intracavernosal pressure reaches around 100 mm Hg in the full erection phase.
- Further engorgement and intracavernosal pressure increase occurs during the *rigid erection* phase.
  - Contraction of the ischiocavernosus and bulbocavernosus muscle → compression of the corpus spongiosum → increases pressure in the glans
- cGMP is broken down by *phosphodiesterase 5* (target of phosphodiesterase inhibitors, PDE5i) to 5-GMP, causing smooth muscle contraction, vasoconstriction and subsequent *detumescence*.

## Detumescence

- Under sympathetic control.
- Cavernosal nerves release NA, which inhibits adenylate cyclase to decrease cAMP and raise inositol triphosphate levels ($IP_3$).
- $IP_3$ causes:
  - Calcium release from the sarcoplasmic reticulum.
  - Opening of calcium channels to increase intracytosolic calcium.
- Calcium–calmodulin complex activates myosin-light chain kinase (MLCK).
  - MLCK phosphorylates MLC, causing smooth muscle contraction and detumescence.
- Another pathway of smooth muscle contraction involves RhoA and Rho-kinase.

- Expressed in higher levels in cavernosal smooth muscle than vascular smooth muscle.
- Rho-kinase phosphorylates and inhibits MLC phosphatase (MLC-P).
- Normally, MLC-P dephosphorylates MLC, causing smooth muscle contraction.

## Central Neurotransmitters Involved in Erection

- Dopamine – excitatory
- Serotonin – generally inhibitory
- GABA – inhibitory
- Oxytocin – excitatory
- NO – excitatory
- Prolactin – inhibitory

## Recommended Reading

1. Yiee, JH, & Baskin, LS. Penile embryology and anatomy. Scientific World J. 2010;10:1174–9.
2. Sadler, TW, Langman J. Langman's Medical Embryology 12th Edition. Philadelphia, PA: Wolters Kluwer Health/ Lippincott Williams & Wilkins; 2012.
3. Wein, AJ, Kavoussi, LR, Campbell, MF. Campbell-Walsh Urology 10th Edition. Philadelphia, PA: Elsevier Saunders; 2012.
4. Mahadevan, V. Surgical anatomy of the male external genitalia. In Atlas of Male Genitourethral Surgery 1–7. Oxford: John Wiley & Sons, Ltd; 2013.
5. Bella, AJ, & Shamloul, R. Functional anatomy of the male sex organs. In Cancer and Sexual Health 3–12. Humana Press; 2011.
6. Tanagho, EA, & McAninch, JW. Smith's General Urology 17th Edition. United States: McGraw-Hill Medical; 2008.
7. Dean, RC, & Lue, TF. Physiology of penile erection and pathophysiology of erectile dysfunction. Urol Clin North Am. 2005;32(4):379–95.
8. Omar M. Aboumarzouk. Blandy's Urology, 3rd Edition. United States: John Wiley and Sons; 2019.
9. Brackett, NL, Lynne, CM, Ibrahim, E, Ohl, DA, & Sønksen J. et al. Treatment of infertility in men with spinal cord injury. Nat Rev Urol. 2010; 7(3)162–172.
10. Wein, Kavoussi, Novick, Partin, Peters. Campbell-Walsh Urology, 10th Edition. Chapter 2. Anatomy of the lower urinary tract and male genitalia. Philadelphia, Elsevier; 2012.

# 13 Anatomical and Physiological Changes in Pregnancy

*Joanna Shepherd and Stephen Radley*

## Pregnancy

- *Pregnancy* is a state in which a fertilised ovum develops into a foetus over a period of ~40 weeks.
- There are *three stages* (or trimesters) of pregnancy:
  - First (0–12 weeks)
  - Second (13–28 weeks)
  - Third (29–40 weeks)
- Full-term at 37–42 weeks.
- *Human chorionic gonadotrophin* (hCG) is detected in urine and blood samples in the 1st trimester.
  - A glycoprotein secreted by the placental syncytiotrophoblast.
  - Present in maternal blood from ~three days post-implantation.
  - Level rises until ~10 weeks, then begins to plateau.
- *Pregnancy gestation*
  1. Estimation based on the date of the *last menstrual period* (LMP).
  2. *Ultrasound* is used between 11 and 14 weeks to accurately date pregnancies:
     - Measurement of the crown-rump length.
  3. *Clinical examination:*
     - 12th week – uterus felt above the pubic symphysis.
     - At 20 weeks – fundus felt at the umbilicus.
     - Term (38–42 weeks) – fundus reaches the xiphisternum.

## Physiological Changes

- The majority of the physiological changes observed in pregnancy are established in the first trimester (Table 13.1).

## The Kidney

### Anatomy

- Increased blood flow results in:
  - 10–15% renal enlargement
    - ~1–1.5 cm by week 20

- Renal size may also increase as a result of:
  - Compressive forces on the ureters, or the dilatation of the pelvicalyceal system.
  - *Progesterone,* which reduces ureteral tone, peristalsis, and ureteric contraction pressure.

## Glomerular Filtration Rate (GFR)

- Increases from ~6 weeks gestation as a result of:
  - Vasodilation and increased plasma volume.
  - Increased plasma volume decreases the oncotic pressures in the glomeruli – increases GFR.
- By the end of week 12, GFR increases to >50%, which is maintained until delivery.
- As GFR rises:
  - Creatinine falls to ~44 mmol/L and urea to 3.2 mmol/L.
  - Creatinine >80 mmol/L may indicate renal impairment.

## Vasculature, Chemical Filtration, and Body Water Maintenance

- During pregnancy:
  - Proximal tubules and collecting ducts are less effective at reabsorption.
  - Urinary excretion of 1–10 g of glucose/day.
  - Increased GFR and capillary permeability to albumin cause:
    - Increase in protein excretion of up to 300 mg/day.
    - At >300 mg/day, be cautious of pre-eclampsia.
- Sodium excretion: mediated by progesterone, atrial natriuretic factor, and some prostaglandins.
- Sodium retention: mediated by aldosterone and oestrogen.
- Increased GFR further promotes sodium excretion.
  - Aldosterone increases to counterbalance this deficit.
  - Aldosterone acts on $Na^+/K^+$ pumps in the collecting tubule:
    - Overall increased total body sodium of ~1 g.
    - Increased fluid increased fluid by to ~5–8 L.

| Table 13.1 Summary of Physiological Changes of Pregnancy | |
|---|---|
| **System** | **Changes** |
| **Neurological** | ↑ CSF pressure |
| | Engorgement of epidural veins |
| | ↓ Minimum alveolar concentration for inhaled anaesthetics |
| | ↓ Local anaesthetics volumes required |
| **Respiratory** | ↑ Minute volume (↑ tidal Vol. and ↑ respiratory rate) |
| | ↓ $PaCO_2$ |
| | ↑ $PaO_2$ |
| | ↓ Functional residual capacity |
| **Cardiac** | ↑ Cardiac output |
| | ↑ Stroke volume |
| | ↑ Heart rate |
| | Left ventricular hypertrophy |
| | Regurgitant murmurs |
| | ↓ Systemic vascular resistance |
| **Renal** | ↑ Renal blood flow |
| | ↑ Glomerular filtration rate |
| | ↓ Plasma urea and creatinine |
| | ↑ Urinary protein and glucose |
| **Gastrointestinal** | ↓ Lower oesophageal sphincter tone |
| | ↑ Risk of aspiration |
| | ↓ Liver enzymes (AST, ALT, GGT) |
| | ↑ ALP |
| **Musculoskeletal** | ↑ Ligamentous laxity |
| | ↑ Risk of dislocation |
| | ↑ Lumbar lordosis |
| **Endocrine** | ↑ Progesterone and oestrogen |
| | Placenta secretes relaxin, human placental lactogen and HCG |
| | Thyroid hyperplasia |
| | Transient hyperthyroidism |
| | Insulin resistance |
| | ↑ Cortisol secretion by adrenal glands |

*Abbreviations:* ALP, alkaline phosphatase; ALT, alanine transaminase; AST, aspartate transaminase; CSF, cerebrospinal fluid; GGT, γ-glutamyl transferase; HCG, human chorionic gonadotrophin.

- 40% reflects the expansion of plasma volume.
- The remainder is attributable to the foetus, placenta, and amniotic fluid.

- The *increased respiratory rate* results in a respiratory alkalosis.
- Compensated by increased renal bicarbonate excretion.

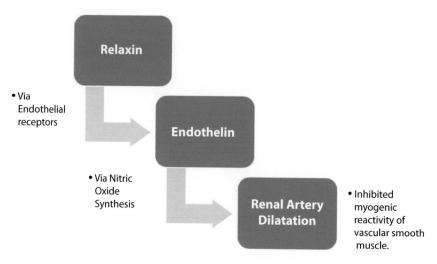

Figure 13.1 Mediators involved in vasodilatation.

## Cardiovascular Changes

- Reduced systemic vascular resistance from ~week 6.
- Hormones involved in vasodilation are shown in Figure 13.1.

## Renin–Angiotensin–Aldosterone (RAA) System

- Triggered early in pregnancy.
- *Angiotensin II resistance* develops:
  - Counteracts the vasoconstrictive effect → results in vasodilation
  - Resistance is linked to:
    - Progesterone
    - VEGF-mediated prostacyclin production
    - Changes to angiotensin I receptors during pregnancy
- Arterial underfilling (despite the increase in plasma volume) stimulates arterial baroreceptors, leading to the activation *of RAA and sympathetic nervous systems:*
  - Anti-diuretic hormone (ADH) from the hypothalamus increases.
  - *ADH* acts on the collecting tubules:
    - Mobilisation of aquaporins.
    - Water reabsorption from urine into the bloodstream.
    - Overall hypo-osmolar, hypervolemic state.
- *Pro-renin* from the ovaries and placenta further stimulates RAA.
- The placenta produces *oestrogen:*
  - Triggers the synthesis of angiotensinogen in the liver.
  - Results in much higher levels of aldosterone compared with renin.
- High levels of *aldosterone* result in plasma volume increase.

## The Ureter

- The ureters and calyceal systems dilate in most pregnancies.
  - *Physiological:* progesterone (reduces ureteric tone and peristalsis).
  - *Anatomical: m*ore marked on the right side.
- 75% are right-sided dilatation, while 33% are left
  - Calyceals dilate to ~15 mm on the right and 5 mm on the left.
- *Anatomical* causes for right-sided predominance:
  - The right ureter crosses the ovarian and iliac vessels at an angle before entering the pelvis.
  - Compression by the gravid uterus due to dextrorotation.
  - Relative protection of the left ureter by the sigmoid colon.

## Renal Failure

- Pregnancy has adverse effects on already compromised maternal renal function.
  - May cause obstetric complications such as,
    - Pregnancy failure
    - Intrauterine growth restriction
    - Pre-term birth (most commonly iatrogenic for maternal reasons)
    - Hypertension, pre-eclampsia
- *Post renal obstructive* causes of acute renal failure:
  - Gravid uterus
  - Urinary tract calculi (or tumour)

# The Bladder

- Bladder compression by the gravid uterus causes:
  - Reduced bladder capacity
  - Urinary frequency
  - Nocturia
  - Hesitancy
  - Urgency (~62%)
  - Urge incontinence (~18%)
  - Stress incontinence (~85%)
- Increased fluid intake in early pregnancy also increases urinary frequency.
- In the nulliparous, the prevalence of stress incontinence is:
  - Pre-pregnancy, 3%
  - Antenatally, 36%
  - Post-partum, 12%
- *Urinary retention* in the post-partum: ~1–18 in 100 pregnancies.
  - Attributable causes or associations include:
    - Prolonged labour
    - Instrumental delivery
    - Epidural anaesthetic
    - Enlarging retroverted uterus
    - Fibroids or other pelvic masses
  - May require intermittent self-catheterisation or an indwelling catheter.

# Urinary Tract Infection (UTI)

- Similar incidence in pregnant and non-pregnant women.
- Asymptomatic bacteriuria (ABU) detected in 4–10%.
  - 20–40% increase in the development of pyelonephritis with ABU.
  - Associated with pre-term birth and low birth weight.
- Cystitis: 1–4%
- Pyelonephritis: 1–2%
- *Risk factors:*
  - Obstruction/stasis of urine due to the gravid uterus
  - Physiological hydronephrosis
  - Decreased immune system (foetal protective)
  - 'DR family' *E. coli* – antibiotic-resistant organism with the ability to invade renal tissue and persist in epithelial tissues.
  - Upregulation of CD55
- *Two components* may impact the course of a UTI:
  - *Nitric oxide* (NO)
    - Keeps the uterus in a dormant state.
    - Helps destroy or impede invasive organisms.
  - *Toll-like receptor 4* (TLR4)
    - Recognise particular danger signals from endotoxins.

- Produces an inflammatory response (cytokines and prostaglandins).
- Could prove disadvantageous to a foetus and potentiate pre-term labour.
- *CD55* complement regulator protects the foetus from maternal complement injury.
  - Expression is increased by progesterone.
  - CD55 is favourable for DR *E. coli* colonisation.
- Decreased NO and TLR4 activity and increase in CD55 → DR *E. coli* can use this opportunity to cause infection
- *Antibiotics:*
  - Amoxicillin or cephalosporin are safe.
  - Trimethoprim: avoid during the 1st trimester.
    - Anti-folate properties increase the risk of neural tube defects.
  - Nitrofurantoin: avoid during the 3rd trimester.
    - Increases risk of neonatal jaundice.
  - Gentamicin: not routinely recommended.
    - Cranial VIII nerve damage in the foetus.

# Renal Calculi

- Incidence in pregnancy is similar to that of non-pregnant women.
- 1 in 1,500.
- Majority are calcium-based, with an increase in struvite stones.
- Increase in calcium excretion → increases risk
  - However, this is counteracted by increased *citrate* filtration.
- Diagnosed with USS (to identify hydronephrosis) or MR urogram (to detect change in ureteric calibre).
- CT scans (radiation) are associated with:
  - Congenital malformations
  - Foetal death
  - Childhood cancers
  - Developmental issues and growth restriction
- Stones resolve with conservative management in ~60% (ureteric dilatation by progesterone effects).
- Risk of *NSAIDs*:
  - Foetal kidney injury
  - Oligohydramnios
  - Premature closure of the ductus arteriosus
- Nifedipine and tamsulosin expulsion therapy in pregnancy are considered 'off-label'.

# Urethra

- Absolute urethral length increases by ~6.7 mm.
- Functional length increases by ~4.8 mm.
- The urethral closing pressure reaches a maximum of:

- ~93 cmH$_2$O at 38 weeks.
- ~69 cmH$_2$O at post-partum (similar to pre-pregnancy).

- The causes of increased urethral closing pressure include:
  - Increase in urethral sphincter volume, secondary to increased blood flow.
  - Amplified vascular pulsations in the urethral wall, most pronounced during the first 16 weeks.

## Recommended Reading

1. Talbot L and Maclennan K. Physiology of pregnancy. Anaest Intensive Care Med. 2016;17(7):341–45.
2. Peters A. Global library of women's medicine (ISSN: 1756-2228) 2008. doi: 10.3843/GLOWM.10093. https://www.glowm.com/section_view/heading/The%20Diagnosis%20of%20Pregnancy/item/93.
3. Conrad KP, Lindheimer MD. Renal and cardiovascular alterations. In: Lindheimer MD, Roberts JM, Cunningham FG. Chelsey's Hypertensive Disorders in Pregnancy, 2nd Edition. Stamford, CT: Appleton and Lange; 1999. pp. 262–326.
4. Soma-Pillay P, Nelson-Piercy C, Tolppanen H, Mebazaa A. Physiological changes in pregnancy. Cardiovasc J Afr. 2016 Mar-Apr;27(2):89–94.
5. Reynard J et al. Oxford Handbook of Urology. Urological Problems in Pregnancy, 4th Edition. Oxford University Press. pp. 657–68.
6. Nowicki B, Sledzinska A, Samet A, Nowicki S. Pathogenesis of gestational urinary tract infection: urinary obstruction versus immune adaptation and microbial virulence. BJOG 2011;118:109–12.
7. Chaliha C and Stanton S. Urological problems in pregnancy. BJU Int. 2002;89:469–76.

# Section III

## BENIGN PATHOLOGY

# 14 Pain

*Karl H. Pang and Sam H. Ahmedzai*

## Pain

International Association for the Study of Pain (IASP) definition: An unpleasant sensory and emotional experience associated with, or resembling that associated with, actual or potential tissue damage.

- Pain is always a personal experience that is influenced to varying degrees by biological, psychological, and social factors.
- Pain and nociception are different phenomena.
- Pain cannot be inferred solely from activity in sensory neurons.
- Through their life experiences, individuals learn the concept of pain. A person's report of an experience as pain should be respected.
- Although pain usually serves an adaptive role, it may have adverse effects on function and social and psychological well-being.
- Verbal description is only one of several behaviors to express pain; inability to communicate does not negate the possibility that a human or a non-human animal experiences pain. Note that emotional, cognitive, behavioural, and sexual responses can all influence how a patient expresses pain.
- There is a complex interplay between signalling systems, modulation from higher centres, and the psychosocial characteristics of the individual.
- Pain lasting up to 3 months is classified as 'acute' and beyond 3 months as 'chronic' (or persistent').

*Aetiological classification:*
- Nociceptive, somatic (skin, musculoskeletal), and visceral (smooth muscle); often initiated by inflammatory processes such as infection, surgery, trauma.
- Referred pain reflects development of embryonic pain (e.g. distal ureteric stone → groin/testis pain).
- Neuropathic (associated with nerve damage at peripheral or central (spinal, cerebral) level).
- Many disease processes give rise to both nociceptive (inflammatory) and neuropathic (nerve damage) pain at the same time.
- Chronic primary pain is chronic pain in one or more anatomical regions, and is characterised by significant emotional distress or functional disability and can include forms of chronic pelvic pain.

*Nerve fibres mediated pain pathways:*
- *A-delta fibres (~20–30%):* myelinated nerves – high conduction speed (5–15 m/s) and large diameter (2–5 μm) → sharp pain.
- *C-fibres (70–80%):* unmyelinated nerves – lower conduction speed (0.5–2 m/s) and smaller diameter (<2 μm) → longer-lasting dull pain.

## Pain Transmission and Drug Modulation

- *Transduction*
  - Production of electrical impulses
  - Tissue damage → nociceptors (free nerve endings) → inflammatory substances (e.g., prostaglandin, histamine, substance P) → electrical impulses → transmitted along sensory nerves
  - Paracetamol and non-steroid anti-inflammatories (NSAIDs) inhibit prostaglandin production.

- *Transmission* (Figure 14.1)
  - Pain sensation along A-delta and C-fibres → synapse in the dorsal horn with second-order neurons → spinal cord → thalamus → sensory cortex in the brain
  - Local anaesthetics prevent the conduction of action potentials in these fibres.

- *Peripheral and central sensitisation*
  - In animal and human pain models and clinically, it can be shown that once acute pain pathways have been initiated, there can be development of sensitisation of the nervous system, leading to heightened pain expression.
  - Sensitisation of pain pathways is accompanied by upregulation of receptors, neurotransmitters and changes in astrocytes and glial cells especially in the spinal cord.
  - Sensitisation accounts for some of the changes in pain expression and in animal

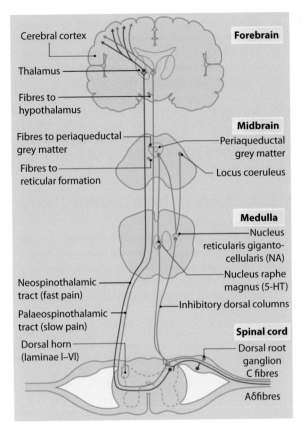

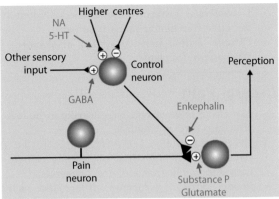

Figure 14.2 Excitatory and inhibitory interactions at the spinal cord level. NA, noradrenaline; 5-HT, 5-hydroxytryptamine; GABA, γ-aminobutyric acid. (Reprinted with permission from Elsevier [1])

Figure 14.1 Spinal and supraspinal pathways of pain. Ascending nociceptive fast (red) and slow (green) pathways; Descending inhibitory tracts (blue); NA, noradrenaline; 5-HT, 5-hydroxytryptamine. (Reprinted with permission from Elsevier [1])

models, such as hyperaesthesia and allodynia (see below).

- *Modulation* (Figure 14.2)
  - *'Gate Control Theory'*
  - A-beta fibres stimulation in the periphery is involved in inhibiting transmission to higher centred- stimulation centres through spinal cord stimulation, which reduces pain (theoretical basis for transcutaneous electrical nerve stimulation (TENS)).
  - Descending spinal pathways (inhibitory or excitatory) can modulate pain signal transmission in the dorsal horn of the spinal cord.
    - *Inhibitory* inputs arise from the periaqueductal grey matter and nucleus raphe magnus (release serotonin - largely excitatory) and locus coeruleus (releases noradrenaline – largely inhibitory).
- *Opioids* (acting via mu, kappa and delta opioid receptors) inhibit peripheral and spinal pain

pathways and stimulate descending inhibitory signalling to spinal cord, via increased noradrenergic activity.
- *Local anaesthetics* act on sodium channels on nerve fibres to reduce neurotransmission (lidocaine, bupivicaine).
- *Anti-depressants* which inhibit noradrenaline reuptake (e.g., selective noradrenaline reuptake inhibitors such as duloxetine, tricyclics) can alleviate pain independent of any action on depressed mood.
- *Anti-convulsants* act on calcium channels on nerve fibres and at synapses to reduce neurotransmission (carbamazepine, gabapentin, pregabalin).
- Local anaesthetics, anti-depressants, and anti-convulsants when used in pain management, are sometimes referred to as 'adjuvants'

*Dorsal horn* – divided into *laminae*
- C-fibres terminate in lamina II.
- A-delta fibres terminate in lamina I and V.
- A-beta fibres (light touch and vibration) terminate in lamina III–V.
- Lamina II and V are important areas for modulation and pain localisation.

## Pain Expression
- Involves emotional, cognitive, behavioural, and sexual responses and mechanisms.
- *Allodynia*: pain due to a visceral stimulus that does not normally provoke pain.
- *Hyperalgesia*: increased sensitivity to painful visceral stimuli.
- *Hyperpathia*: exaggerated and prolonged response to stimulation.
- *Hyperaesthesia*: increased sensitivity to stimulation.

- *Dysaesthesia*: evoked or spontaneous altered sensation (discomfort rather than pain).
- *Chronic*: central nervous system involvement, sensitisation (see later).

## Visceral Pain

- Arise from internal organs — usually in hollow structures (ureter, bladder).
- Colicky in nature.
- Caused by distention (e.g. obstructing urinary tract stone), inflammation, and ischaemia.
- Poorly localised compared to somatic pain because the density of nociceptors on viscera is lower and afferent fibres are less well represented.
- Visceral pain pathways are shared with somatic pathways in the same ascending tracts.
- Visceral and somatic afferents terminate on the same dorsal horn neurons in the spinal cord – viscera-somatic convergence → 'referred' pain to the corresponding somatic tissue.

- Pain is accompanied by motor and autonomic reflexes as visceral afferents which travel together with afferents of the autonomic nervous system:
  - *Example*: renal colic may be associated with nausea and vomiting (Figure 14.3).

## Neuropathic Pain

- Initiated or caused by a lesion or dysfunction of the nervous system.
- Can be sensory, motor, or autonomic.

## Mechanisms of Neuropathic Pain

- *Nerve injury*
  - Results in inflammatory response around damaged nerves → *observed in animal models as upregulation of pain receptors and pathways = plastic changes (neuroplasticity)*.
  - Peripheral nociceptors become sensitised by injury:

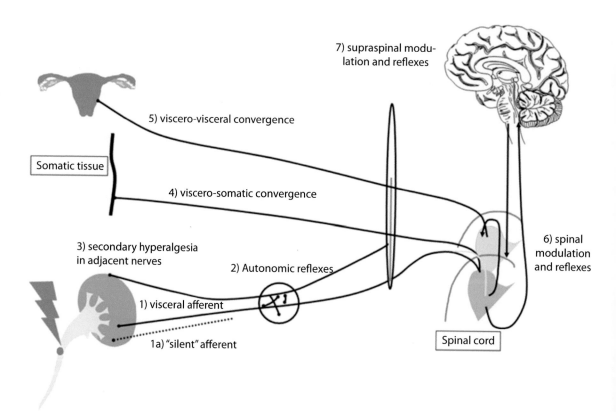

**Figure 14.3** The multiple nervous pathways involved in visceral pain. Visceral nociceptive stimuli can lead to action potentials in true visceral afferent (1), or the inflammation can activate 'silent' afferents (1a) that are not normally active. Autonomic reflexes (2) will typically contribute to the pain. ongoing stimulation can sensitise the nerves and lead to secondary hyperalgesia (3). Viscero-somatic (4) and viscero-visceral (5) convergence between neurons at the spinal cord may give referred pain and visceral allodynia in areas remote from the original lesion. Spinal (6) and supraspinal (7) modulation and hyperexcitability may influence the pain and discomfort experienced. (Reprinted with permission from Elsevier [2])

- Lower threshold of firing.
- Increased response to noxious stimuli.
- Fire in response to non-noxious stimuli.
- Focus of hyperexcitability and ectopic discharge.
- Changes occur in the Schwann cells and glia that surround axons.
- *Central sensitisation*
  - Nerve injury may cause changes to occur in the dorsal horn of the spinal cord.
  - Repetitive C fibre activation → prolonged dorsal horn response
  - Reduction in local inhibition (by GABA and glycine) in the dorsal horn.
  - Increased excitatory synaptic connections.
  - Lowered sensory threshold for pain signalling.
  - Mechanisms leading to enhanced visceral input to the spinal cord level → neuroplastic changes → amplification of the effects of further signals coming from the affected viscus
  - Linked to the phosphorylation of the N-methyl-D-aspartate (NMDA) receptor, leading to phenomenon of 'wind-up', which may mediate hyperalgesia and allodynia.

## Upper Urinary Tract Pain

- Nociceptive afferent inputs from different areas of the upper urinary tract are processed in different regions of the spinal cord — L2-3 and S1-2.
- *Kidney* pain – ipsilateral costovertebral angle just beneath the 12th rib.
  - Radiate across the flank anteriorly towards the upper abdomen and groin.
  - Mechanoreceptors – activated by increased renal pressure.
  - Chemoreceptors – activated by inflammation/ischaemia.
- *Mid-ureteric* pain – referred to the lower left and right quadrant, and to the testis/labia.
- *Lower ureteric* pain – bladder irritability (frequency, urgency) and suprapubic pain → may radiate along the urethra or medial thigh.
- *Pain relief:*
  - NSAIDs inhibit prostaglandin and decreases pain and ureteric peristalsis/pressure. Also reduce renal blood flow and glomerular filtration rate (afferent arteriole constriction) → risk of acute kidney injury.
  - Alpha-blockers and Ca-antagonists relax ureteric smooth muscle and decrease the renal pelvic pressure.

## Lower Urinary Tract Pain

- Sensory innervation of the bladder and urethra originates in the S2-4 region → travel via the parasympathetic pelvic nerves

- Some afferents also originate at the T11-L2 region → sympathetic hypogastric nerves
- External urethral sphincter – somatic pudendal nerve (S2-4).
- Sensory nerves in the bladder are identified submucosally and in the detrusor muscle.
- Acetylcholine and noradrenaline neurotransmitters predominate, but others include:
  - ATP, substance P, neurokinin A, calcitonin gene-related peptide (CGRP), prostaglandin, nitric oxide, vasoactive intestinal peptide (VIP), enkephalins
- *Physiological* sensation – bladder filling and sensation during micturition.
- *Pathological* sensation – urgency, pain (bladder pain syndrome).

## Scrotal Pain

- Perceived in the testes, epididymis, or the vas deferens.
- *Innervation:* L1-2, S2-4 nerve roots through the ilioinguinal, genitofemoral, pudendal nerves.
  - *Ilioinguinal* – innervates the inner thigh, penile base, upper scrotal skin.
  - *Genitofemoral* – inside of the thigh (femoral), cremaster muscle, tunica vaginalis, antero-lateral scrotal skin (genito).
- *Causes:* nerve injury, inflammation, ischaemia
- *Two main syndromes:*
  - Post-vasectomy scrotal pain syndrome (2–20%)
  - Post-inguinal hernia repair pain
- *Mechanisms*
  - Scrotal/testes injury → nerve sensitisation → modulation → hypersensitivity and spontaneous firing
- Referred pain from 'shared' nerve roots, such as:
  - Back pain (T10-L1) → testis
  - Inguinal hernias may stretch the genitofemoral/ilioinguinal nerves
  - Lower ureteric pathology (obstructing stone)

## Management of Pain

- Level 1 (for mild acute and chronic pain): non-opioids +/- adjuvants
- Level 2 (for moderate-severe acute and chronic pain: weak opioids +/- non-opioids / adjuvants
- Level 3: (for severe acute and chronic pain): strong opioids +/- non-opioids / adjuvants
- *Non-opioids:*
  - NSAIDs (inhibit cyclo-oxygenase and subsequently prostaglandin), paracetamol
- *Opioids:*
  - Modulate inhibitory peripheral and central pathways.
  - *Weak:* (dihydro)codeine, tramadol

- *Strong:* morphine (oral, subcutaneous, intramuscular, intravenous), buprenorphine, methadone, oxycodone, fentanyl
- Notes on opioids:
  - Dihydrocodeine and tramadol are pro-drugs and have to be metablised into active agents – this is dependent on individual pharmacogenomic factor
  - Diamorphine (heroin) is a pro-drug for morphine; its only therapeutic advantage is that it is more hydrophilic (soluble in water) than morphine
  - Buprenorphine and fentanyl are highly lipophilic (soluble in fat) and consequently are well absorbed transmucosally and transdermally than morphine and other opioids
- *Neuropathic pain:* SNRIs (duloxetine), tricyclics (amitriptyline); anticonvulsants (gabapentin, pregabalin)

## Local Anaesthetics

- Lidocaine, (levo)bupivacaine, Prilocaine.
- Local infiltration.
- Membrane-stabilising drugs.
- Inhibit sodium influx and generation of action potential → inhibit excitation of nociceptors.

## Metastatic Bone Pain

- Radiotherapy to bone lesion.
- Chemotherapy.
- Hormone therapy (androgen deprivation) in prostate cancer.
- Denosumab: RANK ligand inhibitor → inhibits maturation of osteoclasts.
- Bisphosphonates – inhibit osteoclastic bone resorption.
- Dexamethasone – anti-inflammatory (short-term role only), e.g. for metastatic spinal cord or cauda equina compression.

## Recommended Reading

1. Steeds CE. The anatomy and physiology of pain. Surgery (Oxford). Elsevier 2016;34(2):55–59.
2. Pedersen KV, Drewes AM, Frimodt-Moller PC, Osther PJS. Visceral pain originating from the upper urinary tract. Urol Res. Elsevier 2010;38:345–355.
3. Wybdaele JJ, De Wachter S. The basics behind bladder pain: a review of data on lower urinary tract sensations. Int J Urol. 2003;10 Suppl:S49–S55.
4. Patel AP. Anatomy and physiology of chronic scrotal pain. Transl Androl Urol. 2017:6(Suppl 1): S51–56.

# 15 Acute Kidney Injury and Chronic Kidney Disease

*Lynne Sykes, Ibrahim Ali, and Philip A. Kalra*

## Anatomy and Physiology (see Chapter 8)

### Functions of the Kidney

- Filtration of waste products (e.g., urea and creatinine)
- Electrolyte homeostasis (e.g., sodium and potassium)
- Water balance
- Acid–base balance
- Erythropoietin (EPO) secretion (increases red blood cell production)
- Vitamin D metabolism (involved in bone metabolism)
- Renin secretion (up-regulates renin–angiotensin–aldosterone [RAA] system)
- Metabolism of drugs

### Gross Kidney Structure

- Receive 20% of the cardiac output (~1 L/min) via renal arteries
- Outer renal region – cortex
- Inner region – medulla
- Nephrons – functional units

### Nephron Physiology

- ~1.2 million nephrons per kidney.
- Filtering unit of the kidney.
  - ~180 L of plasma is filtered per day, producing ~2 L of urine.
- Fluid balance homeostasis achieved through cardiac and arterial receptors detecting pressure.
  - Causes a change in sympathetic neural tone.
  - Release of renin and antidiuretic hormone (ADH).
- *Volume depletion:*
  - Arteriolar constriction of renal, splanchnic, and musculocutaneous vessels.
  - Retention of salt and water.
  - Preserve blood flow to the heart and brain.

### Functional Anatomy of the Nephron

- Comprised of the glomerulus, proximal tubules, Loop of Henle (LOH), distal convoluted tubule (DCT), and collecting ducts (CD) (Figure 15.1).

### The Glomerulus

- A tuft of capillaries formed by an afferent arteriole separated from the Bowman's capsule by the glomerular basement membrane (GBM).
- The *Bowman's capsule:*
  - Continuous with renal tubules and CD.
  - Carries away filtrate (urine) into the ureter.
- GBM is a size- and charge-selective barrier.
  - It is where blood filtration commences.
  - Podocytes are situated on the urinary side of the GBM.
    - These are specialised epithelial cells with '*foot processes*'.
    - Provide a further layer of filtration.
- The glomerulus is supplied by afferent arterioles and is drained by efferent arterioles.
- In *low* circulating volume:
  - efferent arteriole constriction limits blood outflow.
  - glomerular pressure increases to maintain filtration.
- Intrinsic and extrinsic mechanisms regulate glomerular filtration.
  - *Intrinsic*
    - The kidney adjusts dilatation or constriction of afferent and efferent arterioles to counteract fluctuations in blood pressure.
  - *Extrinsic*
    - In *low* circulating volume, the RAA system causes constriction of the efferent arteriole.
    - With high blood pressure or volume overload, atrial natriuretic peptide (ANP) is secreted to increase urine production.

### Proximal Tubules

- Filtrate from the Bowman's capsule drains into the proximal convoluted tubule (PCT).

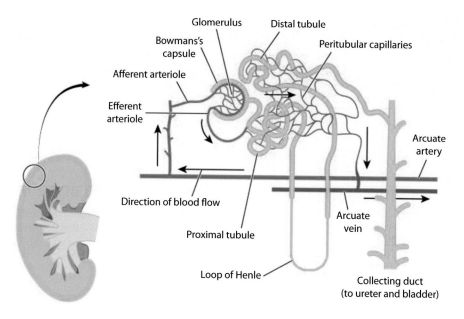

Figure 15.1 Anatomy of the nephron.

- Most metabolically active part of the nephron.
- Almost all filtered glucose, amino acids, and vitamins are reabsorbed.

## Loop of Henle

- Includes descending and ascending limbs.
- High osmolarity in the interstitial environment around the descending loop promotes water reabsorption.
- ~30% filtered sodium is absorbed in the ascending limb (site of loop diuretic action).
- The limbs act as a counter-current multiplier to increase osmolar concentration in the renal medulla.

## Distal Convoluted Tubule

- DCTs are tortuous with many mitochondria.
- Highly metabolically active.
- ~90% of water is reabsorbed prior to the CD.
- ~10% of filtered sodium is reabsorbed (site of thiazide diuretic action).

## Collecting Ducts

- Continuous with the nephron.
- CDs have receptors for ADH.
- ADH stimulates insertion of aquaporin channels into the luminal surface cell membranes.
  - Allows water to pass from the duct lumen into the interstitial spaces and the circulation via the vasa recta.
- CD actively pumps urea into the medulla to further increase osmolarity.

- Aldosterone stimulates sodium reabsorption in exchange for potassium (site of potassium-sparing diuretic action).

## Biomarkers for Renal Function – GFR Estimation Techniques

- *Creatinine:*
  - Creatinine is a waste product from muscle metabolism when creatine is metabolised to generate energy.
  - Freely and exclusively filtered through the kidneys.
    - Considered a measure of filtering capacity.
    - Serum levels are considered with age, sex, and body size when estimating glomerular filtration rate (eGFR).
  - Normal eGFR is at 90–120 mL/min/1.73 m$^2$.
  - *eGFR is* based upon the CKD-EPI (Chronic Kidney Disease Epidemiology Collaboration) equation.

## Limitations to Using Creatinine as a Marker of Renal Function

- ~10% creatinine is secreted by the proximal tubule (not filtered through the glomerulus) – can overestimate GFR.
- Levels vary due to dietary protein intake or muscle mass.
- Variation in secretion.
  - Acute kidney injury – compensatory mechanism

with enhanced proximal tubular secretion (process becomes saturated).

- Extrarenal secretion develops in advanced renal failure via intestinal bacterial overgrowth and increased bacterial creatininase activity.
- Measurement limitations.
  - Some substances (e.g., bilirubin or aceto-acetate in diabetic ketoacidosis [DKA]) interfere with colourimetric assay and artificially inflate creatinine measurement.

# Acute Kidney Injury (AKI)

## Definition and Classification

- Defined as a rapid decline in renal function.
- Divided into *three stages* based upon changes in creatinine or urine output.
- Classification (Table 15.1) is according to:
  - Relative creatinine change in comparison to baseline;
  - Absolute creatinine value; or
  - Urine output.

## Risk Factors

- Infants and older adults over 65 years of age
- Previous AKI
- Known chronic kidney disease
- Symptoms or history which suggest the risk of urinary tract obstruction
- Co-morbidities (e.g., heart failure, liver disease, diabetes mellitus, hypertension)
- Dependence on prompts or physical help for fluid intake
- Sepsis
- Hypovolaemia
- Recent use of medications such as NSAIDs, diuretics, or toxins
- Intravenous contrast
- Cancer and therapy for cancer
- Immunocompromised
- Surgery, particularly urinary tract surgery
- Table 15.2 summarises the causes of AKI according to pre-renal, renal, and post-renal insults.

**Table 15.1** Kidney Disease Improving Global Outcomes (KDIGO) Classification of AKI

| AKI Stage | Serum Creatinine Criteria | Urine Output Criteria |
|---|---|---|
| Stage 1 | Increase of more than 0.3 mg/dL (≥26.4 µmol/L) or increase of 1.5- to 2-fold from baseline | <0.5 mL/kg per hour for 6–12 h |
| Stage 2 | Increase 2- to 3-fold from baseline | <0.5 mL/kg per hour for >12 h |
| Stage 3 | Increase 3-fold or serum creatinine of more than or equal to 4.0 mg/dL (>354 µmol/L) or initiation of renal replacement therapy | Less than 0.3 mL/kg per hour or anuria for >12 h |

**Table 15.2** Summary Table for Causes of AKI

| Type of AKI | Cause |
|---|---|
| Pre-renal (85%) | **Reduced circulating volume** – hypovolaemia or hypotension due to sepsis, liver failure, dehydration or haemorrhage<br>**Reduced cardiac output**<br>**Medication** – any that reduce blood pressure, renal blood flow, or circulating volume in at-risk patients — e.g., ACE inhibitors or ARBs, NSAIDs, diuretics |
| Intrinsic or renal (5%) | **Vascular** – vasculitis, thrombosis<br>**Glomerular** – glomerulonephritis<br>**Tubular** – acute tubular necrosis, rhabdomyolysis, myeloma<br>**Interstitial** – interstitial nephritis, pyelonephritis<br>**Medication** – gentamicin, IV contrast |
| Post-renal (10%) | **Mechanical obstruction** – urinary tract stones, enlarged prostate, urological, or gynaecological malignancies, phimosis, posterior urethral valves, ureteric/urethral strictures, fibrosis (e.g., retro-peritoneal), trauma, blocked catheters/nephrostomies<br>**Neurological obstruction** – interruption of the sensory or motor supply to the detrusor muscle<br>**Medication** – anticholinergic drugs decrease bladder sensation and detrusor contractility or sympathomimetic drugs increase smooth muscle near the bladder neck<br>**Infection** – prostatitis or ureteric/urethral inflammation and oedema |

## Creatinine and eGFR

- eGFR overestimates renal function in critically unwell patients.
- Creatinine is a better reflection of change (more dynamic marker).
  - However, it lags true changes in filtration by 24–48 hours.
- In anuric AKI with no pre-existing chronic kidney disease (CKD):
  - Creatinine takes at least four hours to rise by 50%.
- In pre-existing CKD stage 4, serum creatinine can take up to 23 hours to rise by 50%.
- Novel biomarkers to help earlier detection of AKI are under evaluation.
  - *Examples*: NGAL, KIM-1, L-FABP.
- Creatinine clearance is preferred to calculate drug dosing.

## Transplant Acute Kidney Injury

- Must be considered differently as these patients are immunocompromised.
- *Prone to:*
  - Opportunistic infections (e.g., cytomegalovirus [CMV], *pneumocystis jirevocii,* fungal infections or Epstein-Barr virus [EBV])
  - Re-occurrence of their original primary disease
  - Urinary tract obstruction
  - Transplant rejection

## Pathophysiological Changes

### Pre-Renal: Aetiology and Pathophysiology

- Caused by decreased renal perfusion without damage to renal parenchyma.
- Occurs in hypovolaemic or low cardiac output.
- Prolonged under-perfusion which leads to ischaemic damage.
  - Ranges from reversible changes to severe ischaemic damage with oligo-anuric acute tubular necrosis (ATN) and the risk of non-recovery.
- Kidney response – reabsorbs sodium and concentrates urine.
  - Increases intra-vascular volume and improves renal perfusion.
- In reduced perfusion, depletion of ATP leads to:
  - cytoskeleton disruption of the endothelium;
  - apoptosis and necrosis of cells;
  - cytokine release, inflammation, and leucocyte activation; which
  - results in shedding of tubular cells.
    - Causes tubular obstruction and back leak of urinary filtrate.
    - Affects kidney to concentrate urine and excrete sodium, further reducing GFR.

### Intrinsic or Renal: Aetiology and Pathophysiology

- Affects tubules, glomeruli, interstitium, and blood vessels.
- Occurs at the corticomedullary junction and outer medullary region.

### Tubular Damage

- *Ischaemic* from severe or prolonged reduction in renal perfusion.
- *Nephrotoxic:*
  - Exogenous (aminoglycosides or cisplatinum)
  - Endogenous (haemoglobin in haemolysis, myoglobin in rhabdomyolysis)
- Results in necrosis, denuding of epithelium, and occlusion of tubular lumen by casts or cell debris.

### Glomerular Damage

- Caused by acute *glomerulonephritis* (GN).
  - Primary renal disease (e.g., IgA nephropathy)
  - Secondary GN (e.g., systemic lupus erythematosus, endocarditis, or granulomatosis with polyangiitis—previously known as Wegener's granulomatosis).

### Interstitial Damage

- Caused by *medication:* penicillin, cephalosporins, proton–pump inhibitors, or an infection (bacterial illnesses, e.g., leptospirosis, legionella, and pyelonephritis).

### Vascular Damage

- Caused by decreased renal perfusion.
  - Malignant hypertension
  - Atheroembolic disease
  - Pre-eclampsia/eclampsia and haemolytic uraemic syndrome/thrombotic thrombocytopenic purpura

### Post-Renal: Aetiology and Pathophysiology

- Obstruction in any location of the urinary tract can cause post-renal AKI.
- May be acute or chronic, partial or complete, unilateral or bilateral.
- For AKI to occur, both kidneys usually must be affected.
- May develop in unilateral obstruction in patients with severe insults, superadded infection, or those with pre-existing kidney disease.
- *Pathological changes in obstruction:*

- Vasoconstriction due to increased RAA activity.
- Urine accumulation in renal pelvis → increases retrograde interstitial pressure → increases hydrostatic pressure → tubular distention → epithelial tubular cells damage
- Inflammatory response → macrophage infiltration and myofibroblast accumulation in the interstitium → inflammatory cytokine response → irreversible interstitial fibrosis and renal tubular atrophy

## Early Management in AKI

- Principles of management:
  - Treat the cause.
  - Ensure euvolemia.
  - Prevent complications.
- There is a good chance for recovery of eGFR if obstruction is relieved.
- eGFR usually returns to the baseline despite some nephron loss, due to hypertrophy and hyperfiltration in other nephrons.
- Superadded infection makes full recovery less likely.
- Post obstructive diuresis can cause AKI again → volume loss → hypoperfusion and pre-renal AKI

### Fluid Balance

- In *normal* circumstances, kidneys respond and adapt to maintain an effective circulating volume, electrolyte concentration, and plasma osmolality.
- Obligatory water losses such as sweat, respiratory loss and via the stool amounts to ~500 mL per day.
- Increased losses are seen in:
  - Sepsis (Increased respiration and pyrexia)
  - Diarrhoea and vomiting.
  - Surgery needs consideration for the composition of losses.
- Markers of volume repletion:
  - Absolute values and trends in body weight, blood pressure, heart rate, jugular venous pressure, urine output.
  - Skin turgor and thirst.
- Decreased urine output is the first sign of decreased renal function.

### Optimisation of Intra-vascular Fluid

- Fluid replacement to maintain euvolemia.
- Vasopressor therapy should be considered in unresponsiveness to fluid challenges (excess mortality with fluid overload).
- Fluid composition is also an important consideration.

- >2 L 0.9% saline can cause hyperchloraemic acidosis and can worsen the clinical state of acidaemic patients.
- Balanced crystalloids are preferred; however, NICE recommends against the use of colloids.

## Complications of AKI

### Electrolyte Complications

- *Hyperkalaemia*
  - Develops due to decreased renal excretion and shifts of potassium from the intra to extra-cellular compartments due to acidaemia.
  - Leads to muscle weakness, cardiac arrhythmias, and cardiac arrest.
- *Hypo/hypernatraemia*
  - Due to fluid imbalances.
  - Mild hyponatraemia is the inability of the kidney to excrete free water in AKI.
  - Hypernatraemia is dehydration or iatrogenic after IV fluid.
- *Hyperphosphotaemia*
  - Phosphate – small water-soluble compound which is not excreted in AKI when there is oligo-anuria.
- *Hypocalcaemia* due to:
  - Hyperphosphataemia
  - Change in affinity of calcium–albumin binding
  - Reduced renal production of 1,25-dihydroxycolecalciferol-
  - In surgery, large volume blood transfusion may also cause hypocalcaemia due to the citrate used as anticoagulant in packed red cells chelating the calcium.

### Acid–Base Complications

- Reduced ammonium excretion leads to:
  - Metabolic acidosis
  - Hyperventilation and circulatory collapse (if pH <7.10)

### Fluid Balance Complications

- Pulmonary/peripheral oedema due to failure to maintain euvolemia.

### Waste Product Accumulation

- Uraemia can lead to confusion, lethargy, and altered levels of consciousness.

## Indications for Acute Dialysis

- Oligo-anuria with no evidence of clinical

recovery (e.g., improving urine output) and one or more of the following:
- Development of uraemic symptoms
- Refractory hyperkalaemia
- Refractory fluid overload
- If the patient is fluid, replete, and *normotensive*, haemodialysis can occur on a ward setting via the renal team.
- If the blood pressure is *low*, continuous venovenous haemodiafiltration (CVVH) occurs in a critical care setting with vasopressors to support blood pressure.
- Failure to achieve dialysis-independence post-AKI is rare (5%).

# Chronic Kidney Disease

## Definition and Classification

- Abnormal kidney structure or function of ≥3 months.
- Classified according to eGFR and albuminuria category (Table 15.3).
- Categories provide prognostic information.
  - Worsening kidney function and albuminuria increases the risk of progressive renal decline, AKI, end-stage renal failure (ESRF), cardiovascular mortality, and all-cause mortality.

## Pathophysiology

- CKD arises due to:
  - Persistent risk factors (e.g., hypertension, hyperglycemia); or
  - Specific disease processes that mediate kidney damage.

**Table 15.3** Classification of CKD Based on Level of GFR and Albuminuria

| GFR Category | GFR (mL/min/1.73m$^2$) |
|---|---|
| G1 | >90 |
| G2 | 60–89 |
| G3a | 45–59 |
| G3b | 30–44 |
| G4 | 15–29 |
| G5 | <15 |
| **Albuminuria category** | **Albuminuria (mg/mmol)** |
| A1 | <3 |
| A2 | 3–30 |
| A3 | >30 |

Example: eGFR 36 mL/min/1.73 m$^2$, albuminuria 55 mg/mmol = stage G3bA3.

- Progressive injury triggers an inflammatory process.
  - Results in irreversible fibrosis due to deposition of collagenous extracellular matrix (ECM) within the renal architecture (Figure 15.2).
  - Affects all functional components:
    - Glomeruli, tubules, interstitium, and blood vessels.
    - Causes histological features of glomerulosclerosis, tubulointerstitial fibrosis, and vascular sclerosis.

### Glomerulosclerosis

- Key mechanism of glomerular damage arises from hyperfiltration.
- Once nephrons become scarred, remaining viable renal parenchyma hyperfiltrate to maintain GFR.
  - This is mediated by afferent arteriole vasodilation, which increases intra-glomerular pressure.
- Over time, hyperfiltration causes glomerular endothelial cell injury, which creates an inflammatory milieu:
  - The inflammatory cell infiltrate is mainly lymphomonocytic but also includes neutrophils, macrophages, eosinophils, and dendritic cells.
  - Cells are directly cytotoxic or mediate damage.
  - Release cytokines (e.g., TNF-α) and drive a pro-inflammatory, pro-proliferative, pro-oxidant, and pro-coagulant state.
- Mesangial cells become hypertrophied and proliferate, causing ECM to accumulate.
  - (Mesangial cells provide structural integrity to the glomerulus and are involved in ECM-turnover)
- Pro-fibrotic cytokines (e.g., TGF-β1 and FGF) also activate ECM-producing myofibroblasts and fibroblasts, promoting glomerulosclerosis.

### Tubulointerstitial Fibrosis

- Its mechanism is similar to glomerulosclerosis.
- Inflammatory cascades stimulate end-stage fibrosis.
- Disturbed peritubular perfusion → chronic ischaemia
  - Tubular cells sensitive to hypoxic injury → activate fibroblasts to deposit ECM.
  - Peritubular capillary damage → further hypoxia and ischaemia.

## Complications of Progressive Disease

- Uraemic syndrome, hyperkalaemia, acidosis
- Fluid overload, hypertension
- Anaemia, mineral bone disease
- Cardiovascular disease

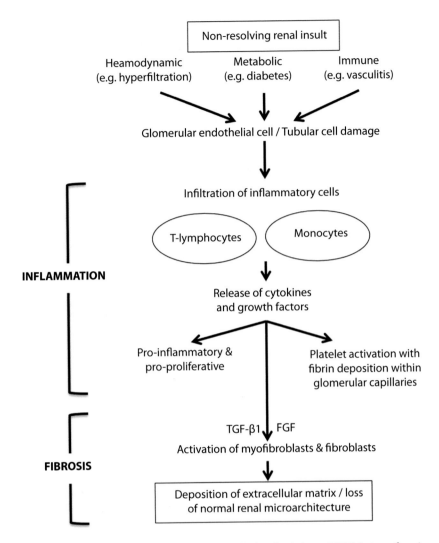

Figure 15.2 Overview of the mechanisms underlying CKD Pathophysiology. TGF-b1, transforming growth factor beta 1; FGF, fibroblast growth factor.

## Anaemia

- Normocytic, normochromic anaemia.
- Main mechanism is reduced EPO from renal interstitial fibroblasts.
  - EPO prevents apoptosis of erythroid progenitor cells.
- Uraemic metabolites also reduce red blood cell survival and production.
- CKD also causes anaemia of chronic disease:
  - Upregulation of hepcidin in inflammation → reduced intestinal absorption of iron → iron sequestered in macrophages → less iron for haemoglobin synthesis.

## Mineral Bone Disease (CKD-MBD)

- Renal osteodystrophy relates specifically to a spectrum of abnormal bone morphology encountered in CKD.

## Secondary Hyperparathyroidism and Osteitis Fibrosis Cystica

- Reduced renal 1α-hydroxylase → decreased $1,25(OH)_2D_3$ (1,25-dihydroxycholecalciferol, calcitriol)
- Low $1,25(OH)_2D_3$ and high phosphate (from reduced excretion in CKD) may cause low serum calcium → stimulates parathyroid gland to secrete PTH.
  - To normalise calcium, PTH causes:
    - Increased osteoclast and osteoblast activity → bone resorption and formation → increases the release of calcium and phosphate from bone turnover.
    - Increased calcium reabsorption by kidneys (reduced phosphate absorption).
    - Increased production of $1,25(OH)_2D_3$, which increases:

- osteoclast activity;
- calcium reabsorption in the kidney; and
- calcium and phosphate absorption in the intestine.
- 'High-turnover' phenotype *(osteitis fibrosa cystica)* → overall weakening of bone architecture.

### Other Forms of Renal Osteodystrophy

- 'Low-turnover' or adynamic bone disease. Over-correction of secondary hyperparathyroidism with vitamin D → reduces PTH → reduces bone turnover.
- Osteomalacia is seen in conjunction with adynamic bone disease.
  - Due to low $1,25(OH)_2D_3$.
  - Causes poor bone mineralisation.
  - Systemic metabolic acidosis can also contribute.

# Renal Replacement Therapy (RRT) for CKD

- 3 RRT methods:
  - Haemodialysis (HD)
  - Peritoneal dialysis (PD)
  - Transplantation (see Chapter 5)
- Usually indicated in CKD stage 5:
  - Symptoms of uraemia which affect quality of life.
  - Medically refractory fluid overload.
  - eGFR of 5–7 mL/min/1.73m$^2$ if asymptomatic.
- Dialysis:
  - Aim – to remove waste products and restore electrolyte, acid–base, and fluid homeostasis.
  - Main mechanisms (HD and PD):
    - *Diffusion* – solute clearance
    - *Convection* – water removal

## Haemodialysis

- Haemodialysis circuit:
  - *Dialyser*
  - *Dialysate* – solution of ultrapure water and various concentrations of electrolytes.
  - *Anticoagulation* – prevents clotting in the extracorporeal circuit.
  - *Vascular access* – removes blood from the patient and have it returned after passing through the dialyser.
- The dialysis machine pumps blood and dialysate fluid in separate compartments through the dialyser (semi-permeable membrane).
- Blood and dialysate flow in opposite directions (counter-current).
- High flow rates maximise *diffusion* of solutes

down the concentration gradients across the semi-permeable membrane.
- The removal of fluid (ultrafiltration) is achieved by *convection*.
  - Water moves across the semi-permeable membrane by osmotic forces and due to the pressure gradient (controlled by the dialysis machine).

## Long-Term Vascular Access

Options include:

- *Arterio-venous fistula* – preferred option
  - Ideally in the non-dominant arm.
  - Surgical anastomosis between an artery and vein.
  - Vein dilates and arterialise (6–8 weeks to fully mature).
  - Common sites: radiocephalic, radiobasilic, brachiocephalic, and brachiobasilic.
- *Graft* – usually PTFE to connect an artery and vein
- *Tunnelled cuffed dialysis catheter*
  - Used as a bridging access for pending fistula or graft formation.
  - Can provide permanent access if fistulas/grafts are not feasible.
  - 2 separate single lumen catheters / or a dual-lumen catheter.
  - Inserted into a large central vein.
    - Commonly through the right internal jugular vein since it is a straighter route to the right atrium.
  - Tunnelled subcutaneously to reduce the risk of infection.
    - Increases distance between the skin exit site and vein entry.
  - A cuff provides anchorage for the catheter subcutaneously and provides a barrier from infection.

## Peritoneal Dialysis

- *Components* – peritoneal dialysis catheter and peritoneal dialysate fluid.
- Solute and fluid transfer across a peritoneal semipermeable membrane between the dialysate and peritoneal capillary bed.

### CAPD (Continuous Ambulatory Peritoneal Dialysis)

- One cycle or 'exchange':
  - The peritoneal cavity is filled with dialysate (~2 L bag) via a catheter.

- This is left for a few hours (dwell) for solute transfer and fluid removal.
- The waste dialysate is emptied via the catheter.
- 3–5 exchanges are performed over 24 hours (including long dwell overnight).

## APD (Automated Peritoneal Dialysis)

- Same principles of solute and fluid transfer as CAPD.
- Instead of performing manual exchanges during the day,
  - a PD catheter is connected to a machine overnight;
  - exchanges are performed to pre-defined desired settings; and
  - a long day-time dwell is performed following overnight APD.

## Transplantation (see Chapter 5)

- Instances where urological input may be needed pre-transplant:
  - Relieving bladder outlet obstruction to ensure adequate drainage post-transplant.

- Native nephrectomy for recurrent pyelonephritis/pyonephrosis.
- Removal of polycystic kidney(s) to make space for transplant.

## Recommended Reading

1. Kellum JA, Lameire N, Aspelin P, Barsoum RS, Burdmann EA, Goldstein SL, et al. Kidney Disease: Improving Global Outcomes (KDIGO) Acute Kidney Injury Work Group. KDIGO Clinical Practice Guideline for Acute Kidney Injury. Kidney Int. 2012;2:1.
2. Waikar SS, Bonventre JV. Creatinine kinetics and the definition of acute kidney injury. J Am Soc Nephrol. 2009;20(3):672–679.
3. National Institute for Health and Care Excellence (NICE), Intravenous fluid therapy in adults in hospital. Clinical Guideline [CG174]. 2017. Available from: https://www.nice.org.uk/guidance/cg174.
4. KDIGO. Clinical practice guideline for the evaluation and management of chronic kidney disease. Kidney Int. 2013; 3(1):i–150.
5. Steddon S, Ashman N. Oxford Handbook of Nephrology and Hypertension. Oxford, UK; 2014.
6. Johnson RJ, Feehally J, Floege J. Comprehensive Clinical Nephrology. Elsevier Saunder, London, UK; 2010.
7. Romagnani P, Remuzzi G, Glassock R, et al. Chronic kidney disease. Nat Rev Dis Primers. 2017;3:17088.

# 16 Inflammation and Infection

*Judith Hall and Christopher K. Harding*

## Urinary Tract Infections (UTIs)

- UTI - inflammatory response of urothelium to micro-organism invasion, usually associated with bacteriuria and pyuria.
- Commonly associated with Gram-negative and Gram-positive bacteria:
  - *Escherichia* (typically *Escherichia coli*, –ve bacillus)
  - *Pseudomonas* (typically *Pseudomonas aeruginosa*, –ve bacillus)
  - *Klebsiella* (typically *Klebsiella pneumoniae*, –ve bacillus)
  - *Staphylococcus* (typically *Staphylococcus saprophyticus*, +ve coccus)
  - *Enterococcus* (typically *Enterococcus faecalis*, +ve coccus)
  - *Proteus* (typically *Proteus mirabilis*, –ve bacillus)
  - Group B *Streptococcus* (+ve coccus) and fungal pathogens including Candida (Figure 16.1)
- Uropathogenic *Escherichia coli* (UPEC) is the main cause for both uncomplicated and complicated UTIs (up to 75%).
- Majority of uropathogens originate in the bowel.
  - Exist as gut commensals.
  - Infect the bladder via an ascending route, involving contamination and colonisation of the urethra (Figure 16.2).
- Uropathogens can avoid bladder host defences and multiply and ascend to the kidneys (pyelonephritis).
  - Infect via virulence factors:
    - Flagella, fimbriae/pili, toxins and enzymes, and iron acquisition systems
  - Initiate bacteraemia by crossing renal tubular epithelial barrier.

## Microbial Virulence Factors (Table 16.1)

- Within 24 hours of infection, UPEC have fewer flagella (reduced motility).
- *Flagella:* swim then translocate from the meatus to the bladder and beyond.
- *Type 1 fimbriae* (also known as Type 1 pili):

- Allow bacterial attachment, bladder colonisation, and persistence.
- *Mannose-sensitive*
- *Characteristics*:
  - Tipped by the adhesion protein, FimH.
  - Bind to mannose containing glycoproteins such as Uroplakin 1a and 1b.
  - Coat umbrella cells of urothelium.
- *Adhesion* or attachment
  - Protects bacteria from being flushed away during micturition.
  - Triggers apoptosis and exfoliation of bladder epithelial cells (BECs).
  - Urine of those with UTI are generally rich in exfoliated BECs.
- *Pyelonephritis*
  - Type 1 fimbriae are replaced by P fimbriae/pili (mannose insensitive) defined by PapG adhesin.
  - Bind galactose containing glycolipids present on renal cells.
  - P fimbriae secure bacterial attachment → result in ceramide release:
    - Activates TLR4 signalling → inflammatory response involving host cytokine and antimicrobial peptide release
    - Inhibits secretory IgA transport into kidney lumen → bacterial colonisation of kidney
- Uropathogens display other fimbriae such as *S fimbriae* and *F1C fimbriae*.
  - *S. fimbriae* associate with *E. coli* strains.
    - Cause sepsis and bind to sialic acid residues through SfaS adhesion protein, which facilitates bacterial dissemination.
  - *F1C fimbriae* bind to glycolipids on kidney cells, causing pro-inflammatory IL-8 response.
- Toxins and enzymes damage the host tissues and release nutrients.

## Lipoprotein α-Haemolysin (HlyA)

- Often linked to pyelonephritis and renal scarring.
- Induces cell apoptosis and exfoliation of BECs.
- At high concentrations, lyses host cells which allow uropathogens to cross the epithelial barrier

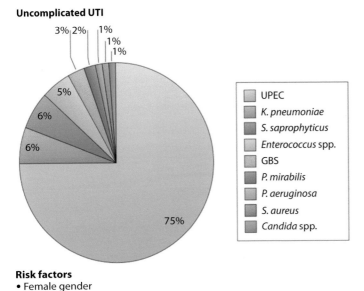

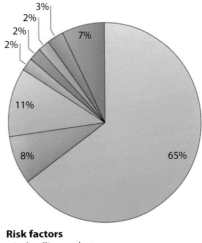

**Uncomplicated UTI**

3% 2% 1%
1%
1%
5%
6%
6%
75%

UPEC
*K. pneumoniae*
*S. saprophyticus*
*Enterococcus* spp.
GBS
*P. mirabilis*
*P. aeruginosa*
*S. aureus*
*Candida* spp.

**Complicated UTI**

3%
2%
2% 7%
2%
11%
8% 65%

**Risk factors**
- Female gender
- Older age
- Younger age

**Risk factors**
- Indwelling catheters
- Immunosuppression
- Urinary tract abnormalities
- Autibiotic exposure

Figure 16.1 Epidemiology of urinary tract infections. (Reprinted by permission from Springer Nature [1])

and gain access to host iron stores that are necessary for growth.

## Cytotoxic Necrotising Factor 1 (CNF1)

- Also secreted by pyelonephritis-associated strains.
- Induces apoptosis and increases BEC exfoliation.

## Urease

- An enzyme synthesised by a number of uropathogens, including:
  - *P. mirabilis, K. pneumoniae, P. aureginosa, S. saprophyticus*

  *P. mirabilis* urease is expressed during growth in urine:
- Hydrolysis of urea to carbon dioxide and ammonia.
- Creates alkaline urine → calcium crystal (apatite) formation and magnesium ammonium phosphate precipitates (struvite)
- Crystals become trapped within polysaccharides produced by attached bacterial cells → crystalline biofilms on tissues/catheters
- Ammonia is toxic to urothelial cells.
- The urinary tract is limited in iron (an essential element for bacterial growth).
  - Uropathogens synthesise *siderophores* to scavenge, chelate, and transport iron ($Fe^{3+}$).
  - Siderophores synthesised include the proteins aerobactin, yersiniabactin, and enterobactin.

## Host Defences

- The host deploys constitutive and induced innate defence mechanisms which interfere with colonisation (Figure 16.3):
- *Urine* – high osmolality and acid pH discourages bacterial growth.
- *Micturition* – flushes away infected, apoptosed BECs and non-adherent microbes.
- *Urothelial barrier:*
  - Comprised of specialised umbrella cells (superficial facet cells).
  - Characterised by uroplakin.
  - Reinforced by a surface mucus or a glycosaminoglycan (GAG) layer.
    - An antibacterial coating impeding microbial attachment.
    - The GAG layer consists of chondroitin and dermatan sulphates; heparins and heparan sulphates; hyaluronate; and keratan sulphate.
- *Commensal flora:*
  - Lactobacilli convert glycogen to lactic acid.
  - Lowers vaginal pH.
- The *BEC layer* is characterised by specific pathogen activated receptors—*toll-like receptors* (TLRs), particularly by TLR5:
  - TLRs are involved in detecting potential uropathogens.
  - Activated by pathogen activated membrane patterns (PAMPs).

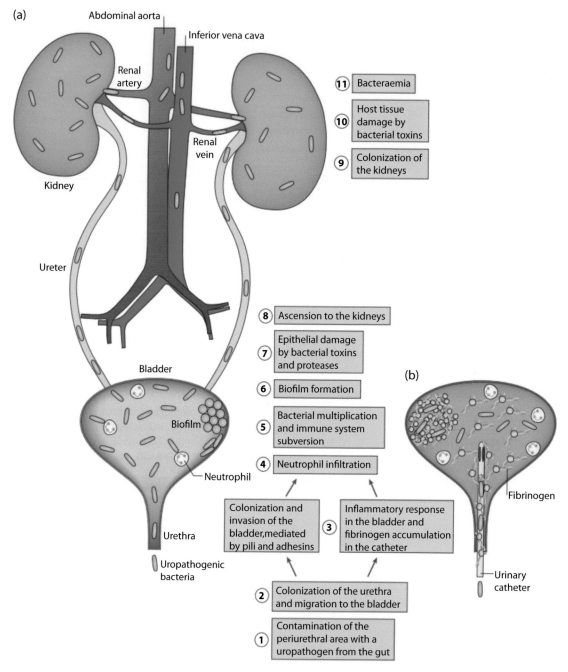

**Figure 16.2** Pathogenesis of urinary tract infections. (a) Uncomplicated UTIs: Step 1, Contamination; Step 2, Colonisation and migration via pili and adhesins; Step 3, Host inflammatory responses; Step 4, Neutrophil infiltration to clear extracellular bacteria; Step 5, Some bacteria evade the immune system, through host cell invasion or morphological changes. become resistant to neutrophils and these undergo multiplication; Step 6, Biofilm formation; Step 7, Toxins and proteases induce host cell damage, releasing essential nutrients that promote bacterial survival; Step 8, Ascension to the kidneys; Step 9, Kidney colonisation; Step 10, Bacterial toxin production and host tissue damage; Step 11, If left untreated, Progress to bacteraemia if crosses renal tubular epithelial barrier. (b) Complicated UTIs: Follow same initial steps (Steps 1–2) as those described for uncomplicated infections (2a). In order for the pathogens to cause infection, the bladder must be compromised. The most common cause of a compromised bladder is catheterisation. Step 3, Fibrinogen accumulates on catheter, provides an environment for the attachment of uropathogens that express fibrinogen-binding proteins. Progression to Steps 4–11. (Reprinted by permission from Springer Nature [1])

**Table 16.1** Virulence Factors of Common Uropathogenic Bacteria

| Uropathogen | Virulence Factors | | | |
| --- | --- | --- | --- | --- |
| | Adherence | Toxin | Iron Acquisition | Other |
| UPEC | Type 1 pili<br>P pili<br>S pili | HlyA<br>CNF1 | Aerobactin<br>Enterobactin | Flagella (Motility) |
| *Klebsiella pneumoniae* | Type 1 pili | | Aerobactin<br>Enterobactin | |
| *Proteus mirabilis* | *Proteus mirabilis-liks* fimbriae | Haemolysins | Proteobactin | Flagella<br>Urease |

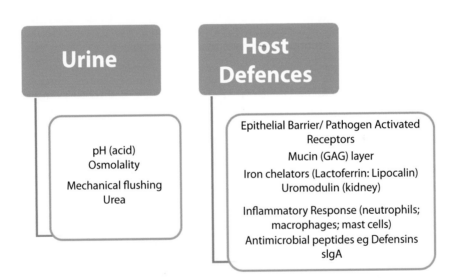

Figure 16.3 Urine characteristics and host defences against UTI.

- Lipopolysaccharide (LPS) and peptidoglycan PAMPS are detected by TLRs 2 and 4.
- Flagellin (constituent of UPEC flagella) PAMP is detected by TLR5.
- *Genetic susceptibility factors:*
  - TLR polymorphisms are linked to adult UTI susceptibility.
  - TLR5 polymorphism encoding a receptor variant that restricts flagellin-induced host signalling responses is associated with an increased risk of recurrent UTI in women.
  - HLA-A3 antigen associated with four times more risk of recurrent UTI.
- ABO group antigen non-secretors, Lewis non-secretor, and P blood group secretors.
- *Host antimicrobial proteins and peptides* (Figure 16.4):
  - Constitutively synthesised or induced in response to infection.
    - Secretory IgA
    - NGAL (neutrophil gelatinase-associated lipocalin)
    - Lactoferrin
    - Defensins and anti-adherence molecules (e.g., Uromodulin or the Tamm–Horsfall Protein).

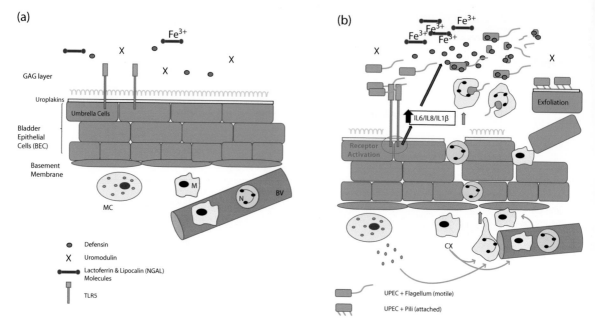

**Figure 16.4** (a) Host innate defences; (b) and their response to UTI. MC, mast cell; M, macrophage; N, neutrophil; BV, blood vessel; CX, chemokine; GAG, glycosaminoglycan; Fe3+, Iron; IL, interleukin, TLR5, toll-like receptor 5; UPEC, *Uropathogenic Escherichia coli*; NGAL, neutrophil gelatinase-associated lipocalin.

# Inflammatory Responses

- Neutrophils, macrophages and mast cells clear infecting bacteria.
- First recruited cells are neutrophils:
  - Often associated with prolonged inflammation and tissue damage.
  - High numbers are cytotoxic to tissues.
- Innate immune cell responses are tightly regulated.
  - Contain and prevent inflammatory damage and maintain the functional integrity of the urinary tract.

## Neutrophil Recruitment: Cytokines

- BEC activation via TLRs recognition of PAMPs:
  - Pro-inflammatory cytokine release.
  - IL-6, IL-8, and IL-1β are detectable in urine within 2–6 hours of infection.
  - Cytokines trigger recruitment and influx of immune cells—specifically, neutrophils from the blood vessels to the epithelial surface (Figure 16.4b).
- *Neutrophils*:
  - Engulf and degrade bacteria intracellularly (phagocytosis).
  - Mediated through pentraxin (PTX3) secretion and functions as an opsonin, which facilitates bacterial uptake.
  - Increased local numbers of neutrophils can be damaging due to:

- Synthesis of reactive oxygen species (ROS) and other products (e.g., cyclooxygenase-2 [COX2]) causing severe inflammatory damage.
- *COX2 inhibition* disrupts neutrophil transmigration, which reduces pyuria and mucosal damage and helps protect against chronic and recurrent UTIs (mice research).

## Neutrophil Recruitment: Macrophages

- Macrophages promote neutrophil influxes into the bladder epithelium.
- Resident LyC6⁻ macrophages (located in bladder lamina propria) secrete:
  - Chemokines (CX) CXCL1 and MIF which recruit neutrophils.
  - CCL2, which recruits Ly6C⁺ macrophages from circulation into urothelial tissues.
- Newly recruited Ly6C⁺ macrophages produce TNF.
  - TNF stimulates resident macrophages to secrete CXCL2.
  - CXCL2 induces circulatory neutrophils to produce metalloproteinases, which allows them to penetrate basement membranes and move transepithelially.
- Macrophages moderate neutrophil response by ingesting and removing apoptotic neutrophils.

## Mast Cells

- Found in bladder lamina propria.
- Relocate and multiply in response to infection.
- Sentinel cells initiate early immune responses.
- Function as pro-inflammatory cells during the early phase of UTI.
- Display pathogen activated receptors and CD48 receptor.
  - Receptors bind to UPEC FimH adhesion protein.
- Contain granules pre-packed with pro-inflammatory mediators, including:
  - *Histamine* – found in urine within an hour of a bacterial infection.
  - *TNF* – involved in stimulating early neutrophil response.
- *Damage-associated molecular patterns* (DAMPs):
  - Including ATP, DNA, and defensin HBD2.
  - Secreted by damaged or stressed urothelial cells.
  - Can activate mast cells.
- Mast cells synthesise anti-inflammatory cytokine *IL-10*:
  - Secreted at later stages.
  - Associated with urothelial cell shedding and tissue damage.
  - Curtails inflammation to re-establish homeostasis and promote tissue recovery.
  - Coordinated innate immune responses ensure efficient bacterial clearance and minimise inflammatory damage.

## Asymptomatic Bacteriuria (ABU)

- 'The presence of bacteria in urine in the absence of clinical symptoms normally associated with an UTI'.
- Prevalent in:
  - *Diabetes, pregnancy, spinal cord injury, catheterisation, older adults*
  - Older adults (particularly institutionalised elderly):
    - ~25–50% nursing-home residents present with bacteriuria at one point.
    - Adjusting for other co-morbidities, older patients with ABU do not show increased mortality.
    - Antibiotics do not reduce rates of subsequent complications but can increase the risk of symptomatic UTI (sUTI) via selection of drug-resistant bacteria and pathogens, including *Clostridium difficile*.
- Bacteria include:
  - *E. coli* (dominates)
  - *P. mirabilis, Klebsiella, Pseudomonas*
  - *Streptococcus agalactiae* is most associated with pregnancy.

## Bacterial Detection

- Analysis of 'clean-catch' urine samples by culture-based methods.
- Significance determined by $\geq 10^5$ Colony Forming Units (CFU)/mL.
- The $\geq 10^5$ CFU/mL threshold was proposed by Stamm in the 1950s.
  - Has high specificity, but sensitivity is at ~50%.
- The $\geq 10^2$ CFU/mL lower threshold was proposed by Kass in the 1980s.
  - Has better sensitivity without a significant loss of specificity.
- A $\geq 10^4$ CFU/mL threshold is used by most microbiology laboratories.
  - Automated counting of bacteria using flow cytometry.
  - Specimens exceeding threshold will be cultured.
- Bacterial counts in specific groups:
  - $\geq 10^3$ in acute *uncomplicated* cystitis in women.
  - $\geq 10^4$ in:
    - Acute *uncomplicated pyelonephritis* in women
    - Straight catheter sample in *complicated* UTI in women
    - Men
  - $\geq 10^5$ in:
    - *Complicated* UTI in women
    - Asymptomatic bacteriuria
- Prognostic markers to differentiate between ABU and sUTI:
  - Pyuria and leucocyte esterase are traditional markers of sUTI (less useful in diabetic and elderly).
  - Dipstick and direct microscopy show poor positive and negative predictive values for ABU.
  - Urinary cytokines (especially IL-6 and IL-8) are used in prognostic value, particularly in the elderly.

## Clinical Aspects of Urinary Tract Infections

### Complicated Versus Uncomplicated UTI

- A *complicated* UTI is associated with factors that increase colonisation and decrease the efficacy of therapy.
- Include any structural or functional urinary tract abnormalities such as:
  - Urinary tract obstruction
  - Duplex kidney, horseshoe kidney
  - Renal insufficiency
  - Immunocompromise
  - Presence of a foreign body including calculi

- Pregnancy
- Multi-resistant organisms
- Advancing age
- Male gender

## Infective Cystitis

- Inflammation/infection of the bladder.
- Acute uncomplicated cystitis is the most common.
  - Can present with dysuria, urgency, increased frequency, suprapubic pain, offensive smelling urine, and haematuria.
- *S. saprophyticus* may be introduced during sexual intercourse in young sexually active women.
- *Recurrent UTI* (rUTI) may require investigations:
  - ≥2 episodes in 6 months; or
  - ≥3 in a year.

## Pyelonephritis

- Infection involving the renal parenchyma and renal pelvis.
- Results from:
  - Ascending infection of the lower urinary tract.
  - Haematogenous spread of infection from other sites.
- Predominated by *E. coli* (60–90% of cases).
- *Typical symptoms:*
  - Flank pain, fever, nausea/vomiting
  - Antecedent history of cystitis
- Complications of pyelonephritis:
  - Sepsis, renal abscess, renal scarring, and emphysematous pyelonephritis
- *Emphysematous pyelonephritis (EPN).*
  - Severe infection of the renal parenchyma.
  - Caused by gas-forming enterobacteriaceae such as *E. coli, Klebsiella*, and *Proteus*.
  - Associated with fermentation of glucose (diabetes) by bacteria to form carbon dioxide, nitrogen, oxygen, and hydrogen.
  - Gas accumulation in the tissues can be seen on x-ray or CT.
  - There are two types of EPN based on CT appearances.
  - *EPN type 1* (up to 60% mortality)
    - Greater than one-third of renal parenchymal destruction
    - Streaky or mottled appearance of gas
    - Intra- or extrarenal fluid collections are characteristically absent
    - Usually more aggressive
  - *EPN type 2* (~20% mortality)
    - Destruction of less than one-third of the parenchyma
    - Renal or extrarenal collections associated with bubbly or loculated gas, or gas within pelvicalyceal system or ureter

- Emergency nephrectomy is indicated if there is no response to IV antibiotics.

## Renal and Perirenal Abscess

- *Abscess:* pus-containing cavity.
- Abscess formation is more common in:
  - Severe or recurrent infections
  - Vesico-ureteric reflux
  - Urinary tract obstruction
  - Urolithiasis
  - Diabetes and those immunocompromised
- The distinction between renal and perirenal abscesses is made via CT scanning.
- *Renal abscesses*
  - Also termed renal cortico-medullary abscesses.
  - Can occur during or after an episode of pyelonephritis.
  - Range from focal lobar nephronia to significant pan-renal infections (e.g., EPN and xantho-granulomatous pyelonephritis [XGP]).
  - Renal abscesses can be exclusively cortical.
  - Haematogenous spread commonly with *Staphylococcus aureus* (~90% of cases).
- *Xanthogranulomatous pyelonephritis*
  - Chronic destructive granulomatous process of the renal parenchyma.
  - Associated with *urolithiasis* and urinary tract obstruction.
  - Microscopically: xanthoma cells (lipid-laden foamy macrophage) infiltration and haemorrhagic necrosis.
  - CT may show an enlarged poor-functioning kidney, pus-containing cavities, and calculi (bear's paw sign).
- *Perirenal abscess*
  - Collection of suppurative material in the space between the renal capsule and Gerota's fascia.
  - Associated with an obstructing stone, although it can arise from a renal cortico-medullary abscess.
- The treatment of renal and perirenal abscesses depends on the severity:
  - Supportive care with IV fluids and antibiotics.
  - Radiological or surgical drainage (of abscess and/or obstructed kidney).
  - Nephrectomy in severe cases.

## Genito-Urinary (GU) Tuberculosis

- *Mycobacterium tuberculosis* is the most common.
- Slow-growing, non-motile, non-flagellated aerobic bacteria.
- Second most common form of extrapulmonary TB, after lymphatic.

- Other implicated Mycobacterial species:
  - *M. bovis, M. leprae,* and *M. africanum*
- Over 90% of cases occur in developing countries.
- Most common sites include the kidneys, followed by the bladder and the epididymis.
- Usually arises following a primary pulmonary infection and subsequent haematogenous spread.
- *Microscopically:*
  - Caseating granuloma contains Langhans giant cells surrounded by lymphocytes and fibroblasts.
  - Healing of lesions leads to fibrosis and calcification.
- *Signs and symptoms:*
  - Sterile pyuria with storage lower urinary tract symptoms (LUTS).
  - Systemic: fever, weight loss, anorexia, night sweats
- *Renal TB* can be advanced at presentation:
  - Destruction of renal anatomy.
  - Cortical granuloma formation and caseous necrosis.
  - Release of bacilli to the lower urinary tract.
  - Usually followed by healing and extensive fibrosis.
  - CT and IV urography appearances:
    - Calyceal calcification and distortion, infundibular stenosis, ureteric strictures, and small, scarred bladder (thimble bladder).
- *Bladder TB*
  - Can be caused by intravesical immunotherapy with BCG (Bacillus Calmette–Guérin).
  - Presents with storage LUTS.
  - Video urodynamics may reveal small, poorly compliant bladder.
  - Ulceration in acute phase and fibrosis in chronic phase can be seen on cystoscopy, with *golf-hole* appearance of ureteric orifices.
- *Epididymis*
  - Most common site in the male genital tract.
  - Discrete focal strictures cause an appearance of a *string of beads* to the spermatic cord.
- *Fallopian tube*
  - Most common site in the female genital tract.
  - Stricturing can be seen on contrast radiography (salpingography).
- *TB diagnosis*
  - At least three early morning urine (EMU) samples for staining.
    - Three samples, since TB is excreted in urine intermittently.
    - EMU, since overnight urine increases the chance of positive yield.
  - Urine reveals acid-fast bacilli using *Ziehl–Neelsen* staining (bright red).

- TB contains a high lipid content in the cell wall which is not suitable for Gram staining.
- Urine cultures require 6–8 weeks in *Lowenstein–Jensen* culture media.
- Modern diagnostic methods available to avoid treatment delay include:
  - Radiometric culture (2–3 days)
  - PCR to amplify bacterial DNA (2–3 hours)
- Long-term combination therapy with antibiotics is the usual treatment.
  - Isoniazid, rifampicin, pyrazinamide, and ethambutol
  - Surgery may be required to reconstruct the urinary tract in the longer term.

# Prostatitis

- Infective or non-infective inflammation.
- Infected urine is refluxed into prostatic ducts → acute prostatitis → obstructed ducts → chronic infection/prostatitis (5%)
- Affects one in 20 men. Most frequent urological diagnosis in men under 50 years.
- *Symptoms:*
  - LUTS (dysuria, urinary frequency, urinary urgency)
  - Perineal discomfort
  - Referred pain – genitalia, perineum, lower back, or suprapubic areas
  - Pain during ejaculation
  - Systemic: fever, malaise
- *Digital rectal examination:* acutely tender or boggy prostate.
- *Risk factors:*
  - UTI
  - Catheterisation
  - Accessory gland infections (e.g., epididymitis)
  - Dysfunctional voiding/bladder outflow obstruction leading to intraprostatic duct reflux
  - Transurethral surgery
  - Phimosis
  - Prostatic calculi
- Non-infective prostatitis: unclear aetiology.
- Infective prostatitis:
  - 90% gram-negative bacteria
    - *E. coli* is the most common
    - *Proteus, Klebsiella, Pseudomonas, Chlamydia trachomatis*
  - <10% gram-positive organisms (e.g., enterococci).
- *Chronic prostatitis (CP):* symptoms present for >3 months.
- *Histologically:*
  - Chronic inflammatory infiltrate of leukocytes and lymphocytes into prostatic ducts and periprostatic tissue.
- Investigation and classification based on *Meares-Stamey 4-glass test*

- Segmented urine microscopy and culture with four specimens:
  - *VB1:* first 10 mL voided urine (reflect bacterial colonisation of the prostate/urethra).
  - *VB2:* midstream specimen of urine (reflect colonisation of the bladder).
  - *EPS:* expressed prostatic secretions from prostate massage (reflect prostatic bacterial colonisation).
  - *VB3:* first 10 mL urine voided following prostatic massage (reflect prostatic bacterial colonisation).
- Prostatitis is classified according to the US National Institutes of Health (NIH) *Chronic Prostatitis Symptom Index:*
  - *Category I:* acute bacterial prostatitis
  - *Category II:* chronic bacterial prostatitis (recurrent bacterial infection)
  - *Category III:* chronic non-bacterial prostatitis/ chronic pelvic pain syndrome (CPPS)
    - *Category IIIA:* inflammatory CPPS (white cell in EPS/VB3 10-fold increase over VB1/2)
    - *Category IIIB:* non-inflammatory CPPS (no white cell in EPS or VB3)
    - *Category IV:* asymptomatic inflammatory prostatitis (e.g., on prostate biopsy)
- *Segmented urine culture:*
  - Aims to localise bacteria to the specific area of the urinary tract.
  - Not universally undertaken since low diagnostic yield may be due to preceding antibiotic treatment.
  - Alternative is the *2-glass test* (Nickel):
    - Pre- and post-prostate massage urine samples.
    - Positive post-prostate massage urine indicates CP/CPPS.

## Scrotal Infections

- Epididymitis and orchitis are the most common.
- *Isolated orchitis:*
  - Mumps orthorubulavirus: rare in pre-pubertal
    - Develops 4–8 days post parotitis.
    - Up to 50% of post-pubertal have reduced testes size with abnormal semen analysis.
  - *Non-infective:*
    - Auto-immune (e.g., polyarteritis nodosa)
- Isolated epididymitis:
  - More common than isolated orchitis.
  - Unilateral is more common than bilateral.
- *Epididymo-orchitis:* inflammation of both epididymis and testis.
  - Most common cause of acute scrotal pain.
  - The main differential diagnosis is testicular torsion.
    - USS: poor sensitivity (~80%)

- Surgical exploration may be performed if in any doubt.
- *Infective aetiology:* sexually-transmitted or non-sexually-transmitted.
  - *Sexually-transmitted* pathogens:
    - *Chlamydia trachomatis* (gram-negative coccus)
    - *Neisseria gonorrhoeae* (gram-negative intracellular diplococcus)
    - Diagnosis with urinary nucleic acid amplification test (NAAT) and urethral swab and culture.
    - Treated with antibiotics based on culture results.
  - *Non-sexually-transmitted:*
    - Gram-negative enteric (e.g., *E. coli, Klebsiella, Pseudomonas*)
    - Mumps virus, tuberculosis, candida
  - *Non-infective:*
    - Idiopathic, trauma, auto-immune
    - Medication (e.g., Amiodarone)
- *Complications* of epididymo-orchitis:
  - Abscess formation, Fournier's Gangrene
  - Testicular infarction
  - Chronic testicular pain
  - Subfertility (up to one in three cases)

## Fournier's Gangrene

- Necrotising fasciitis of the perineum, peri-anal region, external genitalia.
- Synergistic combination of aerobic and anaerobic bacteria, such as:
  - *E. coli, Streptococci, Staphylococci, Proteus,* and other anaerobes
- *Pathophysiology:* obliterative endarteritis and vessel thrombosis.
  - Causes tissue ischaemia and encourages anaerobic bacterial proliferation.
  - Spread is along fascia planes – dartos (scrotum), Buck's (penis), Colle's (perineum), Scarpa's (abdominal wall).
- *Risk factors* (immunocompromised):
  - Diabetes, obesity, HIV, alcohol abuse, malnutrition
  - Recent urethral or perineal surgery
  - Urethral catheters, paraphimosis
  - Lower socio-economic status
- *Signs:*
  - Sepsis
  - Painful swelling of scrotum or perineum
  - Foul-smelling exudate
  - Areas of tissue necrosis and crepitus on palpation
- *Management:* resuscitation and immediate surgical debridement.

- Surgical debridement follows general principles of resection to bleeding tissue.

## Sepsis and Shock

- The 3rd International Consensus definitions for sepsis and septic shock (Sepsis-3, 2016) defined sepsis as:
  - Life-threatening organ dysfunction due to a dysregulated host response to infection.
  - *Septic shock:* persisting hypotension requiring vasopressors to maintain mean arterial pressure of >65 mmHg and blood lactate >2 mmol/L despite adequate volume resuscitation.
- *Pathophysiology:*
  - Endotoxins released by gram-negative bacteria.
  - Inflammatory cells infiltration (neutrophils, macrophages, plasma cells).
  - Cytokine release: TNFα, IL-2, IL-6, IL-8.
  - Activation of kinin complement and the fibrinolytic system.
  - Anaerobic respiration and lactic acid accumulation.
  - Metabolic acidosis → vasoconstriction and cellular membrane dysfunction
  - Microvascular injury and tissue ischaemia.
  - Hypotension (shock) from cytokine-mediated vasodilatation.
- The clinical sepsis definition historically included >2 of the Systemic Inflammatory Response Syndrome (SIRS) parameters in the presence of an infection.
- *>2 SIRS* (1991 consensus conference).
  - Temperature of >38 °C or <36 °C
  - Tachycardia >90 beats per minute
  - Tachypnoea >20 respirations per minute or $PaCO_2$ of <4.3 kPa

- White cell count of >12,000/mm$^3$, <4,000/mm$^3$, or >10% immature forms on blood film
- The Sepsis-3 2016 criteria includes:
  - A *'quick sequential organ failure'* (qSOFA) tool:
    - Alteration in mental state, Glasgow coma scale <15
    - Decrease in systolic blood pressure <100 mmHg
    - Respiratory rate ≥22 breaths/minute
- *Treatment:* Sepsis 6 bundle within the first hour of recognition (golden hour).
  1. Oxygen
  2. Blood cultures and relevant bloods
  3. IV antibiotics
  4. IV fluids
  5. Serial lactate
  6. Measurement of urine output
- Septic shock will need critical care input and vasopressors.

## Recommended Reading

1. Flores-Mireles, AL, et al. Urinary tract infections: epidemiology, mechanisms of infection and treatment options. Nat Rev Microbiol. 2015;13(5):269–84.
2. Abraham, SN and Y Miao. The nature of immune responses to urinary tract infections. Nat Rev Immunol. 2015;15(10):655–63.
3. Lewis, AJ, AC Richards, and MA Mulvey. Invasion of host cells and tissues by uropathogenic bacteria. Microbiol Spectr. 2016;4(6). doi:10.1128/microbiolspec.UTI-0026-2016
4. Hayes, BW and SN Abraham. Innate immune responses to bladder infection. Microbiol Spectr. 2016;4(6). doi:10.1128/microbiolspec.UTI-0024-2016
5. Singer M, Deutschman CS, Seymour CW, et al. The third international consensus definitions for sepsis and septic shock (Sepsis-3). JAMA. 2016;315(8):801–10.
6. Cecconi M, Evans L, Levy M, Rhodes A. Sepsis and septic shock. Lancet. 2018;392(10141):75–87.

# 17 Urolithiasis

*Jade Harrison and Ken Anson*

## Epidemiology

- Increasing incidence – current lifetime incidence of ~15%.
- Recurrence rate: ~50% at five years and ~80% at 10 years.
- Epidemiological studies demonstrate associations between urolithiasis and gender, geographical area, genetics, and lifestyle.

## Risk Factors for Urolithiasis

- General factors, diseases, genetic, drug-induced and anatomical abnormalities (Table 17.1).
- *Age:* peak incidence at 20–50 years.
- *Gender:* male > female (gap is closing).
  - Testosterone may increase oxalate production in the liver.
  - Women have higher urinary citrate levels.
- *Ethnicity:*
  - Uncommon in Native Americans, Black African, and American Blacks.
  - More common in Caucasians and Asians.

## Mechanism of Urolithiasis

### Urine Saturation

- *Saturation point* = point at which a solvent/urine cannot dissolve any more solute.
  - Altered by urinary pH.
  - Some solutes are more soluble in alkaline or acidic urine.
- *Supersaturation* = more solute is added beyond the critical saturation point.
  - Solution holds more solute within it than theoretically possible.
  - The potential for solid crystal formation increases.
- *Solubility product* (Ksp) = point where the solute e.g. calcium oxalate (CaOx), dissolves within solution. i.e. reduces urolithiasis.

### Nucleation and Aggregation

- *Formation product* (KF) = point where a solute (e.g., calcium oxalate [CaOx]), can no longer be held in the solution.

- Free ions associate and form microscopic crystal particles through nucleation (Figure 17.1).
- *Homogenous nucleation* = spontaneous crystal formation within a pure solution of a *single* type of solute.
- *Heterogeneous nucleation* = crystallisation encouraged by debris, bacteria, urinary casts, and epithelial cells.
  - Occurs in less saturated urine as debris acts as a nidus for crystallogenesis.
  - Occurs when a crystal of one substrate (e.g., uric acid) acts as a nidus for ongoing heterogeneous nucleation of another solute (e.g., CaOx).
  - Results in a crystalline substrate with a heterogeneous composition.
- *Aggregation* = individual microcrystals binding together and increasing in size.
  - Numerous individual microcrystals may bind together; or
  - A solitary microcrystal can act as a focus for secondary nucleation to occur upon it.

## Inhibitors and Promoters

- Urine saturation and the degree of stone formation is not a linear relationship.
  - Stones may not form in supersaturated urine.
  - >30% stone-formers have normal ion concentrations during 24 hour urine collections.
- Macromolecules ('modifiers') influence the likelihood of crystal formation.
  - Subdivided into *promoters* or *inhibitors* of crystal formation.

## Inhibitors

- Act as buffers.
- Allow high solute concentrations without nucleation occurring.
- *Metastable urine* = supersaturated urine *without* stone formation.
  - Concentration between solubility product and formation product.
  - If more solute is added to metastable urine, which cannot be counteracted by inhibitors, then microcrystals will form.

**Table 17.1** Risk Factors for Urolithiasis

**General factors**

Low fluid intake

Dietary (salt, oxalate, protein)

Supplements (Vitamin C and D)

**Diseases**

Renal tubular abnormalities (hypercalciuria)

Urinary tract infection

Hyperparathyroidism

Metabolic syndrome, gout

Nephrocalcinosis

Polycystic kidney disease

Gastrointestinal diseases (intestinal resection, inflammatory bowel disease, malabsorptive conditions, enteric hyperoxaluria, absorptive hypercalciuria)

Increased levels of vitamin D

Sarcoidosis

Spinal cord injury, neurogenic bladder

**Genetic**

Cystinuria (type A, B and AB)

Primary hyperoxaluria

Renal tubular acidosis type I

2,8-Dihydroxyadeninuria, Xanthinuria

Lesch–Nyhan syndrome

Cystic fibrosis

**Drug-induced (see Table 17.3)**

**Anatomical abnormalities**

Horseshoe kidney

Medullary sponge kidney (tubular ectasia)

Pelviureteric junction obstruction

Calyceal diverticulum, calyceal cyst

Ureteral stricture

Vesico-uretero-renal reflux

Ureterocoele

- Increasing solute concentrations within metastable urine results in unstable urine and increased nucleation potential.
- *Inhibitors of calcium urolithiasis:*
  - Citrate, magnesium, pyrophosphate, and glycoproteins.
  - No specific inhibitors for uric acid calculi have been identified.

- *Citrate*
  - Complexes with sodium, magnesium, and calcium at physiological pH.
  - Calcium bound to citrate is no longer free to complex with oxalate or phosphate.
  - Citrate alkalinises urine → increases the solubility of solutes
  - ~50% of stone formers have hypocitraturia.

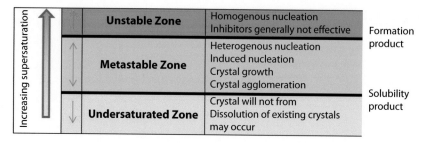

**Figure 17.1** Three degrees of urinary saturation and the crystallisation processes that may occur within each zone. (Reused with permission from Informa UK Limited [2])

- Reabsorption of citrate is influenced by the serum pH.
  - *Acidosis:* increases citrate reabsorption while lowering urinary citrate.
  - *Alkalosis:* reduces citrate reabsorption while increasing urinary citrate.
- Following a high protein meal, transient serum acidosis occurs.
  - Results in increased citrate renal reabsorption.
  - Urinary citrate level decreases → the risk of crystal formation increases
- *Magnesium*
  - Forms complexes with *oxalate.*
  - Oral magnesium reduces oxalate absorption from the gastrointestinal tract.
  - Limited evidence to support magnesium supplementation in stone formers.
- *Pyrophosphates*
  - Occur naturally within the urine at physiological levels.
  - Theoretically should inhibit crystal growth by 50%.
  - Reduce aggregation of calcium phosphate (CaP).
  - Alter the enteric absorption of calcium.
- *Glycoproteins*
  - Tamm–Horsfall protein (THP), osteopontin, and inter-α-trypsin
  - THP- produced by cells of the thick ascending loop of Henle
    - Inhibitory in alkaline urine (inhibitory role is lost in acidic urine).
  - *Osteopontin* (uropontin):
    - Prevents nucleation and aggregation of CaOx.
    - However, osteopontin provides a matrix structure for crystalline structures to adhere to, aiding urolithiasis.
  - *Inter-α-trypsin:*
    - Protease inhibitors with two heavy chains and one light chain made up of bikunin.
    - Has an inhibitory effect on CaOx nucleation, aggregation, and growth.
    - Urinary bikunin levels are ~50% less in CaOx stone formers compared with controls.

## Promoters

- *Matrix calculus*
  - Comprised of aggregated crystals and a non-crystalline organic material 'matrix'.
  - Matrix binds microcrystals together and acts as a platform for *nucleation* to occur.
  - Matrix weight is ~10% of a calculus.
  - Biochemical structure:
    - ~2/3 protein
    - ~1/3 organic ash, bound water, non-amino sugars, and lipids

## Free-Flowing or Fixed Particle Urolithiasis

### Free Particle Growth

- Crystallogenesis in the free-flowing solution within nephrons is debatable.
  - Occurs in the most supersaturated urine—at the end of the descending Loop of Henle.
- Chemically possible, but it is likely that microcrystals will adhere to an intrarenal structure to allow sufficient time to enlarge – *fixed particle nucleation.*
- Mechanism that facilitates adherence is not fully understood.
- One theory = mass precipitation/intranephronic calculosis:
  - Microcrystals plug the distal tubule or collecting duct → stasis of tubular fluid flow → aggregation and crystal growth

### Fixed Particle Theory

- First deduced by Randall in 1937.
- *Hypothesis:* a plaque comprising of crystalline CaP are deposited within the suburothelial layer of the renal papillae.
- CaP deposits act as a focus for crystal aggregation.
- Suburothelial plaques erode through the renal papillae and into the collecting system as renal stones.
- Papillary deposits are eponymously named *Randall's plaques.*

- CaP occurs, following a vascular injury to the vasa recta.
  - During the repair, calcified deposits are laid down — similar to atherosclerosis.
  - *Epidemiological studies:* risk factors for atherosclerosis (obesity, diabetes, hypertension) are all risk factors for urolithiasis.
  - Obesity increases the relative risk of urolithiasis by >20%.

## Metabolic Syndrome, Urinary pH, and Urolithiasis

### Metabolic Syndrome

- Collection of cardiometabolic risk factors.
  - Central obesity, hypertension, dyslipidaemia
  - Glucose intolerance (some definitions requiring evidence of insulin resistance).
- *Epidemiological studies:* obesity, diabetes, hypertension, or metabolic syndrome are risk factors for urolithiasis.
- Increasing incidence due to obesity.
- Relative risk of urolithiasis increases by 20% per five-unit increase in the BMI.
- *Obese patients* have higher concentrations of oxalate, uric acid, and phosphate within lower pH in a 24-hour urine.

### Urinary pH

- Normal urinary pH = 4.5–7.8

- Formation product of a solute is influenced by the pH of a solution.
- *Alkaline urinary pH* promotes calcium and phosphate crystallisation.
- *Acidic urinary pH* promotes the formation of uric acid and cystine stones.
- The kidney is fundamental in maintaining acid–base balance.
  - Almost all bicarbonate ($HCO_3^-$) is reabsorbed at the proximal renal tubule.
  - Excess $H^+$ is removed via the kidney through its binding to phosphate and ammonia, which is then excreted.
- *Renal tubular acidosis* (RTA):
  - Defective distal renal secretion of $H^+$ (Type 1); or
  - Defective proximal $HCO_3^-$ reabsorption (Type 2).
  - This results in metabolic acidosis, hyperchloraemia, impaired urinary acidification, and urolithiasis.
  - *Distal RTA* – defect of the apical $H^+/K^+$-ATPases of α-intercalated cells:
    - Inability to secrete $H^+ \rightarrow$ serum acidosis
    - Acidic urinary pH does not fall below 5.3.
    - Acidic urine favours CaP precipitation.
    - Increased proximal reabsorption of citrate $\rightarrow$ lowers urinary citrate $\rightarrow$ reduces inhibition of urolithiasis

## Urinary Stone Composition

- Stone composition (Table 17.2) is influenced by:

**Table 17.2** The Mineral Composition of Renal Calculi Within the Adult Population

| Stone | Mineral Name | Chemical Formula | Crystal Shape | Formation in Urinary pH | Incidence |
|---|---|---|---|---|---|
| Calcium oxalate monohydrate | Whewellite | $CaC_2O_4.H_2O$ | Ovals, dumbbells, hourglass | Wide range, acidic | 70–80% |
| Calcium oxalate dihydrate | Weddellite | $CaC_2O_4.2H_2O$ | Envelopes, octahedrons | Wide range, acidic | |
| Calcium hydrogen phosphate | Carbonate apatite | $CaC_2O_4.2H_2O$ | Pointing finger, rosettes | Alkaline | 10–15% |
| Calcium phosphate | Apatite | $Ca_{10}(PO_4)_6.(OH)_2$ | Powder-like, cloudy urine | Alkaline | |
| Uric acid | Uricite | $CaC_2O_4.2H_2O$ | Double-headed arrows, rosettes | Acidic | 10% |
| Magnesium ammonium phosphate | Struvite | $MgNH_4PO_4.6H_2O$ | Coffin lids, needle | Alkaline | 5–10% |
| Cystine | | $[SCH_2CH(NH_2)COOH]_2$ | Hexagons | Acidic | 1–2% |

- Climate, gender, age, genetics, and co-morbidities (e.g., obesity)
- *CaOx* stones: 75–80% of all urinary tract calculi.
  - Heterogeneous composition with CaP and uric acid within them.
  - CaP at 10–15% and Ca carbonate at 3%.
- *Infection* stones: (historically known as struvite stone): 5–10% of all calculi.
  - Magnesium, ammonium, phosphate components
- *Uric acid:* 5–15% of all calculi.
- *Cystine, xanthine,* and *drug metabolite* stones: 1–3% of all stones.

## Calcium Metabolism and Calcium-Based Calculi

- ~1/3 of ingested calcium is absorbed in the gastrointestinal (GI) tract at ~300 mg/day.
- Calcium is only absorbed in the ionic state.
- Reduction in free calcium absorption if enteric calcium forms complexes with phosphate, citrate, or oxalate.
- Ionised calcium is filtered at the glomerulus.
  - >95% reabsorbed; and
  - 1–2% is excreted in the urine.
- *Hypercalciuria:* ~50% of calcium stone formers.
  - Excretion of >7 mmol/day in men and >6 mmol/day in women.
- EAU guidelines: consider treatment if urinary calcium levels are at >5 mmol/day.
- *Hypercalciuria:* three mechanisms.
  - Absorptive
  - Renal-induced
  - Resorptive hypercalciuria

1. *Absorptive hypercalciuria*
   - Enhanced enteric calcium absorption → suppresses parathyroid hormone (PTH) → reduces calcium reabsorption from the distal convoluted tubule and collecting duct → hypercalciuria
     - *Type I:* independent on dietary intake. Can result during physiological normal or restricted calcium intake.
     - *Type II:* dependent on calcium dietary intake. Resolves when calcium intake is restricted to ~400–600 mg/day.
     - *Type III:* inappropriate loss of phosphate from the kidney.
       - Depletion in serum phosphate → increases 1,25-dihydroxyvitamin D synthesis → increases phosphate and calcium GI absorption and increases urinary calcium excretion
2. *Renal-induced hypercalciuria*
   - Ineffective reabsorption of calcium from tubules → increases urinary calcium →

hypocalcaemia → increases calcium bone reabsorption and increases enteric absorption of calcium → secondary hyperparathyroidism
- These mechanisms increase serum calcium.
- Undergoes glomerular filtration and is subjected to the dysfunctional calcium homeostasis mechanism in the renal tubule.

3. *Resorptive hypercalciuria*
   - Composes ~5% of all hypercalciuria.
   - Primary hyperparathyroidism is the most common cause.
   - Rarer causes: sarcoidosis, thyrotoxicosis, and malignant hypercalcaemia.

- *Salt and hypercalciuria*
  - Low salt diets are advised, which reduce recurrent stone rates at ~50% over five years.
  - Calciuria is influenced by dietary and urinary sodium levels.
  - Calcium is reabsorbed passively in the proximal renal tubule because of $Na^+$ and $Cl^-$ movement.
    - High sodium diets → reduces renal $Na^+$ reabsorption → reduces passive reabsorption of calcium
  - High dietary sodium reduces urinary citrate levels.

## Oxalate Metabolism

### Serum Oxalate

- Majority formed as a by-product of glyoxylate metabolism.
- 10–20% is dietary.
  - Nuts, chocolate, spinach, animal protein, and tea
- 10% of dietary oxalate is absorbed.
- Enteric absorption of oxalate can be *decreased* by:
  - *Oxalate binders:*
    - $Ca^{2+}$ and $Mg^{2+}$ reduces the bioavailability of oxalate ions.
    - Hence, stone formers are *not* advised to have a low calcium diet.
  - *Non-pathogenic commensal anaerobic bacteria:*
    - *Oxalobacter formigenes* (colon) colonisation is lower in CaOx formers.
    - Degrades oxalate via oxalyl-CoA decarboxylase → reduces absorption
- Absorbed oxalate is not metabolised any further.
  - Excreted predominantly within proximal tubules.
  - Renal reabsorption is negligible.

### Hyperoxaluria

- Urinary oxalate at >40 mg/day.

- Sub-classified into three groups: *primary, enteric,* and *idiopathic.*
- *Primary hyperoxaluria*
  - Autosomal recessive inheritance.
  - *Type 1:* Mutation *AGXT* gene (chromosome 2q)
    - Deficiency of hepatic alanine-glycoxylate aminotransferase (AGT).
    - Glycoxylate to glycolate conversion failure.
  - *Type 2:* Mutation *GRHPR gene* (chromosome 9q)
    - Deficiency of glycoxylate and hydroxy-pyruvate reductase (GRHPR).
    - Glycoxylate to glycolate conversion failure.
  - *Type 3:* Mutation *HOGA1* gene (chromosome 10q)
    - Deficiency of 4-hydroxy-2-oxoglutarate – (HOGA).
    - Failure of HOGA break down.
  - Increased glycoxylate build up → oxidation into *oxalic,* glycolic, glyoxylic acids
  - 50% have end-stage renal failure by early adulthood.
- *Enteric hyperoxaluria*
  - Disruption of enterohepatic circulation of bile acids.
    - Inflammatory bowel disease (IBD)
    - Bowel resection
    - Gastric bypass
  - Terminal ileum reabsorbs >95% of bile acids.
    - Impaired ileum (e.g., IBD) → reduction in bile reabsorption
    - Non-absorbed enteric fatty acids bind calcium → less ionised calcium available to bind oxalate → increased bioavailability and absorption of free oxalate
- *Idiopathic hyperoxaluria*
  - Most common type of hyperoxaluria.
  - Associations:
    - High dietary oxalate intake.
    - Restricted calcium diet (less oxalate binding).
  - CaOx calculi occur in pure form — CaOx monohydrate/dihydrate — or constitute part of a mixed calculus.
    - Influences clinical management (CaOx monohydrate are 'harder').

## Calcium Phosphate

- Pure CaP stones are uncommon.
- ~15% of the stone composition is commonly in combination with CaOx.
- *Forms of phosphate:*
  - Basic CaP (apatite)
  - Calcium hydrogen phosphate dihydrate (brushite)
  - Rarely tricalcium phosphate (whitlockite)
- Dietary phosphate from meat, dairy, and vegetables alters urinary phosphate levels.
- Phosphate is a urinary buffer.

- Filtered by the glomerulus and reabsorbed in the proximal tubule.
- *Hyperparathyroidism*
  - PTH prevents renal reabsorption → increases urinary phosphate → increases risk of CaP stones
- *Renal tubular acidosis*
  - Urinary phosphate excretion increases with urinary acidosis.

## Uric Acid Calculi

- Uric acid (UA) is a product of purine metabolism.
- UA pH = 5.3
- In healthy urine (pH 7.2), >50% of UA is held in its more soluble state of urate.
- Urate is ~20x more soluble than UA in urine.
- More acidic urine → less UA to be held in solution → UA stone formation
- UA stone formation is promoted by high urinary UA.
  - Can also form with normal UA levels through normouricosuria.
  - Form pure UA stones or act as a nidus for CaOx stones.
- *X-ray:* radiolucent (but seen on CT).
- *Medical management:*
  - Urine alkalisation (potassium citrate, sodium bicarbonate)
    - Increases pH by holding UA in its soluble state urate.
  - Xanthine inhibitor (allopurinol)
    - Inhibits the conversion of xanthine to UA.
- *Causes:*
  - Metabolic syndrome
    - Alters urinary pH via insulin resistance → higher incidence of UA calculi
  - High protein diet with low volume urine
  - Lesch–Nyhan Syndrome
    - Deficiency of hypoxanthine-guanine phosphoribosyl transferase.
    - Increases xanthine and UA production.
  - Gout
  - Myeloproliferative disorders
  - Chronic diarrhoea
  - Rare congenital abnormalities of UA metabolism and transportation (e.g., collagen storage disease)

## Cystine Calculi

- Cystinuria: autosomal recessive disorder.
- Defect in tubular reabsorption of '*COLA*' amino acids:
  - *C, Cystine, O, Ornithine, L, Lysine, A, Arginine*
  - Mutation in heteromeric amino acid transporter genes.
    - *Type A: SLC3A1* gene (chromosome 2)
    - *Type B: SLC7A9* gene (chromosome 19)

- Cystine is relatively *insoluble* in urine (ornithine, lysine, and arginine are soluble).
- Makes up ~1–2% of all urolithiasis.
- Peak incidence in adolescence and young adulthood.
- The risk of cystine calculi is correlated with the urinary cystine concentration.
- *Forms:*
  - Heterozygous, 1:200
  - Homozygous, 1:20,000
- Normal cystine excretion is at <100 mg/day (solubility limit ~250–300 mg/day).
  - Heterozygotes: 150–300 mg/day
  - Homozygotes: >400 mg/day
- The solubility is influenced by urinary pH.
  - At pH 7, cystine solubility is ~250 mg/L in urine.
  - At pH 7.5, solubility doubles to 500 mg/L.
- *Cyanide-nitroprusside urinary spot test (Brandt's test).*
  - Cystine + sodium cyanide = cysteine (pink)
  - Cysteine + nitroprusside = *purple* discolouration
  - Positive when urinary cystine is >75 mg/L
- Ground glass appearance on plain x-ray (disulphide bonds).
- Hexagonal shape on microscopy.
- *Medical management:*
  - Reduce urinary saturation via high fluid intake of >3 L/day (~250 mg will dissolve in 1L of fluid).
  - Manipulation of urinary pH (potassium citrate).
- *Chelating agents:*
  - D-penicillamine (forms disulphide bonds with urinary cystine – Penicillamine-cysteine disulfide is 50 times more soluble in urine than cystine).
  - Alpha mercaptopropionylglycine (Thiola)
- Captopril (angiotensin-converting enzyme inhibitor – reduces urinary cystine excretion).

# Infection-Related Stones

- Recurrent urinary tract infections (UTI) is a risk factor.
- *Mechanisms:*
  1. *Urea-splitting bacteria:*
     - Gram-negative: *proteus, providencia, klebsiella, pseudomonas*
     - Gram-positive: *staphylococcus*
     - *Ureaplasma urealyticum*

| Table 17.3 Medications Which Increase the Risk of Urolithiasis Formation and the Underlying Mechanism | | |
|---|---|---|
| **Alteration of Normal Physiology** | | |
| **Drug Class** | **Action** | **Calculi Composition** |
| Loop diuretics e.g., Furosemide | Inhibit Na and Ca resorption in ascending LoH. Diuresis and hypercalciuria. | Calcium oxalate |
| CA inhibitors e.g., Acetazolamide Topiramate | Inhibits proximal sodium bicarbonate reabsorption. Hyperchloremic metabolic acidosis with increased urinary pH and hypocitraturia. | Calcium phosphate |
| Laxatives | Chronic diarrhoea: Low urine volumes and acidic pH. | Ammonium acid, urate stones |
| **Accumulation of drug metabolites** | | |
| Indinavir | Renally excreted. Poor solubility at physiologic pH. | Indinavir |
| Fluoroquinolone e.g., Ciprofloxacin | Insoluble in alkaline or neutral pH. In acidic urine, ciprofloxacin crystalluria has been reported. | Ciprofloxacin |
| Triamterene | Mechanism not fully understood. Provide a matrix for nucleation to occur. | 20% pure triamterene, 80% mixed |
| Sulphonamides | Poor urine solubility – crystalline aggregates. Solubility improves if urine alkalinised. | |
| Allopurinol | Inhibits Xanthine oxidase. Reduces xanthine conversion to UA. | Xanthine |
| Vitamin C (ascorbic acid) | Metabolised into oxalate. | Calcium |
| Vitamin D | Increases digestive Ca. | Calcium |

*Abbreviations:* CA, carbonic anhydrase; Na, sodium; Ca, calcium; LoH, Loop of Henle; UA, uric acid.

- *Ureases* break down urea into ammonium bicarbonate and hydroxyl ions.
- $(NH_2)_2CO$ (urea) + $H_2O$ → $2NH_3$ (ammonia) + $CO_2$ (bicarbonate)
- $NH_3 + H_2O$ → $NH_4+$ (ammonium) + $OH^-$ (hydroxyl)
- Increases urine pH and ammonium.
- Increases CaP and magnesium ammonium phosphate (struvite) formation.
2. *Bacteria* – nidus for crystals to form upon.
   - Adhere to microcrystals and promote aggregation.
3. *Escherichia coli, proteus, klebsiella*: citrate lyase.
   - Degrades citrate → reduces its inhibitory activity
- Treatment includes acidification of urine to pH 6 or above and ther eradication of causative organisms.

## Drug Metabolite Calculi

- Makes up <1% all urolithiases.
- Indinavir (treatment of HIV) – incidence of urolithiasis at ~10%.
- Broad categories (Table 17.3):
  - Alteration of normal physiology
  - Predisposition to urolithiasis

## Xanthine Calculi

- Makes up <1% of all urolithiases.
- Xanthine: natural waste product of purine metabolism.
  - Oxidised into UA by xanthine oxidase.
- An autosomal recessive condition which impairs the function of xanthine oxidase. Xanthine is not converted into its more soluble and excretable waste products.
  - Urinary xanthine concentrations rise (UA levels decrease).
  - Form *radiolucent* xanthine calculi.
- *Management:*
  - High fluid intake
  - Low purine diet avoiding fish (mackerel, anchovies), poultry, and pork

# Anatominal Predispositions and Pregnancy

## Anatomical Predispositions

### Medullary Sponge Kidney (MSK)

- Cystic ectasia of the medullary collecting ducts.
- Multiple sac-like structures in which urine can pool.

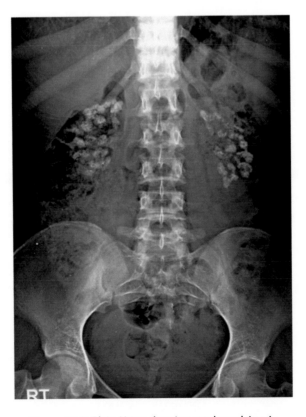

Figure 17.2 Plain X-ray showing nephrocalcinosis.

- Urinary stasis and increased risk of UTI → increase urolithiasis risk
- *Causes* metabolic anomalies:
  - Impaired urinary pH regulation (distal RTA)
  - Hypercalciuria and hypocitraturia
  - Associated with nephrocalcinosis (Figure 17.2)
    - A disorder that occurs when too much calcium is deposited in the kidneys.
    - Caused by any condition that leads to high levels of calcium in the blood/urine.
    - Medullary 95%, cortical 5%

## Pelvic–Ureteric Junction Obstruction (PUJO)

- At 20% risk of urolithiasis.
- Urinary stasis
- Patients with horseshoe kidneys also have an increased risk of urolithiasis.

## Pregnancy

- Incidence 1:250–1:3,000 pregnancies.
- Cardiac output increases in pregnancy → increases renal blood flow → glomerular filtration rate increases (up to 50%) → accumulation of calcium and UA

- Placental 1,25-dihydroxyvitamin D → increases enteric calcium absorption and suppresses PTH
- The increase in filtration of citrate and magnesium restores the balance of urolithiasis risk.

## Recommended Reading

1. Alelign T, Petros B. Kidney stone disease: an update on current concepts. Adv Urol. 2018;3068365.
2. Robertson WG. The scientific basis of urinary stone formation. In: Mundy A, Fitzpatrick J, Neal D, George N, eds, The Scientific Basis of Urology, 2nd edition. London: Taylor & Francis; 1999: 205–29.
3. Ratkalkar VN, Kleinman JG. Mechanisms of stone formation. Clin Rev Bone Miner Metab. 2011;9(3-4):187–97.
4. Pearle M, Antonelli J, Lotan Y. Urinary lithiasis: etiology, epidemiology and pathogenesis. In: Wein A, Kavoussi L, Partin A, Peters C, eds, Campbell-Walsh-Wein Urology, 11th edition. Philadelphia: Elsevier; 2015: 1170–1200.
5. Aune D, Mahamat-Saleh Y, Norat T, et al. Body fatness, diabetes, physical activity and risk of kidney stones: a systematic review and meta-analysis of cohort studies. Eur J Epidemiol. 2018;33:1033–1047.
6. Wiederkehr MR and Moe OW. Uric acid urolithiasis: a systemic metabolic disorder. Clin Rev Bone Miner Metab. 2011;9(3-4):207–17.
7. Matlaga BR, Shah OD, Assimos DG. Drug-induced urinary calculi. Rev Urol. 2003;5(4):227–31.
8. Turk C, Neisius A, Petrik C, et al. Urolithiasis. EAU guidelines. 2020.

# 18 Upper Urinary Tract Obstruction

*Sanjeev Pathak*

## Upper Urinary Tract Obstruction (UUTO)

- *UUTO* – a mechanical or functional impediment of the free flow of urine from the renal pelvis or ureter into the bladder.
- *Hydronephrosis:* dilatation of the renal pelvicalyceal system.
- Classified as congenital or acquired.

## Aetiology

### Antenatal Period

- Congenital pelvic ureteric junction obstruction (PUJO) is the most common cause of unilateral ureteric obstruction (UUO).
  - *Incidence:* 1 in 2,000 live births screened by routine antenatal ultrasound.
  - Males are more commonly affected.
  - Mostly a functional obstruction:
    - Impaired smooth muscle differentiation in the upper ureter/renal pelvis.
  - Aberrant lower pole crossing vessels present in up to 50%:
    - Raises the possibility of a physical obstruction.
    - Supported by studies that show relief of obstruction when the aberrant lower pole crossing vessels are mobilised and 'hitched'.

### Adults

- Ureteric calculus – most common cause of UUO.
- Other causes of UUTO are listed in Table 18.1.

## Clinical Presentation

*Depends on:*
- Aetiology
- Acute or chronic
- Complete or partial obstruction
- Unilateral or bilateral ureteric obstruction (BUO)
- Concomitant urinary tract infection (UTI)

## Antenatal

- Asymptomatic
- Congenital PUJO detected by serial ultrasound scanning.
- The anteroposterior diameter of the renal pelvis (APD) grading system is shown in Table 18.2.

## Childhood

- Fever, abdominal pain, abdominal mass

## Adults

- *Asymptomatic* – may result in irreversible 'silent renal loss'.
  - *Example*: chronic UUO secondary to PUJO resulting in caliectasis and loss of renal parenchyma (Figure 18.1).
- Acute ureteric colic – colicky pain and associated systemic symptoms.
- Chronic BUO or ureteric obstruction of a solitary kidney (UOSK):
  - Symptoms of uraemia, sepsis, and/or multi-organ failure.

## Diagnosis

### Anatomical Imaging

- *USS:* determines hydronephrosis/hydroureter with assessment of renal parenchyma in pregnancy.
- *Non-contrast CT* scan of the abdomen and pelvis is used to diagnose ureteric calculi.
- *Contrast CT* scan of the abdomen and pelvis is used to identify a lower pole crossing vessel.
- *CT Urogram/MR Urogram* determine the level of obstruction.

### Functional Imaging

- *Technetium-99m mercaptoacetyltriglycine* (MAG3) renogram confirms obstruction and relative function.

**Table 18.1** Aetiology of Upper Urinary Tract Obstruction

| Intraluminal | Intramural | Extraluminal |
|---|---|---|
| Ureteric calculus | UTUC | PUJO (crossing vessel) |
| Sloughed renal papilla | PUJO | AAA |
| Blood clot | Benign strictures<br>• Inflammatory<br>• Iatrogenic | Para-pelvic cyst |
| Fungal ball | Ureterocele | Malignant lymphadenopathy<br>• Testicular, ovarian<br>• Lymphoma |
| | | Pregnancy |
| | | Retroperitoneal fibrosis |
| | | Bladder outlet obstruction<br>• BPH<br>• Prostate cancer<br>• Urethral stricture<br>• DSD<br>• PUV |

*Abbreviations:* UTUC, upper tract urothelial carcinoma; PUJO, pelvic ureteric obstruction, AAA, abdominal aortic aneurysm; BPH, benign prostate hyperplasia; DSD, detrusor sphincter dyssynergia; PUV, posterior urethral valve.

**Table 18.2** Anteroposterior Diameter of the Renal Pelvis Grading System (Antenatal)

| Hydronephrosis | Second Trimester | Third Trimester |
|---|---|---|
| Mild | 4–6 mm | 7–9 mm |
| Moderate | 7–10 mm | 10–15 mm |
| Severe | >10 mm | >15 mm |

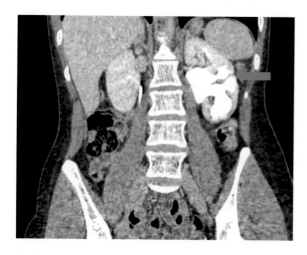

**Figure 18.1** The coronal view of an excretory-phase CT urogram scan. Left PUJO: Radiological Features Confirming Chronic Irreversible Changes with Blunting of the Calyces and Loss of Overlying Renal Parenchyma (Arrow).

- *Whitaker test* (historical test).
  - Role in equivocal cases of obstruction.
  - This invasive, dynamic test measures the pressure gradient between the renal pelvis and bladder.
  - Requires a nephrostomy tube and urinary catheter connected to pressure transducers.
  - The patient is in prone position and diluted contrast media is infused in an antegrade manner at a rate of 10 mL/min.
    - Pressure gradient <15 cmH$_2$O = non-obstructed
    - Pressures gradient between 15–22 cmH$_2$O = equivocal
    - Pressures gradient >22 cmH$_2$O = obstructed

## Pathological Features of UUTO

- Effects are dependent upon the duration of obstruction or the presence of infection.

- The longer complete UUTO continues, the potential for reversible damage decreases.
- Structural and functional changes may persist following relief of the obstruction.
- Most of the evidence discussed is derived from animal experiments (rats, dogs, sheep, and pigs). Caution must be exercised when extrapolating some of the findings to humans.

## Macroscopic Features

- *24–48 hours:* renal pelvis and ureteric dilatation occur.
- *Day 7:* gross swelling and oedema of the kidney.
  - Continues to increase up to three months in UUO.
- *Chronic* changes include:
  - Loss of renal parenchyma
  - Fibrosis
  - Reduction in size compared with the contralateral kidney

## Microscopic Features

- *Tubular apoptosis*
  - *UUO:* increase in pressure → transmitted to the renal tubular cells
  - Mechanical stretching of these cells activates the renin–angiotensin system (RAS).
  - Angiotensin II and tumour necrosis factor-α (TNF-α) promote tubular apoptosis.
  - Seen within hours of UUO. The glomerulus is relatively spared.
  - At 21 days, the disappearance of recognisable renal tubules occurs.
- *Tubulo-interstitial inflammation*
  - Pro-inflammatory chemokines – angiotensin II, TNF-α, and nuclear transcription factor-kappaB (NF-κB) continue to increase → recruit inflammatory cells — predominantly, macrophages
- *Tubular cell death*
  - Ischaemia, oxidative stress, and ATP depletion causes renal tubular cell death.
- *Tubulo-interstitial fibrosis*
  - Major determinant of irreversible loss of renal function post-obstruction.
  - 7–14 days: fibroblast recruitment and diffuse accumulation of extracellular matrix (ECM).
  - Mediated by transforming growth factor-β (TGF-β).

## Physiological Pyeloureteric Peristalsis

- The propulsion of urine from the calyces, renal pelvis, and ureter into the bladder is an active process.
- This coordinated process is dependent upon:
  - Pacemaker cells
  - Adequate mucosal coaptation
  - Peristalsis
  - Renal pelvis/ureteric pressure > intravesical pressure
- Process begins within the *'pacemaker cells'*.
  - Located within the renal pelvis, mostly in the calyceal–pelvic junction.
  - Calcium-dependant pacemaker cells consist of:
    - Atypical smooth muscle cells: low depolarisation potential compared with typical smooth muscle cells and are more excitable, which initiates and promotes peristalsis.
    - Interstitial cells of Cajal.
- At *low* urine flow rates, the renal pelvis contractions outnumber ureteric contractions.
  - Resting ureteric pressure = 0–5 cmH$_2$0
  - Peristatic waves = 20–80 cmH$_2$0
  - Resting potential = –30 to –70 mV
  - Frequency of contractions are 2–6/minutes
- At *high* urine flow rates, the renal pelvis contractions instigate myogenic transfer to the ureter.
  - Results in the coalescing of urine boluses.
  - At this stage, there is no coaptation and urine flows as a continuous column.
- *Neurogenic control* (particularly, distal ureteric peristalsis)
  - *Stimulatory*
    - Cholinergic
    - Alpha-adrenergic
  - *Inhibitory*
    - Beta-adrenergic

## Obstructional Effects on Peristalsis

- Changes in ureteric pressure (UP) and peristalsis are determined by:
  - Complete or partial UUO
  - Duration of obstruction
- Obstruction for *one month*:
  - Marked increase in UP (*in vivo* human renal pelvis and ureter tissue, *in vitro* dog studies).
- Obstruction at eight *weeks* (following relief of obstruction):
  - UP decreases but remains two-fold higher compared with baseline.

### Complete Obstruction

- Increased ureteric pressure by seven-fold
- Increased amplitude
- Aperistalsis

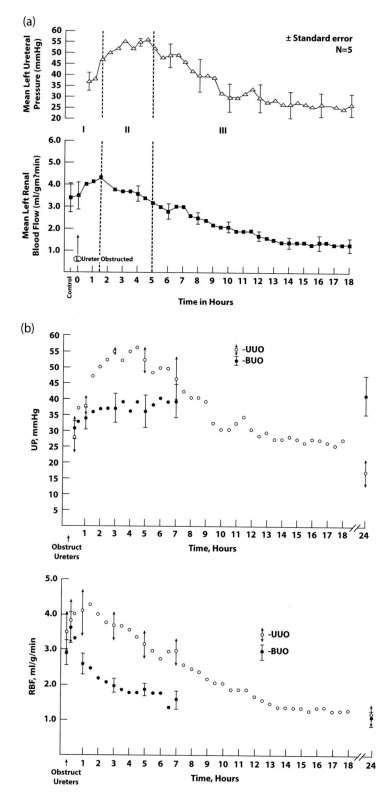

**Figure 18.2** The ureteral pressure and renal blood flow changes seen in (a) unilateral ureteric obstruction (triphasic); (b) bilateral Ureteric Obstruction (biphasic) UUO, unilateral obstruction; BUO, bilateral ureteric obstruction; UP, ureteric pressure; RBF, renal blood flow. (Adapted from Moody et al. [5])

## Partial Obstruction

- Reduction in contractility by ~50%.
- Increased amplitude.
- Continued peristalsis.

## Pathophysiology of UUTO

- Complete UUO, BUO and UOSK have pathophysiological differences.
- Characterised by changes in:
  - Renal pelvis/ureteric pressures
  - Renal blood flow (RBF)
  - Glomerular filtration rate (GFR)
- Structural/functional changes may persist following post-obstruction.

## Haemodynamic Changes in UUTO

- Animal studies demonstrate a *tri-phasic* and *bi-phasic* response to RBF and UP in UOO and BUO/UOSK, respectively.
  - The aim of the haemodynamic response seen is the desperate but failed attempt of the kidney to maintain GFR (Figure 18.2 and Table 18.3).

## Complete UUO

- *Phase I* (0–90 min) – *increase* in both RBF and UP.
  - Fall in the GFR.
  - Pre-glomerular/afferent arteriolar dilatation via the tubule-glomerular feedback, attempting to prevent a fall in the GFR.
  - *Vasodilators* involved:
    - *Nitic oxide* (NO) – the inducible form is increased. Administration of NO inhibitor pre-UUO attenuates the RBF.
    - *Prostaglandin E$_2$* (PGE$_2$) – production is increased in the contralateral kidney and detected in the urine. Indomethacin inhibits PGE$_2$ synthesis and attenuates the response.
- *Phase II* (90 min–5 hours) – *decrease* in RBF but continued *increase* in UP.
  - The continued increase in UP and short-lived afferent arteriolar dilatation is followed by a prolonged post-glomerular/efferent arteriolar constriction, again attempting to prevent a fall in the GFR.
  - *Vasoconstrictors* involved:
    - *Angiotensin II (ATII)* – released via the RAS.
    - *Thromboxane* – derived from inflammatory cells.
    - *Endothelin* – released in response to the stretching of the endothelium.
- *Phase III* (>5 hours) – *decrease* in the RBF and UP.
  - Continues until at least 18 hours.
  - Afferent and efferent arteriolar constriction results in a drastic fall in the RBF and UP causing a decrease in the GFR.
  - There is redistribution of RBF in the kidney from the renal cortex to the juxtamedullary regions.

| Table 18.3 Haemodynamic Changes Seen in UUTO | | |
|---|---|---|
| **Phase** | **UUO Tri-phasic** | **BUO/UOSK Bi-phasic** |
| **Phase 1** 0–90 min | RBF ↑ and UP ↑ | RBF ↑ and UP ↑ |
| | Afferent vasodilation: NO, PGE2 | Afferent vasodilation: NO, PAF |
| **Phase 2** >90 min | RBF↓ and UP ↑ | RBF ↓ and UP ↑ (elevated >24 h) |
| | Afferent vasodilation | Afferent vasodilation |
| | Efferent vasoconstriction: ATII, TX, Endothelin | Efferent vasoconstriction |
| | | GFR ↓ |
| | | (No afferent vasoconstriction phase) |
| **Phase 3** >5 h | RBF↓ and UP ↓ | |
| | GFR ↓ | |
| | Afferent vasocontriction: ATII, TX, Endothelin | |

*Abbreviations:* UUO, unilateral ureteric obstruction; BUO, bilateral ureteric obstruction; UOSK, unilateral; RBF, renal blood flow; UP, ureteric pressure; GFR, glomerular filtration rate; NO, nitric oxide; PGE2, prostaglandin E2; PAF, platelet-activating factor; ATII, angiotensin II; TX, thromboxane.

- Endothelin plays a greater role than ATII and thromboxane.
- Adaptive dilatation of lymphatic and venous channels allows redistribution of urine.
  - >24 hours of UUO, UP falls but remains 50% above the baseline, which limits renal damage.

## Complete BUO or UOSK

- BUO or UOSK has marked differences compared with UUO.
  - Bi-phasic response.
  - Modest increase in the RBF.
  - Marked increase in UP.
  - RBF is increased in the renal cortex but reduced in the juxtamedullary regions; the redistribution is the exact opposite seen in a UUO.
- *Phase I* (0–90 min) – *increase* in both the RBF and UP.
  - Increase in afferent arteriolar dilatation:
    - NO and platelet-activating factor (PAF)
- *Phase II* (>90 min) – *decrease* in the RBF with continued *increase* in UP (>24 hours).
  - Afferent arteriolar dilatation with a marked increase in efferent arteriolar constriction.
  - Mediated via substances that would be excreted via the contralateral kidney in a UOO, e.g., atrial natriuretic peptide (ANP) which promotes diuresis and natriuresis:
  - ANP is released by the cardiac atrium in response to increased intravascular volume.
    - Inhibits the tubulo-glomerular feedback.
    - Inhibits sodium chloride absorption in the ascending Loop of Henle (LoH).
    - Inhibits vasopressin-mediated water permeability.
    - Promotes diuresis and natriuresis via afferent arteriole vasodilatation and efferent arteriole vasocontraction (note: no afferent vasoconstriction phase).

## Effects of UUTO on Tubular Function

- The ascending limb of LoH (sodium reabsorption) and distal collecting tubules (potassium and acid excretion) are vulnerable to ischaemic insults:
  - Loss of energy-dependant ($Na^+/K^+$-ATPase, $H^+$-ATPase) reabsorption of electrolytes and water.
- The proximal tubules and glomeruli are relatively spared of this insult.
- *Complete UUO* – hyperkalaemia and post-obstructional diuresis *do not* occur (due to a normal functioning contralateral kidney).
- *BUO/UOSK* – increase in serum ANP, post-obstructional diuresis, and natriuresis *do* occur.

- Directly proportional to the duration of obstruction.
- The urine has:
  - High sodium content (reduced reabsorption of sodium)
  - Low potassium content (reduced GFR and secretion in distal tubules)
  - Alkaline (inability to secrete hydrogen ions)
  - Low urine osmolality (insensitivity to vasopressin in collecting ducts)

# Post-Obstructional Renal Recovery

- Post-obstructive recovery of renal function is influenced by the duration of obstruction.
- *Renal recovery:*
  - *Partial/short* duration – full recovery:
    - With the loss of renal tubular cells, the remaining renal tubular cells repopulate the tubules.
  - *Prolonged* obstruction – little to no recovery:
    - Significant loss of renal tubular cells and marked interstitial fibrosis.
- A complete UUO has worse prognosis than a partial UUO.
- It has been reported that despite 150 days of complete UUO in humans, functional recovery does occur.
  - May be due to the lymphatic and venous channels conferring greater protection in the human.

## Complete UUO

- 1–3 days of obstruction, full recovery of renal function at 14 days.
- Seven days of obstruction, full recovery of renal function at 14 days.
- 14 days of obstruction, recovery of 70% renal function up to six months.
- Four weeks of obstruction, 'some' recovery of renal function.
- Six weeks of obstruction, no recovery of renal function.

## Partial UUO

- Relief of obstruction at day 14, full recovery of renal function.
- Relief of obstruction at day 28, recovery of 30% renal function.
- Relief of obstruction at day 60, recovery of only 8% renal function.

## Complete BUO

- No clear relationship between duration of obstruction and recovery of renal function.

- The study of 21 men with chronic bladder outflow obstruction showed a two-phased, post-obstructional recovery.
  - *Tubular* phase: increased urea, electrolyte and water excretion that improved at two weeks.
  - *Glomerular* phase: improvement of GFR at three months.

# Recommended Reading

1. Whitaker RH. Methods of assessing obstruction in dilated ureters. Br J Urol. 1973;45(1):15–22.
2. Lang RJ, Tonta MA, Zoltkowski BZ, Meeker WF, Wendt I, Parkington HC. Pyeloureteric peristalsis: role of atypical smooth muscle cells and interstitial cells of Cajal-like cells as pacemakers. J Physiol. 2006;576(Pt 3):695–705.
3. Thulesius O, Angelo-Khattar M, Sabha M. The effect of ureteral distension on peristalsis. Studies on human and sheep ureters. Urol Res. 1989;17(6):385–388.
4. Lennon GM, Ryan PC, Fitzpatrick JM. Recovery of ureteric motility following complete and partial ureteric obstruction. Br J Urol. 1993;72(5 Pt 2):702–707.
5. Moody TE, Vaughn ED, Jr., Gillenwater JY. Relationship between renal blood flow and ureteral pressure during 18 hours of total unilateral uretheral occlusion. Implications for changing sites of increased renal resistance. Invest Urol. 1975;13(3):246–251.
6. Vaughan ED, Jr., Sorenson EJ, Gillenwater JY. The renal hemodynamic response to chronic unilateral complete ureteral occlusion. Invest Urol. 1970;8(1):78–90.
7. Vaughan ED, Jr., Shenasky JH, 2nd, Gillenwater JY. Mechanism of acute hemodynamic response to ureteral occlusion. Invest Urol. 1971;9(2):109–118.
8. Harris RH, Yarger WE. Renal function after release of unilateral ureteral obstruction in rats. Am J Physiol. 1974;227(4):806–815.
9. Nagle RB, Bulger RE. Unilateral obstructive nephropathy in the rabbit. II. Late morphologic changes. Lab Invest. 1978;38(3):270–278.
10. Shapiro SR, Bennett AH. Recovery of renal function after prolonged unilateral ureteral obstruction. J Urol. 1976;115(2):136–140.
11. Leahy AL, Ryan PC, McEntee GM, Nelson AC, Fitzpatrick JM. Renal injury and recovery in partial ureteric obstruction. J Urol. 1989;142(1):199–203.
12. Jones DA, George NJ, O'Reilly PH, Barnard RJ. The biphasic nature of renal functional recovery following relief of chronic obstructive uropathy. Br J Urol. 1988;61(3):192–197.

# 19 Non-Neurogenic Lower Urinary Tract Dysfunction

*Nadir I. Osman and Karl H. Pang*

## Introduction

- Lower urinary tract dysfunction (LUTD) is considered according to two phases of the micturition cycle: *storage* and *voiding*.
  - *Storage* symptoms – due to failure to store urine.
  - *Voiding* symptoms – due to failure to void urine.
- Patients may have a combination of storage and voiding dysfunction.
- LUTD can be due to bladder problem, bladder outlet problem, or a combination.

## Failure to Store Dysfunctions

### 1. Stress Urinary Incontinence

- *Stress urinary incontinence (SUI):* involuntary leakage of urine on coughing, straining, sneezing, and straining.

### Stress Urinary Incontinence in Men

- Two functional sphincter mechanisms:
  - Proximal bladder neck (internal urethral sphincter)
  - Distal urethral sphincter (DUS) (external urethral sphincter)
- *Bladder neck:*
  - Circular smooth muscle continuous with the trigone muscle.
  - Innervated by sympathetic (adrenergic) fibres.
- *Distal urethral sphincter:*
  - Extends from the distal part of the prostate to the membranous urethra.
  - Thicker and longer anteriorly (horseshoe-shaped).
  - Major outer striated component (pudendal nerve, S2-S4).
  - Minor inner smooth muscle component (sympathetic nerves, T10-L2).
- Continence is possible if one mechanism is damaged but the other is maintained:
  - Transurethral resection of the prostate (TURP) damages the bladder neck, yet patients are continent due to the intact DUS mechanism.
  - Pelvic fracture urethral injury (and surgical repair) damages the DUS mechanism, yet patients (without prior bladder neck surgery) are usually continent.
- Radical prostatectomy is the most common cause, where the bladder neck and DUS mechanisms are both disrupted.

### Stress Urinary Incontinence in Women

- One functional sphincter mechanism: DUS.
- Bladder neck mechanisms deficient (completely absent in 40%).
- DUS is thicker and longer anteriorly (horseshoe-shaped), composed of:
- *Major outer striated components*
  - *Three muscles:*
    - Rhabdosphincter, compressor urethrae, urethrovaginal sphincter
  - Act as a single functional unit.
  - Somatic innervation – pudendal nerve (S2-S4).
  - Muscle fibres:
    - *Type I* (slow twitch) – for resting tone.
    - *Type II* (fast twitch) – for sudden pressure rise (e.g., coughing).
- *Minor inner smooth muscle component*
  - *Two layers*: inner longitudinal and outer circular.
  - Extends 4/5 of urethral length (proximal to distal).
  - Sympathetic innervation (T10-L2).
  - Tonic contraction during urine storage.
- *Submucosal venous plexus*
  - Mid to distal urethra.
  - Aids coaptation – 'vascular cushion'
- DUS requires intact pelvic floor support structures to function adequately and continence to be maintained.
- Two mechanisms for SUI which are not mutually exclusive. Most patients have both:
  1. *Urethral hypermobility*

- Weakness in pelvic floor support structures.
- Caused by injury to pelvic floor structures of innervation.
2. *Intrinsic sphincter deficiency*
   - Defective DUS.
   - Caused by injury to the sphincter or innervation.

- Two main theories proposed to explain how *urethral hypermobility* leads to SUI:
  1. *Hammock hypothesis* (Delancey 1994).
     - Urethra rests on the hammock (fused layers of endopelvic and pubocervical fascia attached to the arcus tendinous fascia pelvis and levator ani) (Figure 19.1).
     - ↑ in abdominal pressure transmitted to urethra.
     - Urethra is compressed against a rigid support of the hammock.
     - Loss of compression → leakage
  2. Pressure transmission theory (Enhorning 1961).
     - Normal position of urethra is intra-abdominal (Figure 19.2).
     - Loss of urethral support → descent of urethra out with abdomen
     - Loss of transmission of abdominal pressure to urethra → leakage
     - *Aetiology:* childbirth, ageing, obesity, connective tissue disorders, genetic predisposition, radiation-related injury, and peri-urethral surgery.

- *(Video) urodynamics*
  - *Definition of SUI* – involuntary leakage of urine during increased abdominal pressure, in the absence of a detrusor contraction.
  - *Abdominal leak point pressure* (ALLP) – the lowest value of the intentionally increased intravesical pressure that provokes urinary leakage in the absence of a detrusor contraction.
- *McGuire* described:
  - <60 cmH2O – represent intrinsic sphincter deficiency
  - 60–90 cmH2O – equivocal
  - >90 cmH2O – sphincter competence
- The *Blaivas and Olson* VUDS classification is based on the position of the bladder neck (BN) in relation to the inferior margin of the pubic symphysis (IMPS) on coughing/straining:
  - Type 1 (urethral hypermobility): *Closed* BN at rest. *Normal* position of BN. Leakage and descent of BN *<2 cm* below IMPS.
  - Type 2a (urethral hypermobility): *Closed* BN at rest. *Normal* position of BN. Leakage and descent of BN *>2 cm* below IMPS.
  - Type 2b (urethral hypermobility): *Closed* BN at rest. BN *below* IMPS. Leakage and descent of BN *>2 cm* below IMPS.
  - Type 3: *Open* BN at rest in the *Normal* position above the IMPS. Leakage on coughing.

## 2. Urgency Urinary Incontinence

- *Overactive bladder (OAB)* – symptom complex:
  - Urinary urgency with or without urgency incontinence is usually accompanied by frequency and nocturia.
- *Urinary urgency* – pivotal symptom of OAB: A sudden and compelling desire to void that is difficult to defer.
- Overall prevalence (EPIC study): 11.8% (women: 12.2%, men: 10.8%).
- Prevalence ↑ with age.
- OAB and incontinence (OAB-wet) in 1/3.
- OAB may be associated with underlying detrusor overactivity (DO).
- *Detrusor overactivity* – urodynamic diagnosis:
  - Involuntary detrusor contractions during the filling phase of the micturition cycle.
- OAB is more strongly correlated to underlying DO in men vs women.
- Wet OAB is more strongly associated with DO than OAB without incontinence (OAB-dry).
- *Aetiology:* idiopathic, ageing, BOO.
- Pathogenesis of OAB, four main theories:
  1. *Myogenic:* spontaneous excitation in detrusor muscle spreads to other parts of the bladder.
  2. *Urothelium:* urothelium responds to mechanical, osmotic, inflammatory, and chemical stimuli → ↑ sensory nerve stimulation.
  3. *Neurogenic:* NDO from generalised nerve mediated excitation of detrusor.
  4. *Integrative:* range of triggers generate localised detrusor contractions and spread in the bladder wall via various routers.

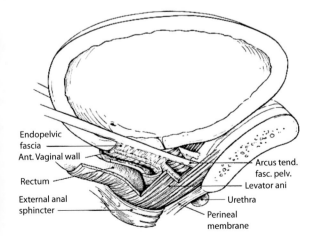

Figure 19.1 Lateral view of the urethral support structures. (Reuse with permission from John Wiley and Sons [1])

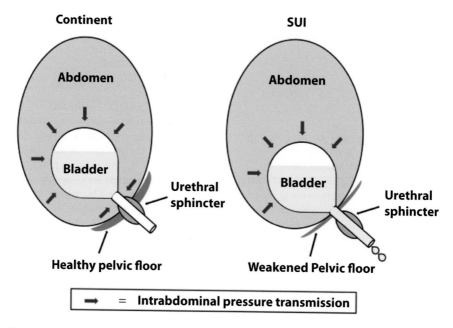

Figure 19.2 Theoretical mechanisms of urethral leakage. Enhorning's theory of urethral hypermobility showing inadequate urethral compression with urethral descent out with the abdominal cavity leading to leakage. SUI, stress urinary incontinence.

# Interstitial Cystitis (IC)/Bladder Pain Syndrome

- *Definition:* chronic (>6 months) pelvic pain, pressure, or discomfort perceived to be related to the urinary bladder accompanied by at least one other urinary symptom such as the persistent urge to void or urinary frequency (ESSIC 2008).
- *Aetiology:* unknown, but likely multifactorial.
- *Possible pathogenic mechanisms:*

1. *Urothelial defects:* deficient glycosaminoglycan (GAG) layer, impaired cell adhesion, aberrant epithelial proliferation, toxic substances in urine, autoimmunity against bladder urothelium. The GAG layer consists of hyaluronic acid and heparin/keratan/dermatan/chondroitin sulphate (forms the basis behind intravesical instillations).
2. *Inflammation:* activation of mast cells (*Hunner's ulcers*) → immunological inflammation.
3. Increased *nociceptive reflex* pathways.
4. Increased *angiogenesis* in urothelium (*glomerulation*).

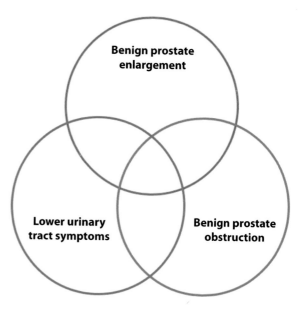

Figure 19.3 Hald diagram.

# Failure to Void Dysfunctions

## 1. Bladder Outlet Obstruction

### Benign Prostatic Hyperplasia

- Benign prostatic hyperplasia (BPH) – histological diagnosis.
- Benign prostatic enlargement (BPE) – clinical diagnosis.
- Benign prostatic obstruction (BPO) – BOO due to BPE.
- Hald's rings describe interaction between BPH, BPE, and BOO (Figure 19.3).

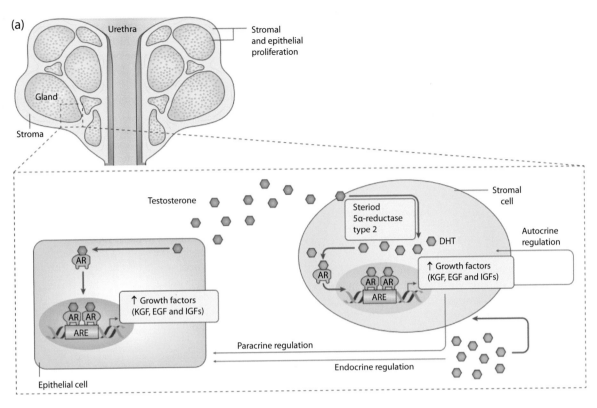

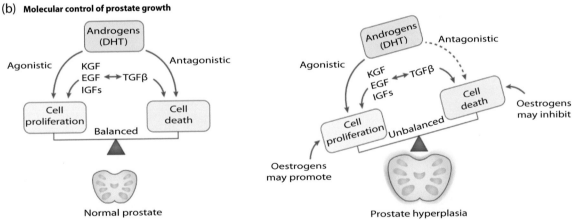

Figure 19.4 Role of testosterone and molecular control in benign prostate hyperplasia. (a) Testosterone diffuses into stromal and epithelial cells of the prostate. Testosterone and its derivatives interact with the androgen receptor (AR), which upon binding translocates to the nucleus and binds to the androgen response element (are), promoting the expression of genes encoding various growth factors (including Keratinocyte Growth Factor (KGF), Epidermal Growth Factor (EGF) and Insulin-like Growth Factors (IGFs). In stromal cells, most of the testosterone is converted to Dihydrotestosterone (DHT), which then acts in an autocrine manner to promote stromal proliferation. DHT can also diffuse into the adjacent epithelial cell to act in a paracrine manner. DHT produced peripherally in the liver and the skin can also diffuse from the circulation into the prostate to act in an endocrine manner. (b) Benign Prostatic Hyperplasia (BPH) probably develops as a result of an imbalance between mechanisms that regulate cell death and cell proliferation. Growth factors such as KGF, EGF and IGFs, which are AR target genes, are probably involved, as is Transforming Growth Factor-β (TGFβ), which is negatively regulated by androgens. In Part b, the dashed arrow indicates a less antagonistic effect. (Reprinted by permission from Springer Nature [5] and [6])

- BPH – increased number of epithelial and stromal cells in the transition zone.
- BPH is primarily a stromal process.
  - Ratio of stroma to epithelium in BPH – 4:1 to 5:1
  - Smooth muscle proportion of the hyperplastic stroma is ~40%.
- *Prevalence:* 20% in 30–40 years, 50–60% in 40–60 years, and >80% in >80 years.
- *Aetiology:* unclear, due to imbalance cell proliferation vs cell death (Figure 19.4).
  - *Androgens:* necessary for BPH development; however, role is unclear but is likely permissive.
  - *Paracrine and autocrine growth factors (GF):* stimulate or inhibit cell growth (e.g., epidermal GF, insulin-like GF, Keratinocyte GF, Transforming GF-Beta).
  - *Inflammation:* common in BPH specimen where inflammatory cytokines may promote cell growth/smooth muscle contraction.
  - *Oestrogens:* may sensitise prostate to androgens.
  - *Genetic:* no specific gene identified but a higher proportion of first-degree relatives of men with BPH develop clinical problems related to BPH.
- *Anatomic-pathologic aspects* (Figure 19.5)
  - *Zones:* BPH develops initially as nodules in the transition zone (TZ), then as the disease develops, nodules in any of the TZ or peri-urethral (PUZ) region develop.

- *Prostatic capsule:* important in the development of BOO and LUTS, which allows increased prostate volume to be transmitted to the urethra (dogs do not develop BOO due to absence of capsule).
- *Median lobe:* derived from the PUZ (no TZ at the bladder neck).
- Smaller resected prostates: mainly fibro-muscular stroma.
- Larger resected prostates: mainly epithelial nodules.

- *Components of BPO:*
  - *Passive* – related to stromal cells, epithelial cells, and extracellular matrix.
  - *Active* – related to smooth tone.
- Smooth muscle tone is regulated by the sympathetic nervous system acting as an alpha-1a adrenoreceptor.
- *Bladder response to obstruction:*
  - Increased work to overcome BOO → DO → detrusor underactivity (DU)
  - *Stages:*
    1. BOO increases outlet resistance.
    2. Compensatory detrusor hypertrophy and hyperplasia. Contractile function preserved.
    3. Bladder smooth muscle dysfunction and fibrosis:
       - Detrusor overactivity
       - Decreased contractile function → bladder emptying impaired

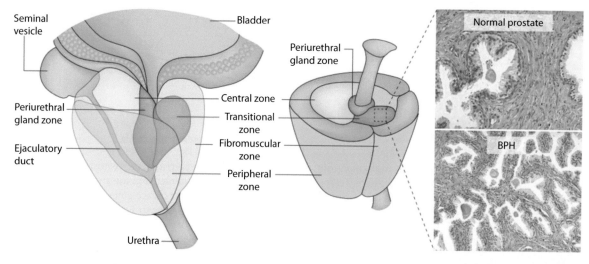

**Figure 19.5** Histological aspects of benign prostate hyperplasia. McNeal introduced the anatomical concept of the transitional zone as the principal site of Benign Prostatic Hyperplasia (BPH). The size of the prostate remains stable until approximately 40 years of age, after which hyperplasia of the prostate gland typically develops. Histological slides of both a normal prostate and BPH Tissue are included. BPH typically exhibits considerable pleomorphism in terms of stromal/epithelial ratio; here, the BPH section shows proliferation of the glandular epithelial cells. (Reprinted by permission from Springer Nature [6])

- *Mechanism of bladder dysfunction:*
  - BOO → increases bladder wall tension during contraction (*Laplace law*) → compression of bladder wall vessels → tissue ischaemia
  - Cyclic ischaemia/reperfusion injury during micturition cycles → damage to cellular/subcellular membranes
  - Impaired myocyte function and denervation → decompensation of detrusor function

## Urethral Stricture Disease

- *Urethral stricture*: a narrowed segment of the anterior urethra due to a process of fibrosis and cicatrisation of the urethral mucosa and surrounding spongiosis tissue (*spongiofibrosis*).
- *Male posterior urethra* – no spongiosis tissue and at this location the term *stenosis* or *contracture* is preferred.
- UK prevalence: 40 per 100,000
- Increases with age.
- *Aetiology:*
  - Idiopathic (penile 15%, bulbar 40%)
  - Iatrogenic (penile 40%, bulbar 40%)
  - Infective/inflammatory (penile 40%, bulbar 10%)
  - Traumatic (penile 5%, bulbar 15%)
  - Congenital/miscellaneous
- *Inflammatory strictures* – often caused by Lichen sclerosis (LS) (historically caused by gonorrhoea).
- *Pathogenesis:*
  - Insult (bacterial, chemical, or physical such as a catheter).
  - Pseudostratified columnar epithelium → stratified squamous epithelium
  - Splits develop in the epithelium.
  - Urine extravasation occurs (no subepithelial layer c.f. muscularis).
  - Fibrosis develops in the spongiosis tissue.
  - Repetitive insults cause more fibrosis.
  - Coalescence of fibrous plaques leads to circumferential fibrosis.
  - Constriction of the urethral lumen.
  - Obstruction leads to squamous metaplasia upstream.
  - Proximal propagation of stricture.
- *Lichen sclerosis*
  - Chronic inflammatory skin condition which leads to scarring.
  - 20% involves the urethra.
  - Most common cause of pan-urethral stricture.
  - Does not pass the external urethral sphincter.
  - *The aetiology* is unknown, but is possibly autoimmune.
  - Associated with uncircumcised, higher body mass index, diabetes mellitus, coronary artery disease, tobacco usage, hyperlipidaemia, and hypertension.

## 2. Detrusor Underactivity

- *Detrusor underactivity (DU)* – urodynamic term:
  - Contraction of reduced strength and/or duration, resulting in prolonged bladder emptying and/or failure to achieve complete bladder emptying within a normal time span.
- If no contraction occurs = 'acontractile detrusor' (AcD)
- DU is associated with a range of storage and voiding symptoms.
- *Men:* DU in 9–28% <50 years and 48% in >70 years undergoing urodynamics.
- *Women:* DU in 12–45% undergoing urodynamics.
- *Aetiologies* of DU classified as:
  - *Myogenic:* affecting function of myocytes or extracellular matrix.
  - *Neurogenic:* affecting sensory nerves, motor nerves, or central circuits.
  - *Role of sensation:* bladder sensory nerves monitor volume during storage and magnitude of detrusor contractions during voiding. Urethral sensory nerves perceive flow through the urethra. Impairment in sensory function → reduce/prematurely end voiding reflex.
- *Important aetiologies:*
  - BOO – see BOO section.
  - Diabetes Mellitus:
    - Myogenic and neurogenic mechanisms → DU
    - *Neurogenic:* hyperglycaemia damages motor and sensory nerves.
    - *Myogenic:* hyperglycaemia → osmotic diuresis → bladder wall stretching → bladder hypertrophy (storage symptoms) → build-up toxic products of oxidative stress → decompensation of detrusor function

## 3. Fowler's Syndrome

- Urinary retention in young women due to failure of the urethral sphincter to relax.
- High urethral pressure.
- Abnormal electromyography (EMG) signals in the urethral sphincter:
  - Complex repetitive discharges (CRD)
  - Decelerating bursts (DB)
- Up to 50% have associated polycystic ovaries.

# Urodynamic Aspects of LUTD

## Storage

- Normal bladder has high compliance.
- Accommodates large rise in volume without a significant rise in pressure.
- Bladder modelled as a thin-walled sphere.
- Pressure/volume characteristics according to the *Law of Laplace*.

- $P = 2\ T/R$, $P$ = pressure, $T$ = wall tension, $R$ = radius (i.e. volume)
- In a normal bladder, as volume increases, R increases and T increases to a similar degree; hence, P remains constant.
- As volume reaches capacity (i.e. R cannot increase further), T continues to rise; hence, P increases.
- At low bladder volume, the elastic properties of the smooth muscle (low stiffness) determine wall tension.

- Towards capacity, elastic properties of collagen (high stiffness) determine wall tension.
- Bladder also has visco-elasticity (features of viscous fluid and elastic solid).
  - If fills fast, exhibits greater stiffness, and pressure rises more rapidly.
  - When filling stops, it loses stiffness exponentially (stress relaxation).
  - It elongates over time if subjected to constant stretch (creep).

## Voiding

- Voiding arises from the balance between contracting detrusor (mechanical energy) and relaxed bladder outlet (passive conduit).
- Relations are important in the urodynamic assessment of voiding:

1. *Bladder outlet relation (BOR)* (Figure 19.6):
   - Considers the contracting bladder for a given bladder volume.
     - Detrusor pressure (Pdet) becomes equivalent to bladder contractility only when a bladder contracts while no flow occurs – *isovolumetric contraction* (Pdet.iso).
   - In a normal bladder, detrusor pressure depends on the rate of flow out of the bladder.
   - In the presence of obstruction leading to low flow, the normal bladder will void at a high pressure.
   - Higher voiding pressures seen in BOO are not due to "compensation".
   - At lower bladder volume or in detrusor underactivity, curves shift to the left (V3).

- *Passive urethral resistance relation (PURR)*

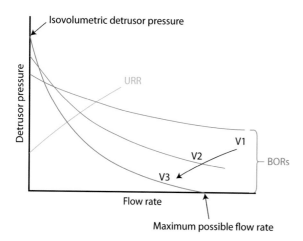

**Figure 19.6** Bladder outlet relation. The BOR is shown as the bladder empties from V1 to V3. Isovolumetric detrusor pressure gradually increases as bladder volume decreases. The detrusor pressure increases as the urethral resistance increase. Bladder outlet relation (BOR); URR, urethral resistance relation. (Reuse with permission from John Wiley and Sons [9])

| Type of BOO | Characteristic During Voiding | Example | CSA of FCZ | Minimal Urethral Opening Pressure | Flow Pattern | Likelihood of Elevated Residual Urine |
|---|---|---|---|---|---|---|
| **None** | Yielding, stretches during voiding | – | High | Low | Bell shaped | Low |
| **Constrictive** | Rigid, minimal stretch during voiding | Urethral stricture | Low | Low | Flat | Low |
| **Compressive** | Yielding, stretches during voiding | Benign prostatic enlargement | High | High | Extended Bell shaped | High |

**Table 19.1** Constrictive Versus Compressive Bladder Outlet Obstruction

*Abbreviations:* BOO, bladder outlet obstruction; CSA, cross-sectional area; FCZ, flow controlling zone.

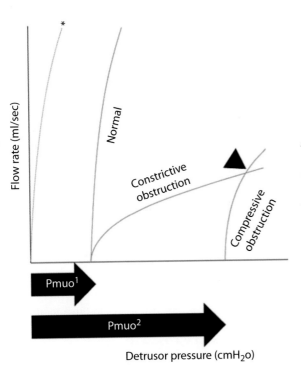

Figure 19.7 Urethral resistance relation. Dashed curve (*) represents URR in a rigid pipe where primarily the CSA of the tube determines URR. Three solid curves represent URR in collapsible/distensible tube where Pmuo, as well as the CSA of FCZ, Is an important determinant for URR. If the CSA is reduced (e.g., urethral stricture), the curve becomes flatter (constrictive obstruction). If Pmuo is elevated from Pmuo$^1$ to Pmuo$^2$ (e.g., BPO), the curve is shifted towards the high pressure (compressive obstruction). Because Pmuo determines the detrusor contraction strength necessary to initiate and maintain voiding, a compressive obstruction is more prone to promote retention or significant residual urine than a constrictive obstruction, even with the same Pdet.qmax (arrowhead). UUR, urethral resistance relation; CSA, cross sectional area; FCZ, flow controlling zone; Pmuo, minimum urethral opening pressure. (Reuse with permission from John Wiley and Sons [9])

- Considers the bladder outlet.
- Describes the relationship between pressure and flow during the period of lowest urethral resistance (between minimum voiding pressure and detrusor pressure at maximal flow).
- Urethra considered as a *collapsible* and *distensible* tube.
- Pressure is required to open lumen before flow can start.
- Flow controlling zone (FCZ): urethral segment which controls flow rate/pattern.
- Parameters characterise outlet function:

  - Minimum urethral opening pressure (Pmuo) reflects the collapsibility of FCZ.
  - Cross-sectional area (CSA) of FCZ reflects the distensibility of FCZ.
- In a normal outflow, FCZ = pelvic floor.
- In BOO, FCZ = site of obstruction.
- Types of BOO: *compressive* and *constrictive* (Table 19.1 and Figure 19.7).

# Urinary Retention
## Acute Urinary Retention (AUR)

- *Definition* – sudden painful inability to void (500–800 mL retained urine).
- Painless AUR is rare and is often associated with central nervous system pathology.
- *Incidence:* 5–25 cases per 1,000 person-years.
- *Aetiology* unclear:
  - *BOO:* static obstruction (e.g., BPO, urethral stricture) or dynamic obstruction (increased α-adrenergic activity such as drugs or post-op pain).
  - *Bladder overdistension* (e.g., post anaesthesia, immobility, drugs, alcohol excess).
  - Neuropathic causes (e.g., diabetic cystopathy).
- *Possible mechanisms:*
  - Prostatic infarction.
  - Increased α-adrenergic activity.
  - Decrease in the stromal-epithelial ratio.
  - Neurotransmitter modulation → decrease nonadrenergic, noncholinergic transmitters (e.g., vasoactive polypeptide [VIP]).
  - Prostatic inflammation.

## Chronic Urinary Retention

- *Definition (ICS):* non-painful bladder which remains palpable or percussable after the patient has passed urine (>800 mL retained urine).
- Classified according to detrusor pressure at the end of micturition.
  - *Low pressure*
    - Normal detrusor pressure at the end of micturition ('end void pressure').
    - Reduced bladder contractility and normal compliance.
    - No upper tract changes and normal renal function.
  - *High pressure*
    - Increased end void pressure.
    - Preserved bladder contractility and impaired compliance.
    - If end void pressure is >25 cm $H_2O$ → upper tract dilation and renal impairment
- *Decompression haematuria*

- Chronic retention causes structural changes in the bladder.
  - Affects the integrity of capillaries and tissues within the wall.
  - Smooth muscle hypertrophy occurs to increase contractility → eventually leading to the thickening, trabeculation, and friability of the bladder wall
- Rapid bladder decompression can drop intravesical pressure to ~50% of the initial value after drainage of ~100 mL of urine.
- The pressure change and 'collapse' of the bladder may induce haematuria (2–16% of cases) from the capillaries.

## Post obstructive diuresis (POD)

- *Definition:* a state of marked polyuria following relief of bilateral ureteric obstruction or obstruction of a solitary functioning kidney.
- 10% of men presenting with urinary retention.
- 60% of cases of obstructive AKI.

### Physiological POD

- Self-limiting response, lasts around 24–48 hours.
- Elimination of accumulated excess water, salt, urea, and solutes.
- Atrial natriuretic peptide (ANP):
  - Released due to intravascular volume expansion.
  - Causes afferent arteriolar dilation and efferent arteriolar vasoconstriction → increasing glomerular filtration pressure and inhibiting renin release
- Promotes diuresis and natriuresis.

### Pathologic POD

- Water and salt elimination continue despite homeostasis being reached.
- May result in hypovolaemia, electrolyte abnormalities, and acid–base imbalance.
- Sodium transporters are down-regulated, resulting in impaired sodium reabsorption.
- Downregulation due to reduced substrate delivery in the period of obstruction.
- PGE2 released due to obstruction → reduces sodium transport in thick ascending limb and collecting duct.
- Reduced expression of water channel proteins (AQP1, AQP2 and AQP3) → nephrogenic diabetes insipidus
- Potassium secretion in the collecting duct increases following the relief of obstruction.
- Excretion of phosphate accompanying natriuresis also occurs.
- Magnesium excretion also increases because of ischaemia to the thick limb of the Loop of Henle.
- Urine acidification may become impaired due to deficits in proton and bicarbonate transport.

## Recovery of Renal Function Occurs in Two Phases

1. Tubular phase: ≤2 weeks.
2. Glomerular phase: two weeks to three months.

## Recommended Reading

1. DeLancey J. Structural support of the urethra as it relates to stress urinary incontinence: the Hammock hypothesis. Am J Obstet Gynecol. 1994;170(6):1713–20.
2. Enhorning G. Simultaneous recording of intravesical and intra-urethral pressure. A study on urethral closure in normal and stress incontinent women. Acta Chir Scand Suppl. 1961;(Suppl 276):1–68.
3. Aoki, Y., Brown, H., Brubaker, L. et al. Urinary incontinence in women. Nat Rev Dis Primers. 2017;3:17042.
4. Irwin DE, Milsom I, Hunskaar S, Reilly K, Kopp Z, Herschorn S, et al. Population-based survey of urinary incontinence, overactive bladder, and other lower urinary tract symptoms in five countries: results of the EPIC study. Eur Urol. 2006 Dec 1;50(6):1306–15.
5. Roehrborn CG. Pathology of benign prostatic hyperplasia. Int J Impot Res. 2008 Dec 10;20(S3):S11–8.
6. Chughtai, B, Forde, J, Thomas, D et al. Benign prostatic hyperplasia. Nat Rev Dis Primers. 2016; 2:16031.
7. Mundy AR, Andrich DE. Urethral strictures. BJU Int. 2011;107(1):6–26.
8. Osman NI, Chapple CR. Fowler's syndrome – a cause of unexplained urinary retention in young women? Nat Rev Urol. 2014;11(2):87–98.
9. Sekido N. Bladder contractility and urethral resistance relation: what does a pressure flow study tell us? Int J Urol. 2012;19(3):216–28.

# 20 Neurogenic Lower Urinary Tract and Sexual Dysfunction

*Karl H. Pang, Nadir I. Osman, and Altaf Mangera*

## Spinal Cord Neuroanatomy

- The spinal cord ends at vertebra level L1/2 (Figure 20.1).
- *Blood supply of the spinal cord*:
  - One anterior spinal artery (from vertebral artery)
  - Two posterior spinal arteries (from vertebral artery)
  - Medullary arteries
  - Radicular arteries
  - Artery of Adamkiewicz (from anterior segmental medullary artery):
    - Supplies the inferior two-thirds.
    - Originates on the left (75%) side of the aorta between the T8-L1 vertebrae.

## Descending Tracts

- Motor signals
- *Pyramidal tracts* originate in the cerebral cortex.
  - Voluntary control of musculature.
- *Extrapyramidal tracts* originate in the brainstem.
  - Involuntary and autonomic control of muscle tone, balance, posture, and locomotion.
- Upper motor neurons (UMN):
  - Cell bodies are located in the cerebral cortex/brainstem.
  - Axons remain within the central nervous system (CNS).
  - Synapse with lower motor neuron (LMN) → muscle

### Corticospinal (Pyramidal) Tract

- Cerebral cortex → divides at the medulla
- *Lateral corticospinal* decussates at the medulla and descends into the spinal cord and synapse with LMNs at the ventral horn.
- The *anterior corticospinal* descends into the spinal cord and decussates and synapses in the ventral horn of the cervical and upper thoracic segment levels.

### Corticobulbar (Pyramidal) Tract

- Cerebral cortex → nuclei of the cranial nerves → LMN → face and neck muscles

## Extrapyramidal Tracts

- *Vestibulospinal*
  - Medial and lateral tracts
  - Arises from the vestibular nuclei.
  - Receives input from the organs of balance.
- *Reticulospinal*
  - The medial tract arises from the pons, which facilitates voluntary movements and increases tone.
  - The lateral tract arises from the medulla, which inhibits voluntary movements and reduces tone.
- *Rubrospinal*
  - Arises from the midbrain red nucleus.
  - In charge of fine control of hand movements.
- *Tectospinal*
  - Begins at the midbrain.
  - Coordinates movements of the head in relation to visual stimuli.

## Ascending Tracts

- Sensory signals

### Dorsal Column-Medial Lemniscal (DCML) Tract

- Fine touch (tactile sensation), vibration, proprioception
- In the *spinal cord*, signals travel in the dorsal (posterior) column.
- In the *brainstem*, signals are transmitted through the medial lemniscus.
- *First-order neuron*
  - Upper limb (>T6) → lateral DC → Medulla nucleus cuneatus
  - Lower limb (<T6) → medial DC → Medulla nucleus gracilis

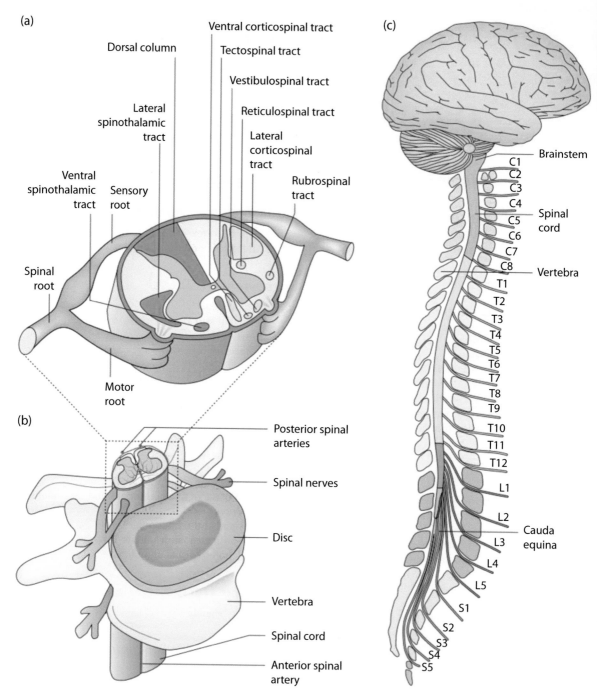

**Figure 20.1** Anatomy of the spinal cord. (a) The spinal cord is organised into grey matter (neuronal cell bodies) and white matter (myelinated axons). The white matter can be subdivided into ascending or descending tracts, which are composed of bundles of axons that originate from and project to specific regions in the brain and periphery. These tracts transmit specific information, such as sensory information (e.g., temperature/itch) or motor information. spinal nerve roots enter the spinal cord and either convey sensory information to the spinal cord (through the sensory/dorsal root) or convey motor information to the periphery (through the motor/ventral root); (b–c) the vertebral column encircles the spinal cord in protective bone and ligament, which is segmented into 7 cervical, 12 thoracic, 5 lumbar and 5 sacral vertebrae. blood is supplied to the spinal cord by the spinal arteries, which are located anteriorly and posteriorly and branch to perfuse the spinal cord parenchyma. (Reprinted by permission from Springer Nature [2])

- *Second-order neuron*
  - Begins at the medulla nucleus cuneatus/gracilis.
  - Decussate → contralateral medial lemniscus → thalamus
- *Third-order neuron*
  - Thalamus → ipsilateral sensory cortex

## Anterolateral System

- *Anterior spinothalamic* tract – crude touch and pressure.
- *Lateral spinothalamic* – pain and temperature.
- *First-order neuron*
  - Sensory receptors → enter the spinal cord and ascend 1–2 vertebral levels → synapse at the dorsal horn (substantia gelatinosa)
- *Second-order neuron*
  - Substantia gelatinosa → decussate within the spinal cord → thalamus
  - Crude touch and pressure fibres → anterior spinothalamic tract
  - Pain and temperature fibres → lateral spinothalamic tract
- *Third-order neuron*
  - Thalamus → ipsilateral sensory cortex

## Spinocerebellar Tracts (Unconscious Sensation)

- Muscles → cerebellum
- *Posterior and anterior spinocerebellar tracts* – proprioception information from the *lower* limbs to the ipsilateral cerebellum.
- *Cuneocerebellar and rostral spinocerebellar tracts* – proprioception information from the *upper* limbs to the ipsilateral cerebellum.

## The Lower Urinary Tract and Neuroanatomy (see Chapter 10)

- *Brainstem*
  - Periaqueductal grey
  - Pontine micturition centre (PMC)
  - *Function:* micturition cycle, libido.
- *Sympathetic:* T10-L2 (hypogastric nerve, inferior pelvic plexus)
  - Ejaculation centre
  - *Function:* micturition cycle (detrusor relaxation, involuntary sphincter contraction), ejaculation, psychogenic erections.
- *Parasympathetic:* S2-4 (pelvic nerve)
  - Sacral erection centre
  - Sacral micturition centre
  - *Function:* micturition cycle (detrusor contraction), erection.

- *Somatic:* S2-4 (pudendal nerve)
  - Onuf's nucleus (guard reflex)
  - *Function:* micturition cycle (voluntary sphincter contraction), ejaculation (bulbospongiosus and ischiocavernosus muscle contraction).
- *Bladder control:* storage and voiding phase
  - The disruption in the cerebral, spinal, and/or peripheral neurological control of the micturition cycle results in a neurogenic bladder.
  - Neurogenic lower urinary tract dysfunction (NLUTD):
    - *Storage symptoms:* urgency, frequency, incontinence.
    - *Voiding symptoms:* incomplete bladder emptying, lack of volitional voiding control.

# Spinal Cord Injury

- The patterns of sensorimotor loss with spinal cord injury (SCI) syndromes can be explained by the damage to specific spinal cord tracts with the sparing of other tracts.
- Damage to the spinal cord can result in partial/complete loss of function below the level of the injury.
- *High-flow (non-ischaemic) priapism* may occur:
  - Loss of sympathetic input to the pelvic vasculature → ↑ parasympathetic input and uncontrolled arterial inflow into the penile sinusoidal space
- SCI is divided into four *phases*.

## Phases of Spinal Cord Injury

1. *Acute (<48 hours)*
   - Oedema, haemorrhage, ischaemia, inflammatory cell infiltration, release of cytotoxic products, cell death.
   - This secondary injury leads to necrosis and/or apoptosis of neurons and glial cells, (oligodendrocytes) → demyelination and the loss of neural circuits
2. *Subacute (14 hours–14 days)*
   - Further ischaemia occurs due to ongoing oedema, vessel thrombosis, and vasospasm.
   - Persistent inflammatory cell infiltration → further cell death
   - Astrocytes proliferate and deposit extracellular matrix molecules into the perilesional area.
3. *Intermediate (14 days–6 months)* and 4. *Chronic (>6 months)*
   - Axons continue to degenerate.
   - Astroglial scar matures to become a potent inhibitor of regeneration.

- Cystic cavities coalesce → restrict axonal regrowth and cell migration

## Shock

### Spinal Shock

- A temporary clinical state of flaccid paralysis post-SCI, including the loss of motor, sensory, autonomic, and reflex function at/below the level of injury.

### Neurogenic Shock

- Hypotensive state caused by loss of sympathetic outflow (↑ vasodilatation).

## Spinal Cord Syndromes (Figure 20.2)

### Central Cord Syndrome

- Disproportionate motor impairment of the upper limbs compared with the lower limbs.
- Complete, non-selective injury to the corticospinal tract, which transmit impulses related to fine hand and finger movements.
- Preservation of the extrapyramidal tracts which control gross leg and proximal arm movements.

### Brown-Séquard Syndrome

- Different levels of sensorimotor, pain and temperature loss.
- Contralateral pain and temperature loss detected

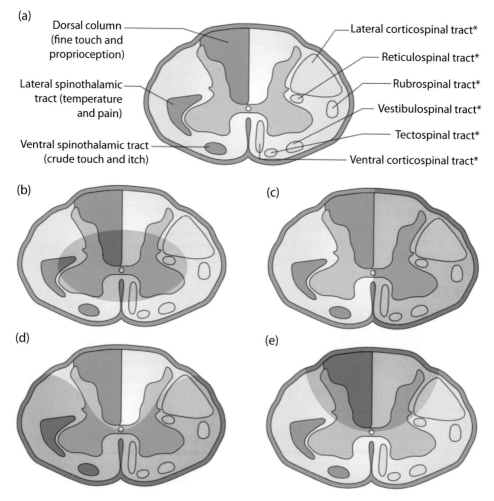

(a)
Dorsal column (fine touch and proprioception)
Lateral spinothalamic tract (temperature and pain)
Ventral spinothalamic tract (crude touch and itch)
Lateral corticospinal tract*
Reticulospinal tract*
Rubrospinal tract*
Vestibulospinal tract*
Tectospinal tract*
Ventral corticospinal tract*

(b)　(c)　(d)　(e)

Figure 20.2 Spinal cord injury syndromes. (a) The major descending motor tracts are in yellow and the major ascending sensory tracts are in blue; (b) Central cord syndrome; (c) Brown-Séquard syndrome; (d) Anterior cord syndrome; (e) Posterior cord syndrome. (Reprinted by permission from Springer Nature [2])

several levels below that of the ipsilateral sensorimotor loss.

- Decussation of the lateral spinothalamic tract over several spinal segments.

## Anterior Cord Syndrome

- Complete motor paralysis due to damage to the corticospinal tract.
- Loss of pain and temperature sensation

secondary to damage of the spinothalamic tract.

- Preservation of light-touch sensation and proprioception (dorsal columns are generally preserved).

## Posterior Cord Syndrome

- Loss of light touch and proprioception.
- Preservation of motor function, pain, and/or temperature sensation.

**Table 20.1** Causes of Neurourological Disorders by Location

| Location | Disorders |
| --- | --- |
| Suprapontine and pontine | Cerebral palsy |
| | Cerebrovascular accident |
| | Head injury |
| | Multiple sclerosis |
| | Parkinson's disease |
| | Multiple System Atrophy |
| | Dementia |
| | Cerebral tumour |
| Spinal | Spinal dysraphism |
| | Myelomeningocele |
| | Spina bifida |
| | Spinal cord injury |
| | Traumatic |
| | Tumour |
| | Infective (tuberculosis) |
| | Multiple sclerosis |
| | Cervical spondylosis |
| Sacral | Spinal cord injury |
| | Spinal dysraphism |
| | Sacral agenesis |
| | Anorectal anomalies |
| Peripheral nerves | Disk prolapses |
| | Cauda equina syndrome |
| | Peripheral neuropathy |
| | Diabetes |
| | Alcohol excess |
| | Vitamin B12 deficiency |
| | Guillain Barre syndrome |
| | Amyloidosis |
| | Pelvic surgery |

# Classification of Neuropathic Lesions

1. Lesions/disease can be classified by *location* (Table 20.1):
2. Suprapontine and pontine.
3. Spinal (infrapontine and suprasacral): UMN-type injury.
4. Sacral and infrasacral: LMN-type injury.

## Functional Outcome

- Bladder function depends on the location of the pathology.
- Bowel and sexual function may also be affected.
- Functional outcome (Madersbacher):
  - *Bladder:* over or underactive, good or poor compliance.
  - *Bladder neck:* failure to relax (can also be caused by non-neurogenic smooth muscle hypertrophy).
  - *Urethral sphincter:* over or underactive.
- Bladder and sphincter function, symptoms, ultrasound (USS), and video urodynamic (VUDS) findings are summarised in Table 20.2.

## Clinical Features

- History, neurological examination, USS, and VUDS (Figure 20.3) are required for full assessment.

- SCI – 70–84% have NLUTD.
  - Possible development of a new spinal reflex mediated by C fibres in an attempt to 'reorganise' synaptic connections.
  - Possible role of neurotrophic hormones (e.g., nerve growth factor) in neuropathic bladder dysfunction.
- Detrusor overactivity on VUDS secondary to neurological disease is termed *'neurogenic detrusor overactivity (NDO)'*.
- Management options for NDO:
  - *Medical:* anticholinergics, intravesical botulinum toxin A (Figure 20.4).
  - *Surgical:* sacral neuromodulation (doesn't work in complete SCI), augmentation cystoplasty.
- Spinal injury/lesions may cause overactivity in both the bladder and urethral sphincter.
  - Uncoordinated contraction/relaxation → detrusor sphincter dyssynergia (DSD)
  - Defined as *involuntary contraction of the urethral rhabdosphincter simultaneously with a detrusor contraction.*
- Management options for DSD:
  - Urethral stent (with sheath catheter)
  - External sphincterotomy
  - Intravesical toxins and intermittent self-catheterisation (ISC)
  - Cystoplasty and ISC
  - Indwelling catheter
- Unsafe, high-pressure bladders (spinal region):
  - *VUDS trace:* DSD (saw-tooth), NDO, high detrusor leak point pressure (DLLP).

**Table 20.2** Patterns of Lower Urinary Tract Dysfunction Following Neurological Disease

| Location | Bladder | Urethral Sphincter | Signs and Symptoms | Potential VUDS Findings (Figure 20.3) |
|---|---|---|---|---|
| Suprapontine Pontine | Overactive Reflexic Safe Low pressure | Nomo-active | Storage symptoms | Insignificant PVR NDO |
| Spinal Suprasacral | Overactive Reflexic Unsafe High pressure | Overactive | Storage Voiding Risk of high renal pressures Autonomic dysreflexia | Raised PVR NDO DSD Poor compliance VUR |
| Sacral Infrasacral | Underactive Areflexic Acontractile Safe Low Pressure | Nomo- or underactive | Voiding Risk of high renal pressures | Raised PVR Acontractile bladder Poor compliance SUI |

*Abbreviations:* VUDS, video urodynamics; PVR, post-void residual; NDO, neurogenic detrusor overactivity; DSD, detrusor sphincter dyssynergia; VUR, vesico-ureteric reflux; SUI, stress urinary incontinence.

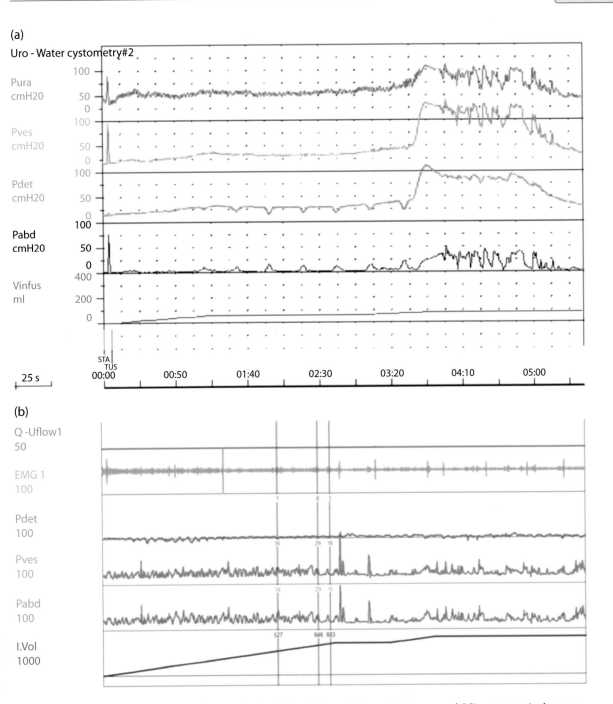

**Figure 20.3** Video urodynamic traces from patients with spinal cord injury. (a) Suprasacral SCI: neurogenic detrusor overactivity with detrusor sphincter dyssynergia (saw-toothed pattern) and reduced bladder compliance; (b) Sacral SCI: detrusor acontractility and a large capacity bladder. (Reprinted by permission from Springer Nature [3])

- DLLP >40 cmH$_2$0 → risk of renal injury, VUR, and hydronephrosis.
- DLLP is defined as *'the lowest pressure at which urine leakage occurs in the absence of detrusor contraction or increased abdominal pressure'.*

- *Cystography:* VUR, contracted urethral sphincter, trabeculated bladder.
- Underactive sphincter or sphincter insufficiency:
- Urinary leakage
- *Management:*

- Catheter sheaths (male)

- Consists of light and heavy chains.

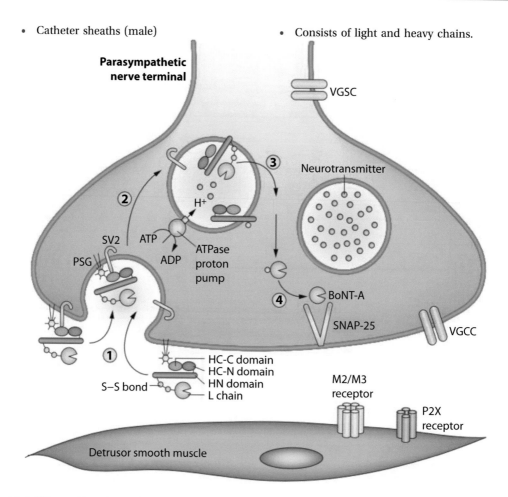

Figure 20.4 Effects of botulinum Toxin A on detrusor smooth muscle contraction. (1) BoTN-A binds to PSG and SV2 receptors; (2) Endocytosis of BoTN-A; (3) Release of BoTN-A light chain; (4) Cleavage of SNAP-25. BoNT-A, botulinum toxin A; HC-C, heavy chain, N-terminal fragment, C-terminal domain; HC-N, heavy chain, N-terminal fragment, N-terminal domain; HN, heavy chain N-terminal fragment; L, light chain; M2, muscarinic acetylcholine receptor subtype 2; M3, muscarinic acetylcholine receptor subtype 3; PSG, polysialoganglioside; P2X, purinergic receptor; SNAP-25, synaptosomal-associated protein 25; SV2, synaptic vesicle associated protein-2; VGCC, voltage-gated calcium channel; VGSC, voltage-gated sodium channel. (Reprinted by permission from Springer Nature [4])

- Urethral bulking agents
- Urethral tapes/slings
- Artificial urinary sphincter
- Management of acontractile bladder:
  - Long-term ISC or indwelling urethral/suprapubic catheters.

## Botulinum Toxin

- Neurotoxin derived from *Clostridium botulinum*.
- Seven serotypes (A-G).
- Botulinum toxin A (BoNT-A) and B (BoNT-B) have been developed for clinical use.

- *Mechanism*:
  - Intravesical injection (LA flexible cystoscopy or GA rigid cystoscopy).
  - NICE guidelines: starting dose is at 200 units.
  - No consensus on technique and the number of injections. Generally:
    - Dilute with normal saline at 10 units per mL.
    - 1mL per intradetrusor/submucosal injections (e.g., 20 injections consisting of 200 units).
    - Trigone sparing.
  - BoTN-A binds to PSG and SV2 receptor → endocytosed → light chain is released →

cleaves SNAP-25 → prevents fusion of pre-synaptic ACh vesicles with the neuromuscular junction → blocks ACh release → reduces stimulation of detrusor muscarinic receptors → reduces detrusor contraction.

## Autonomic Dysreflexia (AD)

- This is considered a medical emergency.
- Sudden and exaggerated autonomic response to various stimuli.
- Occurs in SCI *at/above T6 level* (sympathetic outflow).
- Defined as systolic BP *>20 mmHg.*
- *Causes:* any noxious stimuli below the level of SCI.
  - Bladder distention/irritation (~75–85%) – urinary tract infection (UTI) and blocked catheter.
  - Bowel distention (~13–19%) – faecal impaction.
  - Interventions – catheterisation, urodynamics (ensure slow fill rate 10–20 mL/s), cystoscopy.
  - Urinary tract calculi.
  - Pressure sores, distal skin infection, fractures, ingrown toenails.
- *Mechanism* (Figure 20.5):
  - Noxious stimuli → 1) sympathetic discharge → reflex vasoconstriction below level of SCI → systemic hypertension and pale skin/cool peripheries → carotid bodies detect raised BP → 2) reflex parasympathetic vagal discharge to lower BP → brachycardia and vasodilatation → flushed and sweaty above SCI level
- *Clinical features:*
  - Headache, blurred vision, stuffy nose
  - Piloerection
  - Flushing, sweating (above lesion)
  - Pale, cold skin (below lesion)
- *Untreated* can lead to:
  - Seizures
  - Cerebral haemorrhage
  - Retinal detachment
  - Death
- *Management:*
  - Recognition
  - Treat the cause (e.g., drain bladder, evacuate the bowel)
  - Sit upright to induce orthostatic hypotension
  - Sublingual glyceryl trinitrate, oral nifedipine, intravenous labetalol/phentolamine

## Sexual Function

- *Neurophysiology of erection/ejaculation – See Chapter 12.*
- *Neurosexuality components:*
  - Psychological stimuli
  - Cerebral cortex, brainstem
  - Ejaculation centre: T10-L2 (sympathetic)
- Erection centre: S2–4 (parasympathetic)
- Sensation: S2–4, somatic (pudendal)
- *Spinal cord injury:*
  - Psychogenic erection (sympathetic)
  - Reflex erection (parasympathetic)
- *Erectile dysfunction* treatment:
  - Medications: phosphodiesterase-5 inhibitors, prostaglandin E1
  - Vacuum device
  - Penile prosthesis
- *Ejaculatory dysfunction* treatment:
  - *Vibrator:* stimulates reflex ejaculation
  - *Neural Brindley electroejaculator:* stimulates sympathetic nerves. Spastic lesions with distal (including T10) autonomic cord
  - *Rectal Seager electroejaculator:* all patients
- Patterns of sexual function are summarised in Table 20.3.
- *Sperm parameters:* normal sperm concentration, ↓ motility and viability.
  - *Associations:*
    - Scrotal hyperthermia (prolonged period in wheelchair)
    - Infrequent ejaculation (semen stasis)
    - Seminal plasma
    - Seminal vesicle dysfunction
    - Leucocytospermia
    - ↑ cytokines (IL-1 beta, TNF-alpha, IL6), ↑ reactive oxygen species
    - Endocrinopathy: variable results – some studies showed lower levels of FSH, LH, testosterone in SCI vs control, some showed no difference.

# Specific Neuropathologies
## Dementia

- Alzheimer's (80%), vascular (10%), other (10%).
- *Syndrome complex:* deterioration in memory, thinking, behaviour, and the ability to perform everyday activity.
- Caution with anticholinergics in the elderly (trospium preferred).

## Multiple Sclerosis

- Demyelination of nerve fibres.
- White plaques in the central nervous system and spinal cord.
- Relapsing-remitting in ~85%.

## Parkinson's Disease

- Degeneration of substantia nigra in the basal ganglia.
- Dopamine deficiency.
- *Triad:* resting tremor, bradykinesia, rigidity.

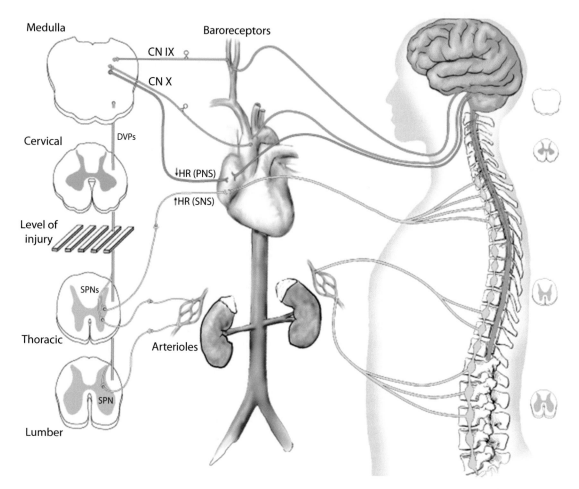

**Figure 20.5** Autonomic dysreflexia. Injury at the cervical level (≥T6) Results in increased sympathetic output (yellow) below the level and increased parasympathetic output (blue) above the level of injury. Parasympathetic afferents (green) from the aortic arch and carotid artery baroreceptors travel to the medulla through the glosso-pharyngeal (CN IX) and Vagus (CN X) Nerves. SPN, sympathetic preganglionic neurons; DVP, descending vasomotor pathway; PNS, parasympathetic nervous system; SNS, sympathetic nervous system; HR, heart rate; CN, cranial nerve. (Reprinted with permission from Wolters Kluwer Health, Inc. [5])

**Table 20.3** Pattern of Sexual Function According to Location of Spinal Cord Injury

| Location | Erection | Ejaculation | Autonomic Dysreflexia | Fertility Treatment Options |
|---|---|---|---|---|
| >T6 *spastic* | Reflex | Reflex | Yes | Vibrator |
| | | Antegrade, propulsive | | Brindley or Saeger electroejaculator |
| T10 *spastic* | Reflex | Absent | No | Saeger electroejaculator |
| | | | | Sperm retrieval |
| T8 *flaccid* | Absent | Absent | No | Saeger electroejaculator |
| | | | | Sperm retrieval |
| L4 *flaccid* or sacral | Psychogenic | Psychogenic | No | Retrograde ejaculation sample from bladder for in vitro fertilisation |
| | | | | Saeger electroejaculator |
| | | | | Sperm retrieval |

## Multiple System Atrophy

- Rare, degenerative neurological disorder
- Formerly called Shy-Drager syndrome
- Alpha-synuclein deposits in oligodendrocytes in the mid brain, basal ganglia, pons and cerebellum
- Affects autonomic functions, such as blood pressure, breathing, bladder function
- Two types:
  - Parkinsonian type
    - Signs and symptoms similar to Parkinson's disease
  - Cerebellar type
    - Ataxia, dysarthria, visual disturbances, dysphagia

## Spina Bifida

- Spina bifida occult
- Spina bifida aperta
  - Meningocele (meninges)
  - Myelomeningocele (meninges and cord)
  - Open or closed
- Sacral agenesis
- *Cause:* failure of neural tube closure.
  - Folate deficiency
  - Mutation of 5,10-Methylenetetrahydrofolate reductase gene
- 25% contractile bladder, 10% acontractile, 65% intermediate

## Cauda Equina Syndrome

- Compression of the cauda equina.
- L4/5, L5/S1

- *Causes:*
  - Disc prolapses
  - Trauma
  - Malignant compression
- Acute back pain, saddle anaesthesia, painless urinary retention, flaccid paralysis
- Emergency management with steroids and referral to spinal surgeons, or oncologists for consideration of radiotherapy for malignant causes.

## Recommended Reading

1. Panicker JN, Fowler CJ, Kessler TM. Lower urinary tract dysfunction in the neurological patient: clinical assessment and management. Lancet Neurol. 2015;14(7):720–32.
2. Ahuja CS, Wilson JR, Nori S, et al. Traumatic spinal cord injury. Nat Rev Dis Primers. 2017;3:17018.
3. Hamid R, Averbeck MA, Chiang H, Garcia A, Al Mousa RT, Oh S-J, et al. Epidemiology and pathophysiology of neurogenic bladder after spinal cord injury. World J Urol. 2018;36 (10):1517–27.
4. Jiang Y-H, Liao C-H, Kuo H-C. Current and potential urological applications of botulinum toxin A. Nat Rev Urol. 2015;12(9):519–33.
5. Furlan JC. Autonomic dysreflexia: a clinical emergency. J Trauma Acute Care Surg. 2013;75(3):496–500.
6. Everaert, K, de Waard, W, Van Hoof, T. et al. Neuroanatomy and neurophysiology related to sexual dysfunction in male neurogenic patients with lesions to the spinal cord or peripheral nerves. Spinal Cord. 2010;48(3):182–91.
7. Ibrahim E, Lynne CM, Brackett NL. Male fertility following spinal cord injury: an update. Andrology. 2016;4(1): 13–26.

# 21 | Penoscrotal Pathology

*Karl H. Pang and Majid Shabbir*

## Penile Disorders

### Phimosis

- The inability to retract the prepuce due to tightness.
- It may be pathological or physiological (Table 21.1).

- *Associated complications:*
  - *Lichen sclerosus (LS):* ~5% of cases may progress to penile cancer, but it has a long latency period (~17 years). Phimosis increases the odd ratio of developing cancer (OR 4.9–37.2). Neonatal circumcision is protective (OR 0.33). LS is associated with well-differentiated and keratinising squamous cell carcinoma subtypes.
  - *Balanitis* (inflammation of the glans penis) and *posthitis* (inflammation of the prepuce, Figure 21.1c) – inflammatory secretions and pus are trapped under the foreskin, not in the foreskin by the phimotic band.
  - *Treatment:* improve hygiene. Antibiotics/anti-fungals dependent on infective cause. Circumcision for recurrent infections
  - Other causes of balanitis include local irritants, Candida fungal infection, psoriasis, eczema, sexually transmitted infection (STI, see below), Zoon's.
  - *Paraphimosis* (Figure 21.1d): prepuce gets stuck in the retracted state → venous congestion → oedema → swelling → arterial occlusion and necrosis
  - *Treatment:* manual reduction but if unsuccessful → surgical reduction, dorsal slit +/- circumcision

### Zoon's Balanitis

- Also referred to as 'plasma cell balanitis'.
- Tends to occur in older, uncircumcised men (Figure 21.1e).
- Well-circumcised, shiny, moist, erythematous plaque on the glans (Cayenne pepper). Typically, corresponding to a 'mirror image' or 'kissing' lesion on the glans.
- Chronic inflammation with plasma cells infiltrating the dermis.

- *Treatment:* Steroid ointments. Circumcision if persists. Biopsy red area if there are any clinical doubts of premalignant/malignant lesions.

### Lichen Planus

- Affects all age groups.
- Affects the skin, mucous membranes, scalp, and nails.
- *On the penis:* red-purple annular plaques on the glans and coronal sulcus (Figure 21.1f).
- *Treatment:* Steroid ointments. Biopsy if there are any clinical doubts.

### Urethritis

- Inflammation of the urethra
- *Presentation:* pain, dysuria, bleeding, itch, discharge.
- May cause urethral stricture and present with weak stream and prolonged flow (see Chapter 19).
- *Causes:* may be infective or non-infective.
- Infective can be associated with STI (see Chapter 16).
  - *Gonococcus*
  - *Chlamydia trachomatis*
  - *Herpes Simplex virus*
  - *Treponema pallidum* (Syphilis)
    - *Primary:* penile chancre (Figure 21.1g) – develop ~3 weeks after exposure.
    - *Secondary:* extensive symmetrical, erythematous rash on the trunk and extremities appearing ~6 week–6 months after infection.
    - *Latent:* untreated disease moves from the secondary stage to the asymptomatic latent stage.
    - *Late:* benign tertiary, neurosyphilis, or cardiovascular syphilis.
    - *Treatment:* penicillin, contact tracing, and serology follow-up.
  - Genital/urethral warts
    - Caused by the human papilloma virus (HPV).
    - Associated with the risk of cancer (HPV types 6, 11 and 16, 18) (see Chapter 27).

**Table 21.1** Features of Pathological and Physiological Phimosis

| Features | Pathological | Physiological |
|---|---|---|
| Appearance | Most commonly due to BXO, also known as genital lichen sclerosis: thickened, scarred, fissured prepuce with pale white ring causing an hourglass or 'waisting' effect. | Carnation flower: inner mucosa pouts through the preputial opening (Figure 21.1b). |
| | Active areas of inflammation (red) with firm white plaques/scar tissue. | |
| | Can lead to complete fusion of the prepuce to the glans (Figure 21.1a). | |
| Pathology | BXO: Hyperkeratosis, atrophic epidermis. Fibrosis and dermal oedema. Infiltration of T lymphocytes. Autoimmune aetiology suggested. Can affect prepuce, glans and urethral mucosa | Preputial adhesions separate by proximal desquamation, may be due to infection of retained smegma. |
| Clinical features | BXO: Affects 1 in 300–1,000 men of all ages. | Phimosis: 8% in 6-7y, 1% in 16-17y |
| | Uncommon under the age of 5 years (~1%). | Preputial adhesion: 63% in 6-7y, 3% in 16-17y |
| | Often associated with post micturition dribble. | |
| | Inability/difficulty/pain on retracting foreskin/ dyspareunia due to splitting of skin. | |
| | Spraying of stream (meatal stenosis) | |
| | Obstructive LUTS (urethral stricture). | |
| | Associated with penile cancer | |
| Treatment | Mild – may benefit from emollient creams/ barrier creams and topical steroids. | Conservative |
| | Moderate – severe or failed medical therapy: Circumcision. | |
| | If BXO is affecting the glans and refractory to medical therapy, may need glans resurfacing. | |
| | If affecting the urethra, may require urethroplasty. | |

*Abbreviations:* BXO, balanitis xerotica obliterans; LUTS, lower urinary tract symptoms.

- Asymptomatic or present with single or multiple 'cauliflower'-shaped lesions (Figure 21.1h).
- *Treatment:* topical cryotherapy, topical imiquimod cream, surgical excision, contact tracing, and consideration of HPV vaccination.
- Non-STI organisms: coliforms, streptococci.

- *Reactive arthritis (formerly known as Reiter's syndrome):*
  - *Triad:* urethritis, conjunctivitis, seronegative arthritis.
  - Tends to present in younger men.
  - Can be caused by *Chlamydia trachomatis.*

# Crohns' Disease of the Penis

- Diagnosed at the same time as intestinal Crohn's in >50%.
- It has an autoimmune aetiology.
- *Features:* ulcers, fissuring. Can also present with penile or penoscrotal lymphoedema.
- *Management:* MDT with colorectal and dermatology. Disease modifying drugs including azathioprine, compressive dressings for lymphoedema and excision of any residual lesion.

Other *benign, premalignant, and malignant* pathologies such as penile intraepithelial neoplasia (PeIN) (previously known as Bowen's disease (BD) and

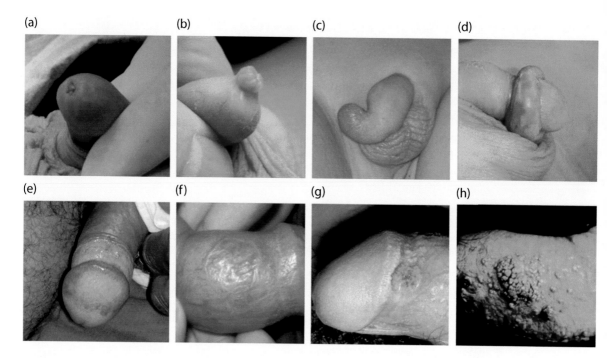

**Figure 21.1** Benign Penile Pathology. (a) Balanitis Xerotica Obliterans; (b) Physiological Phimosis; (c) Posthitis; (d) Paraphimosis; (e) Zoon's Balanitis; (f) Lichen Planus; (g) Genile Chancre; (h) Genital Warts. (a–c) Reprinted from Hindawi [7]; (d–e) Reuse with permission from Wolters Kluwer Medknow Publications [8]; (g) Reprinted with permission from Elsevier [9]; (h) Reuse with permission from John Wiley and Sons [3]

Erythroplasia of Queyrat (EQ)), Human Papilloma Virus (HPV), warty lesions, and squamous cell carcinoma are discussed in Chapter 27.

# Priapism

- Unwanted painful erection of the penis not associated with sexual desire lasting for over four hours.
- Categorised into ischaemic, non-ischaemic and stuttering priapism (Table 21.2):
  - *Ischaemic*
    - Low flow
    - Veno-occlusion
  - *Non-ischaemic*
    - High flow
    - Cavernosal artery and corporal tissue fistula
  - *Stuttering* (recurrent or intermittent)
    - Repetitive ischaemic and painful episodes of prolonged erections typically lasting <1–2 hours.
    - Intervening periods of detumescence.
    - Often self-limiting.
    - Aetiology is similar to that of ischaemic priapism. Often, they are a warning sign and the 'tremors before the earthquake' of a fulminant ischaemic priapism.

- *Aetiology:* same as in ischaemic priapism.
- *Acute management:* treatment of underlying cause. Aspiration and intracavernosal injection with alpha-adrenergic drugs during acute episodes.
- *Prevention:* modification of underlying cause (stop causative medication), optimise management of sickle cell disease (hydration/ oxygenation/warmth/analgesia), reduction of HbS%, consideration of disease-modifying treatment of sickle cell (hydroxyurea). Use of alpha-adrenergic drugs such as Etilefrine, or hormonal suprression with cyproterone acetate.
- Preventive treatments are discussed in Chapter 30.

- Pathophysiology of low flow priapism
  - Veno-occlusion → 'compartment syndrome' → cavernosal smooth muscle anoxia → failure of muscle contraction → persistent erection → continual anoxia and smooth muscle necrosis
  - <12 hours: minimal trabecular oedema.
  - 24–48 hours: endothelial destruction.
  - >48 hours: endothelial denudation, smooth muscle necrosis, fibrosis of trabeculae, smooth muscle cell transformation.

**Table 21.2** Features of Ischaemic and Non-ischaemic Priapism

| Features | Ischaemic | Non-ischaemic |
|---|---|---|
| Mechanism | Low flow | High flow |
| | Veno-occlusion | Unregulated cavernous arterial inflow |
| | Trapping of blood within the corpus cavernosa | Cavernosal artery and corporal tissue fistula. |
| Causes | Haematological disorders | Penile/perineal trauma |
| | Sickle cell disease | Spinal cord injury |
| | Leukaemia | |
| | Thalassaemia | |
| | Pelvic malignancy (rare) | |
| | Penile metastases to corpus cavernosum | |
| | Antiphospholipid syndrome | |
| | Medications (Chapter 30) | |
| | Treatments for erectile dysfunction | |
| | Intracavernosal injections | |
| | Antipsychotics | |
| | Anticoagulants | |
| | Antidepressants | |
| Clinical features | Painful erection | Painless |
| | Rigid corpus cavernosum and a soft glans | Not fully rigid |
| Corporeal blood gas | | |
| $pO_2$ | <30 mmHg | >90 mmHg |
| $pCO_2$ | >60 mmHg | <40 mmHg |
| pH | <7.25 | 7.4 |
| Lactate | Raised | Normal |
| Treatment | <48 h duration:<br>  Aspiration (~50 mL) +/- saline irrigation | Conservative (perineal pressure/ice packs) |
| | Vasoactive injection:<br>  Phenylephrine: 200 mcg every 5–10 min until detumescence at a maximum of 1 mg within 1 h (with cardiac monitoring). | Pudendal angiography with super-selective embolisation of any fistula |
| | Distal surgical shunt if fails:<br>  Winter, Ebbehoj, Al-Ghorab, T-shunt | Open fistula ligation (rare) |
| | >48 h duration:<br>  Aspiration and phenylephrine as above<br>  Distal T-shut +/- tunnelling | |
| | >72 h duration:<br>  Aspiration and phenylephrine as above.<br>  Consider acute placement of penile prosthesis | |

- General management of idiopathic ischaemic priapism:
  - Full haematological and biochemical assessment including vasculitis screen to exclude any underlying cause.
  - CT Chest-Abdo-Pelvis to exclude underlying malignancy.
  - If due to metastases, radiotherapy or penectomy may be required.

# Scrotal Pathology

## Classification

- Benign or malignant
- Pain or painless
- Intra or extra-testicular
- *Clinical manifestations*: infection, pain, mass/swelling, infertility.

## Varicocele

- Dilatation of the pampiniform venous plexus due to incompetent venous valves, creating a 'bag of worms'.
- 90% on the *left* side:
  - The left renal vein is compressed between the aorta and superior mesenteric artery (*nutcracker*).
  - The left testicular drains into the left renal vein (right drain into IVC).
  - The absence of venous valves is more common on the left.
  - 'Fixed' large varicocele (large grade three which does not change with posture) and right-sided varicoceles may be associated with upper renal tract or retroperitoneal pathology, and abdominal USS is advisable.
- *Hudson's Classification:*
  - *Subclinical:* detected on doppler USS only.
  - *Grade 1:* palpable during a valsalva manoeuvre.
  - *Grade 2:* palpable on standing without valsalva manoeuvre. Not visible.
  - *Grade 3:* visible and palpable.
- Clinically significant grades (grades 1–3) are associated with impaired fertility (see Chapter 22).
- *Indications to treat:* impaired fertility, associated hypogonadism or testicular atrophy, pain.
- *Treatment:* embolisation, laparoscopic or open microsurgical sub-inguinal approach.

## Hydrocele

- A collection of peritoneal fluid between the parietal and visceral layers of the tunica vaginalis.
- Painless fluctuate swelling that may trans-illuminate.

- *Congenital*
  - Patent processus vaginalis (PPV) in 2–5% of boys.
  - 90% resolve by one year (surgical ligation performed after two years).
  - Communicating, non-communicating, or hydrocele of the cord (encysted hydrocele).
  - Communicating hydrocele may be associated with an inguinal-scrotal hernia.
- *Primary*
  - Idiopathic
  - Lymph: obstruction of drainage or reduced absorption.
- *Secondary*
  - Production and accumulation of exudate fluid.
  - Associated with inflammation or malignancy.
- *Investigation:* confirmation on USS and exclusion of underlying testicular pathology.
- *Treatment:* conservative if asymptomatic. If bothered by cosmetic appearance or size - open surgical evacuation of fluid with plication (Lord's plication) or excision/eversion of tunical sac (Jaboulay repair) might be necessary.

## Epididymal Cyst

- Arises as diverticula of the vas deferens.
- Contains clear fluid.
- Incidental finding in 30% of men.
- Spermatocele – if the cysts contain spermatozoa, they typically arise due to obstruction.
- May increase in size over time.
- *Investigation:* confirmation on USS.
- *Treatment:* no intervention required unless pinpoint cause of pain, or bothersome due to size. There is a risk of causing epididymal obstruction with surgery. Avoid surgery if preservation of fertility is potentially important.

## Acute Scrotum

- *Trauma*
  - Haematocele (extra-testicular)
  - Testicular rupture/dislocation/avulsion
  - Diagnosed on history, clinical examination, and scrotal USS.
  - *Treatment:* conservative vs early surgical exploration. Explore if there is a tense haematocele or any testicular rupture. Conservative management is associated with a greater risk of infection testis atrophy and subsequent orchidectomy. Key principles of exploration include the evacuation of hematoma and debridement of extruded non-viable tubules + closure of the albuginea (use of vaginalis flap if cannot oppose albuginea).

- *Infection* – testis (orchitis) and/or epididymis (epididymitis) (Chapter 16).
- *Idiopathic scrotal oedema*
  - Paediatric, peak incidence at 5–6 years.
  - Self-limiting
  - Usually unilateral swelling with erythema.
  - Conservative management with anti-inflammatories.
- *Testicular torsion*
  - Twisting of the spermatic cord → vascular compromise → venous congestion and arterial ischaemia → testicular infarction and necrosis
  - The time before testicular necrosis depends on the degree of torsion.
  - *Neonatal:* extra-vaginalis.
    - Incomplete fixation of the gubernaculum to the scrotal wall.
  - Children/adult: intra-vaginalis.
    - 1:4,000, 25–35% of all acute scrotum cases.
    - Bimodal distribution: first year of life and around puberty (when testis increases in volume).
    - Bilateral in ~10%.
    - An undescended testis leads to increased risk.
    - *Bell clapper:* high investment of the tunica vaginalis.
    - High-riding/painful/swollen testis and absent cremasteric reflex.
  - Urgent scrotal exploration for acute presentation (within six hours of onset of symptoms).
    - If confirmed torsion – detort + wrap in gauze with warm saline and perform testicular 3-point fixation. If it does not regain colour despite detorsion and warm swab, incise tunica albuginea of torted testis; fix if bleeding/viable, and

perform an orchidectomy if non-viable. If torsion is confirmed, contralateral testicular 3-point fixation must be performed.

- *Torsion of testicular appendage*
  - Infarction of the hydatid of morgagni (remnant of the Mullerian duct) → discolouration → blue dot sign

## Genital Lymphoedema

- Lymphatic obstruction → protein and interstitial fluid cannot return to the vascular system → accumulates behind the obstruction → local oedema
- *Primary oedema* (Figure 21.2)
  - Aplasia or hypoplasia of lymphatics.
  - *Congenital:* Milroy's disease.
- *Secondary oedema*
  - Infection (Filariasis)
  - Inflammation (Crohn's)
  - Surgery (Inguinal /Pelvic lymphadenectomy)
  - Radiotherapy (Pelvic / genital tumours)
  - Malignant infiltration (pelvic malignancy)
  - Trauma
- *Management:* compression. Prevention of secondary cellulitis. Surgical excision and primary closure or reconstruction of affected areas. Manage as part of MDT with dermatology.

## Hidradenitis Suppurativa (HS)

- Chronic inflammatory skin disease primarily affecting apocrine gland-rich areas:
  - Inguino-scrotal region
  - Perineum
  - Axillae

(a)  (b)

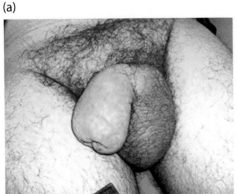 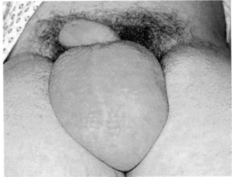

Figure 21.2 Genital Lymphoedema. (a) idiopathic penile lymphoedema in isolation; (b) combined idiopathic penoscrotal lymphoedema. (Reuse with permission from John Wiley and Sons [10])

(a)                                    (b)

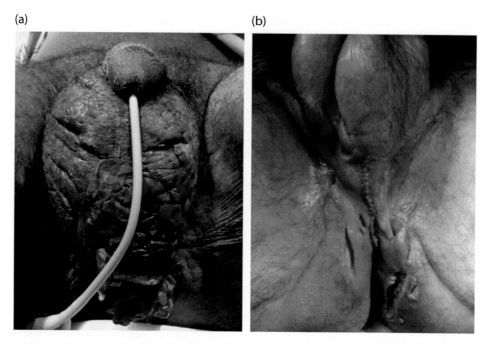

**Figure 21.3** Hidradenitis Suppurativa. (a) Hidradenitis suppurativa involvement of the scrotum with multiple abscesses; (b) Abscesses of perineum have been incised with no resolution. (Reprinted with permission from Elsevier [11])

- Associated with painful nodules, (boils/pimples) abscesses, sinus tracts, and scarring (Figure 21.3).
- Multifactorial causes:
  - *Genetic:* mutations in subunits of gamma-secretase proteins.
  - *Environmental:* obesity, smoking.
  - Bacterial infection can worsen HS.
- Follicular occlusion → follicular rupture → perifollicular lympho-histiocytic inflammation (TNF-alpha, IL-1, IL-17)
- *Management:* MDT management with dermatology, urology (penoscrotal involvement), colorectal (anorectal involvement), and plastics (axilla and all complex reconstruction). Prevention or drainage of recurrent abscesses with complex fistulae laid open. Disease-modifying treatments, including Humira. Antibiotics for infective exacerbations. Resection with skin graft /flap for resistant disease.

## Recommended Reading

1. Thomas, DFM, Duffy PG, Rickwood AMK. Essentials of Paediatric Urology. 2nd Edition. UK: CRC Press; 2008.
2. Omar M. Aboumarzouk. Blandy's Urology, 3rd Edition. UK: John Wiley and Sons; 2019.
3. Buechner SA. Common skin disorders of the penis. BJUI. 2002;90(5):498–506.
4. Shabbir M, Kayes O, Minhas S. Challenges and controversies in the management of penile cancer. Nat Rev Urol.2014;11(12):702–141.
5. BAUS Section of Andrology Genitourethral Surgery, Asif Muneer, Gareth Brown, Trevor Dorkin, Marc Lucky, Richard Pearcy, Majid Shabbir, Chitranjan J. Shukla, Rowland W. Rees and Duncan J. Summerton. BAUS consensus document for the management of male genital emergencies: priapism BJU Int. 2018 Jun;121(6):835–39.
6. Cass AS. Testicular trauma. J Urol. 1983;129(2):299–300.
7. Hayashi, Y et al. Prepuce: phimosis, paraphimosis, and circumcision. Scientific World J. 2011;11: 289–301 (figures 1, 2, 3 and 5).
8. Saraswat, PK  et al. A study of pattern of nonvenereal genital dermatoses of male attending skin OPD at a tertiary care centre. Indian J Sex Transm Dis AIDS. 2014;35(2):129–134 (figures 5 and 8).
9. Sukthankar, A. Syphilis. Medicine. 2010;38(5):263–266 (figure 3).
10. Garaffa, G. The management of genital lymphoedema. BJUI. 2008; 102(4):480–484 (figures 1 and 2).
11. Michel, C. The treatment of genitoperineal hidradenitis suppurativa: a review of the literature. Urology. 2019; 124:105.

# Male Sexual Dysfunction and Male Factor Infertility

*Ian Eardley*

## Erectile Dysfunction (ED)

- *Definition:* inability to achieve or maintain an erection sufficient for satisfactory sexual performance.
- The most common form of ED occurs with ageing.
- Dominant pathology = vascular disease (Table 22.1).
- Increasing prevalence: ~20% of men in their 50s, ~40% in their 60s, and 60% in their 70s.
- A proportion returns to relatively normal erectile function over time – may reflect resolution of 'psychological' ED.

## Erectile Dysfunction at a Cellular Level

- Cavernosal bodies are central to the development of a normal erection.
- Structurally consists of:
  - Blood filled sinusoids
  - Endothelial lined spaces
  - Trabecular network – smooth muscle (SM), connective tissue, nerves
- Damage to these structures will affect erection (vascular endothelium most prone).

## Pathophysiological Processes

- *Smooth muscle function* can be adversely affected by:
  - Uraemia, liver failure, severe hyperglycaemia
  - Drugs (e.g., alpha-adrenoceptor agonists)
- *Smooth muscle loss* occurs with:
  - Arterial disease, hypoxia, prolonged ischaemic priapism
- *Parasympathetic nerves* release nitric oxide (NO), acetylcholine and vasoactive intestinal peptide (VIP).
  - Parasympathetic nerves are lost in:
    - Cavernosal nerve injury
    - Peripheral neuropathy (e.g., diabetic autonomic neuropathy)
- *Endothelium* damage results in reduced NO caused by:
  - Hyperglycaemia, hyperlipidaemia, uraemia, diabetes, hypertension, smoking

## Neurological Erectile Dysfunction

- Neurological control of erection involves (see Chapter 12):
  - Cerebral cortex → descending pathways via hypothalamus → brainstem → spinal cord → sacral nerve (S2–4) → pelvic plexus → cavernous nerve → penis
- Neurological disease at any of the above sites can result in ED:
  - Multiple sclerosis, spinal cord injury, cauda equina syndrome
  - Nerve injury (e.g., pelvic surgery)

### Post-Prostatectomy ED

- Almost all men develop ED in the early postoperative period.
- Even with cavernosal nerve-sparing prostatectomy, nerves are '*bruised*'.
  - This results in a temporary neuropraxia and immediate ED.
  - A proportion regains some erectile function when nerves recover (may take up to 24 months), but some do not regain erectile function.
  - *Neuropraxia* is associated with:
    - Cavernosal SM atrophy
    - Replacement by fibroblasts and collagen
    - Dysfunctional SM when nerves recover
    - Veno-occlusive dysfunction (see below)
- Most normal men get several nocturnal erections each night.
  - Results in regular oxygenation of the corpora.
  - Maintains health of SM and cavernosal tissue.
- Regular nocturnal erections are lost in neuropraxia.
  - The absence of regular oxygenation results in

**Table 22.1** Causes of Erectile Dysfunction

| Category | Causes |
| --- | --- |
| Vascular disease | Atherosclerosis |
| | Hyperlipidaemia |
| | Obesity |
| | Smoking |
| | Hypertension |
| | Diabetes |
| | Cardiovascular disease |
| | Pelvic radiotherapy |
| Neurological disease | Multiple sclerosis |
| | Spinal cord injury |
| | Cauda equina syndrome |
| | Stroke |
| | Multiple system atrophy |
| | Peripheral neuropathy |
| | Radical pelvic surgery |
| Psychological and psychiatric disease | Depression, anxiety |
| Endocrine disease | Hypogonadism |
| | Hyper/hypothyroidism |
| | Hyperprolactinaemia |
| | Hypopituitarism |
| Penile and anatomical causes | Phimosis |
| | Peyronie's disease |
| | Penile cancer |
| | Hypospadias |
| | Penile fracture |
| Mixed causes | Chronic renal failure |
| | Chronic liver failure |
| | Obstructive sleep apnoea |
| | Lower urinary tract symptoms |
| Prescription drugs | Anti-hypertensive agents |
| | Anti-depressants |
| | Anti-psychotic drugs |
| | Anti-androgenic drugs |
| Recreational drugs | Alcohol, Cocaine, Heroin |

SM loss and collagen formation (associated with *TGF-beta-1*).
- There are no convincing evidence that pharmacological and physical approaches (penile rehabilitation) to maintain the presence and function of cavernosal SM are effective.

# Vasculogenic Erectile Dysfunction

- *Atherosclerosis* is the most common cause of ED in the Western world.
- All major risk factors for atherosclerosis are also risk factors for ED:
  - Hypertension, hyperlipidaemia, diabetes (hyperglycaemia), smoking (free radicals), and obesity → cause *endothelial injury*

## *Atherosclerosis – Early Pathophysiology*

- Progressive thickening and hardening of the arterial wall due to fatty plaque.
- Endothelial injury → inflammatory response → monocytes differentiate into macrophages in the intima → macrophage retain lipid (foam cells) → fatty streaks
- Endothelial dysfunction → reduced NO release

## *Atherosclerosis – Late Pathophysiology*

- Smooth muscles migrate from the media to the intima and proliferate.
- Accumulation of lipid and SM in intima → atheroma plaque
- Atheroma reduces arterial inflow → hypoxia (*TGF-beta-1* mediated)
- Hypoxia results in SM loss/dysfunction and cavernosal fibrosis.
  - Veno-occlusive-dysfunction or '*venous leakage*' is the failure of cavernosal bodies to fully relax (decreased SM to collagen ratio).
- In the 1990s 'Venous leak' was considered to be a potential primary cause of ED and potentially curable by surgery.
  - However, results of surgery were inconsistent, and venous leak is thought to be secondary to SM dysfunction or SM loss resulting in:
    - Poor expansion of the cavernosal sinusoids.
    - Uncompressed subtunical plexus and poor closure of emissary veins.
    - Failure of rigid penile erection to occur.
- It became clear that surgical treatment of venous leakage was illogical, and is no longer indicated as a treatment for ED.

## *Penile Doppler Ultrasound*

- Requires intracavernosal injection of prostaglandin E1 to induce an erection.

- Peak systolic velocity at <25 cm/s indicate arterial insufficiency.
- End diastolic velocity of >5 cm/s may indicate venous leak or veno-occlusive dysfunction.
- Venous leak may be seen on cavernosography.

## Hypertensive ED

- Independent risk factor for ED and atherosclerosis.
- Causes endothelial dysfunction.
- Antihypertensives affect erectile function (reduces penile blood flow):
  - Beta-blockers.
  - Thiazide and loop diuretics.
  - Centrally acting antihypertensives.
- Angiotensin II causes arteriole vasoconstriction.
  - Implicated in ED pathogenesis.
- Angiotensin receptor blockers (ARB such as Valsartan or Losartan) are useful to treat hypertension and maintain erectile function.

## Metabolic Syndrome and ED

- *Definition* – a clustering of risk factors including:
  - Central obesity, diabetes, hypertension, and hyperlipidaemia.
- Increased amounts of central adipose tissue results in:
  - Systemic hyperinsulinemia;
  - Increased peripheral insulin resistance;
  - Glucose intolerance.
- Metabolic syndrome is associated with excess cardiovascular morbidity and mortality.
- The mechanisms leading to ED include:
  - Hyperglycaemia, hyperlipidaemia
  - Endothelial dysfunction
  - Hypogonadism (which is more common in metabolic syndrome)
  - Diabetic neuropathy
  - Peripheral vascular disease
  - Oxidative stress
- Some drugs that are used to treat the various components of the metabolic syndrome can also exacerbate ED.

## Hyperlipidaemia, Smoking, and Obesity

- Isolated *hyperlipidaemia* has a more nuanced effect on erectile function compared to diabetes and hypertension.
- *Epidemiological studies* showed that hyperlipidaemia only has an adverse effect in older men.
  - Likely mechanisms: endothelial dysfunction and atherosclerosis.
- *Smoking* – direct toxic effect on endothelial dysfunction.

- Associated with atherosclerosis, diabetes, and hypertension.
- *Obesity* is associated with hyperlipidaemia and metabolic syndrome.

## Endocrine Disease

- Commonest endocrine causes – diabetes, hypogonadism.
- Less common causes – hyperprolactinaemia, hypo/hyperthyroidism.
- *Hyperprolactinaemia* – seen in younger men.
  - Clinical features – ED, infertility, gynaecomastia, and galactorrhoea
  - Slightly low serum testosterone, markedly raised serum prolactin.
  - MRI scan may show a pituitary gland tumour.

## Diabetic ED

- Most common endocrine cause of ED.
- ~2x as likely to suffer from ED vs non-diabetics of the same age.
- Both type 1 and type 2 diabetes are associated with ED.
- *Mechanisms* involved include:
  - Hyperglycaemia and hyperinsulinemia (type 2 diabetes)
  - Glycation of cellular proteins (advanced glycation end-products) impairs endothelial and SM cellular function → endothelial dysfunction
  - Small vessel disease and large vessel atherosclerosis
  - Autonomic neuropathy
- Diabetes is associated with low testosterone levels.
- Often have a more severe form of ED.
- Lower therapeutic response rate to phosphodiesterase 5 (PDE5) inhibitors.
- Greater likelihood of needing more invasive treatments, such as penile implant.

## Testosterone

- Controls sexual arousal at the level of the spinal cord.
- Regulates penile endothelial and SM function.
- Modulates the release of NO and the functioning of NO synthase.
- Modulates the activity of PDE5.

# Psychogenic Erectile Dysfunction

- More common in young men.
- *Predisposing* factors:
  - Lifestyle problems, prior sexual trauma, restricted upbringing, poor education

- *Precipitating* factors:
  - Ageing, infidelity, loss of partner, unrealistic expectations
- *Maintaining* factors:
  - Performance-related anxiety, poor communication, poor education

## Performance-Related Anxiety

- Abnormal interaction between the two components of the autonomic nervous system.
- *Normal physiology*:
  - *At rest* – flaccid:
    - The sympathetic nervous system is dominant.
    - Penile SM is contracted.
    - Parasympathetic nervous system is quiescent.
  - *Erection*:
    - Inactive sympathetic nervous system.
    - Activated parasympathetic nervous system.
    - SM relaxation.
- In *performance-related anxiety*:
  - Sexual stimulus activates the parasympathetic nervous system.
  - However, the sympathetic nervous system does not become inactive.
  - This causes an incomplete SM relaxation and inadequate erectile response.

## Depression and ED

- Mechanisms are poorly understood.
- May reflect abnormalities of central neurotransmission.
- Anti-depressants (e.g., Selective Serotonin Reuptake Inhibitors [SSRIs]) have an adverse effect on:
  - Erectile function, sexual desire, and ejaculatory function.

# Iatrogenic Erectile Dysfunction

- Radical pelvic surgery (e.g., radical prostatectomy) results in neurogenic ED.
  - Cavernous nerve injury
  - Accessory pudendal artery injury
- Pelvic radiotherapy causes:
  - Progressive small vessel endarteritis.
  - Ischaemic damage to the base of the penis and its innervation.
- Pelvic fracture.
- Drugs – multiple, varying mechanisms (Table 22.2).

# Other Causes of Erectile Dysfunction

- *Tight phimosis* – pain during erection leading to ED.
- Early-stage Peyronie's disease – pain associated with an erection with penile deformity. Altered haemodynamics of cavernosal blood flow.

## Peyronie's Disease

- Development of fibrous plaque or scar tissue within the tunica albuginea.
- Curvature deformity occurs.
- *Associations*:
  - Dupuytren's contracture (palmer fascia)
  - Ledderhose's disease (plantar fascia contracture)
  - Diabetes, Paget's disease of bone, tympanosclerosis
  - Beta-blockers, Phenytoin
  - HLA-DQ5, HLA-A1, HLA-DQw2
- *Two phases* of the disease:
  - Acute (pain and deformity) – lasts ~12–18 months.
  - Chronic – stabilisation of the deformity.
- ~40% worsen, ~47% are stable, ~13% are resolved.
- *Pathogenesis* is unclear.
  - Micro-trauma of the tunica albuginea during sexual intercourse.
  - Subtunical bleeding and inflammatory wound healing process.
  - Poor vascularity prevents complete resolution.
  - Retention of *TGF-beta-1* perpetuating inflammatory response.
  - Deposition of abnormal collagen with excessive fibrosis.

# Ejaculatory Dysfunction

- The most common are premature ejaculation and retrograde ejaculation.

# Premature Ejaculation (PE)

- Intravaginal ejaculatory latency time (IVELT) <1 minute.
- *Epidemiological studies* showed that the prevalence of PE is unrelated to age.
- *Two types* of PE:
  - Lifelong or primary
  - Acquired or secondary

## Primary PE

- Mechanisms are poorly understood.
- Disordered central neurotransmission of serotonin (5HT), oxytocin, and dopamine.

## Secondary PE

- *Associated with*:
  - Erectile dysfunction
  - Prostatitis
  - Hyperthyroidism
  - Alcoholism, and withdrawal from opiate addiction

**Table 22.2** Drug-related Sexual Dysfunction

| Drug type | Drug or Class of Drug | Effect |
|---|---|---|
| **Anti-hypertensive drugs** | Diuretics | ED |
| | Beta-blockers | ED |
| | Centrally acting anti-hypertensive agents (e.g., clonidine, methyl DOPA) | ED |
| **Centrally acting agents** | Phenothiazines | ED, reduced libido, ejaculatory dysfunction |
| | Butyrophenones | ED |
| | Serotonin reuptake inhibitors | ED, ejaculatory dysfunction |
| | Tricyclic anti-depressants | ED, reduced libido |
| | Phenytoin | ED, reduced libido |
| **Endocrine drugs** | LHRH analogues | ED, reduced libido |
| | Anti-androgens | ED, reduced libido |
| | Oestrogens | ED, reduced libido |
| **Recreational drugs** | Alcohol | ED, reduced libido, ejaculatory dysfunction |
| | Marijuana | ED |
| | Cocaine | ED |
| | Opiates | ED, reduced libido |
| | Amphetamines | Reduced libido, ejaculatory dysfunction |
| | Anabolic steroids | ED, reduced libido |
| **Other drugs** | Cimetidine | ED, reduced libido |
| | Metoclopramide | ED, reduced libido |
| | Digoxin | ED |

*Abbreviation:* ED, erectile dysfunction.

- Psycho-relational problems (anxiety, relational, marital problems)
- There is an epidemiological association between acquired PE, ED, and prostatitis.
- A true causal relationship has not been proven.

## Retrograde Ejaculation (RE)

- Occurs when the bladder neck fails to close at the time of ejaculation.
- Bladder neck contraction is mediated by sympathetic innervation that releases noradrenaline.
- Confirmed with sperm present on microscopy of post-orgasm urine.
- *Causes* of RE:
  - *Neurological:*
    - Spinal cord injury
    - Multiple sclerosis
    - Myelodysplasia
    - Diabetic autonomic neuropathy
  - *Surgical damage to the lumbar sympathetic outflow:*
    - Retroperitoneal lymph node dissection
    - Sympathectomy
    - Aorto-iliac surgery
    - Abdominal-perineal resection
  - *Bladder neck injury/dysfunction*
    - Transurethral prostatectomy
    - Bladder neck incision
    - Alpha-adrenergic blockers
    - Psychotropic agents
- Medical treatments aim to *close* the bladder neck:
  - Pseudoephedrine, ephedrine (sympathomimetics)
  - Imipramine (tricyclic antidepressant)

## Anejaculation

- Failure of emission.
- Common cause – spinal cord injury.

- Semen analysis – complete absence of antegrade ejaculation.
- Post-orgasmic urine analysis – absence of fructose and sperm.
- Lesions above T10 have intact bulbocavernosus reflex and can use penile vibratory stimulation to stimulate ejaculation.
- Lesions below T10 or failed penile vibratory stimulation can use a rectal probe electroejaculator.
- Sperm quality is usually poor (stasis).

## Hypogonadism

- *Hypothalamic/pituitary origin:*
  - Secondary (hypogonadotropic hypogonadism).
- Testicular origin:
  - Primary (hypogonadal hypogonadism).
- The main causes in each group are listed in the male factor infertility section.
- For urologists, the most common cause of hypogonadism is that seen in older men.

## Age-Related Hypogonadism

- Serum total testosterone gradually declines as men get older.
- ~20% of those aged 60 years have testosterone levels below normal.
- *Mechanisms:*
  - Defect at the hypothalamic (GnRH) or pituitary level (FSH, LH).
  - Obesity, hyperlipidaemia, type 2 diabetes:
    - Low testosterone is a common feature in metabolic syndrome.
  - *Obesity:*
    - Peripheral aromatisation (aromatase) of testosterone in adipose tissue to oestrogen.
      - Less bioavailable testosterone
      - Gynaecomastia
  - Ageing increases the sex hormone-binding globulin.
    - Increased bound testosterone → less bioavailable testosterone
- *Signs and symptoms:*
  - ED, loss of nocturnal erections
  - Loss of sexual interest
  - Fatigue, loss of physical endurance
  - Reduced muscle mass and strength
  - Reduced motivation, depressed mood, irritability, poor concentration
- The mechanism by which low testosterone results in ED is poorly understood.
  - *Testosterone:* Possible modulatory effect on penile SM, and the endothelium are necessary for normal erectile function.

- PDE5 inhibitors are usually ineffective in hypogonadism unless combined with testosterone replacement.
  - May reflect a direct effect of testosterone on NO synthase.
- Effect on sexual interest is likely modulated within the central nervous system.

## Male Factor Infertility

- *Primary infertility:* the inability of a sexually active couple to achieve a pregnancy within 12 months following regular (every 2–3 days) unprotected sexual intercourse.
- Male cause ~20%, female ~50%, mixed ~30%.
- *Commonest causes:*
  - Primary testicular insufficiency (varicoceles ~30–40%)
  - Obstruction (10–15%)
  - Genetic anomalies
  - Endocrine disorders (~2%)

- *World Health Organization* (2010) lowered the reference limits (5th centiles and their 95% confidence intervals) for semen characteristics:

| | |
|---|---|
| Ejaculation volume: | 1.5 mL (1.4–1.7) |
| Sperm concentration: | 15 × 10⁶/mL (12–16) |
| Total sperm number: | 39 × 10⁶ (33–46) per ejaculate |
| Total motility: | 40% (38–42) with progressive and non-progressive motility |
| Motility: | 32% (31–34) with progressive motility |
| Morphology: | 4% (3.0–4.0) normal forms |
| Vitality: | 58% (55–63) |
| pH: | >7.2 |
| White blood cell: | <1 million/mL |

- *Optional investigations:*

| | |
|---|---|
| Mixed antiglobulin reaction (MAR test – motile spermatozoa with bound particles): | <50% |
| Immunobead test (motile spermatozoa with bound beads): | <50% |
| Seminal zinc: | >2.4 µmol/ejaculate |
| Seminal fructose: | >13 µmol/ejaculate |
| Seminal neutral glucosidase: | <20 mU/ejaculate |

- *Oligospermia:* low sperm count ($<15 \times 10^6$/mL).
- *Azoospermia:* absence of sperm.
- *Asthenospermia:* reduced progressive sperm motility ($<32\%$).
  - *WHO (1999) classification of motility:*
    - Rapid progressive, slowly progressive, non-progressive, non-motile
- *Teratospermia:* abnormal morphology ($<4\%$ normal).
- ~30–40% have no clear cause to explain abnormal sperm parameters.
  - Historically termed as idiopathic male infertility.
  - Now believed to be associated with:
    - Generation of reactive oxygen species (ROS)
    - Sperm DNA damage
    - Genetic and epigenetic abnormalities
- *ROS* are the final products of oxidative stress, which results in:
  - Lipid peroxidated plasma membrane.
  - Impaired acrosome reaction and chromatin maturation.
  - Increased DNA fragmentations.
  - Impaired sperm motility.
- *Sperm DNA fragmentation*
  - Increased fragmented DNA or accumulation of single- and double-strand DNA breaks → reduce the chances of natural conception
  - *Associated with:*
    - Poorer assisted reproductive technique (ART) outcomes
    - Impaired embryo development
    - Miscarriage
    - Recurrent pregnancy loss
    - Birth defects
  - *Risk factors* for sperm DNA damage:
    - Hormonal anomalies
    - Varicocele
    - Chronic infection
    - Lifestyle (e.g., smoking)
  - Most common assay to measure sperm DNA:
    - *Sperm chromatin structure assay (SCSA)*
      - Threshold DNA fragmentation index (DFI): 30% (number of cells with DNA damage).
  - Other assays:
    - *COMET assay* (single cell gel electrophoresis assay, SCGE)
      - DNA migration through the electrophoresis gel resembles a *comet.*
    - TUNEL assay (terminal deoxynucleotidyl transferase-mediated deoxyuridine triphosphate nick-end labelling)
      - Labels 3' hydroxy termini in double-strand DNA that breaks from apoptosis.

- Reaction catalysed by terminal deoxynucleotidyl transferase.

## Testicular Insufficiency

- Disease or damage to the testicles which results in low/absent sperm production.
- Can cause low serum testosterone and raised LH/FSH (primary hypogonadism).
- Two testicles provide some extent protection.
- Both testicles need to be affected to cause testicular insufficiency and hypogonadal hypogonadism. Causes include:
  - Bilateral testicular maldescent
  - Bilateral orchitis (e.g., mumps orchitis)
  - Bilateral testicular torsion
  - Bilateral testicular malignancy
  - Radiation to the testicles
  - Systemic cytotoxic chemotherapy
  - Bilateral varicoceles

## *Testicular Maldescent*

- The likelihood of male factor infertility depends on:
  - Whether it is in a bilateral or unilateral condition.
  - The level of the testicle (with higher placed testicles being more likely to be associated with infertility).
  - Timing of surgery (recommended by 12 months of age).
- *Paternity rates:* 80–90% for unilateral inguinal orchidopexy, ~50% for bilateral.
- *Orchidopexy:* <2 years ~90% fertile, 3–4 years ~60%, 9–12 years ~30%.

## *Varicocele*

- Dilatation of the pampiniform venous plexus (~2–3 mm on USS).
- Mechanisms affecting spermatogenesis and fertility:
  - Testicular temperature of 1–2°C higher.
  - Hypoxia and oxidative stress.
  - Reflux of renal and/or adrenal metabolites into the testicular vein.
- Some men may have low serum testosterone.
- *Management:* embolisation, surgical ligation.

## Obstructive Azoospermia

- Bilateral obstruction causes absence of sperm from the ejaculate:
  - Ejaculatory duct obstruction

- Congenital bilateral absence of the vas deferens
- Scrotal (including vasectomy) and inguinal surgery
- Epididymal obstruction

## Ejaculatory Duct Obstruction

- May be congenital or acquired.
- *Congenital:*
  - Mullerian (utricular) and Wolffian (diverticular) cysts
- *Acquired:*
  - Surgical trauma
  - Prostatic calcification
  - Seminal vesicle calculi
  - Infection-related scarring
- *Clinical features:*
  - Low-volume ejaculate (<1.5 mL), low pH (<7.2), low fructose
  - Azoospermia
  - Dilated seminal vesicles - may be seen on transrectal ultrasound
  - Normal hormone profile

## Epididymal Obstruction

- Young's syndrome (rare)
- *Triad includes*:
  - Chronic sinusitis
  - Bronchiectasis
  - Epididymal obstruction with azoospermia

# Endocrine Disorders

- *Hypogonadotropic hypogonadism:*
  - Primary abnormality of the pituitary or hypothalamus.
  - Low levels of LH (and usually FSH).
  - Testicular insufficiency with low testosterone (Table 22.3).
  - Oligozoospermia or azoospermia.
- *Causes:*
  - Kallmann syndrome

- Isolated LH deficiency
- Prader–Willi syndrome
- Laurence–Moon–Biedl syndrome
- Pituitary tumours
- Pituitary infarct
- Craniopharyngioma
- Haemochromatosis
- Neurosarcoid
- Anabolic steroid use

## Kallmann Syndrome

- Congenital hypogonadotropic hypogonadism.
- Malformation of midline cranial structures.
- Defects in the hypothalamic production of GnRH.
- *Clinical presentation* varies but includes:
  - Delayed puberty
  - Anosmia
  - Cleft palate
  - Small testes
  - In more severe cases: congenital deafness, asymmetry of the cranium and face, cerebellar dysfunction, cryptorchidism, renal abnormalities.

## Anabolic Steroid Use (e.g., Bodybuilders)

- Feedback inhibition on the hypothalamic GnRH production.
- Reduced testosterone and sperm production.
- Cessation does not always guarantee the restoration of normal testosterone/sperm production.

# Genetic Infertility

- The most common causes of genetic associated infertility are:
  - Chromosomal abnormalities
  - Congenital bilateral absence of the vas deferens (CBAVD)
  - Y-chromosomal micro-deletions
- Chromosomal abnormalities are identified in both:
  - Oligospermia (~5%)

| Table 22.3 Interpretation of Male Reproductive Hormonal Profile | | | | |
| --- | --- | --- | --- | --- |
| Condition | T | FSH | LH | PL |
| Normal | Normal | Normal | Normal | Normal |
| Primary testis failure | ↓ | ↑ | Normal / ↑ | Normal |
| Hypogonadotrophic hypogonadism | ↓ | ↓ | ↓ | Normal |
| Hyperprolactinaemia | ↓ | ↓ / Normal | ↓ | ↑ |
| Androgen resistance | ↑ | ↑ | ↑ | Normal |

*Abbreviations:* T, testosterone; FSH, follicle stimulating hormone; LH, luteinising hormone; PL, prolactin.

- Azoospermia (~10–15%)
- The most common chromosomal abnormality is *Klinefelter's syndrome.*
- Rarer causes include:
  - XX-Male syndrome, mixed gonadal dysgenesis

## Klinefelter's Syndrome 47XXY

- Affects ~1 in 600 men.
- Most common chromosomal cause of male factor infertility.
- Variety of clinical presentations:
  - Atrophic testicles
  - Gynaecomastia
  - Azoospermia in ~90% and severe oligospermia in the rest
  - Raised FSH and LH
  - Typical reduced serum testosterone (but can be normal in some)
- Microtesticular sperm extraction (TESE) can be a successful treatment in a small number of cases (up to 50%).

## Congenital Bilateral Absence of the Vas Deferens

- Affects ~1 in 1,600 men.
- Associated with cystic fibrosis (CF).
  - Autosomal recessive inheritance.
  - Mutation of the CF transmembrane conductance regulator (CFTR) gene.
  - CFTR gene is on chromosome 7q.
  - The most common mutation is ΔF508del (~2/3 of all CFTR alleles).
- CBAVD is usually diagnosed upon clinical examination.
  - When identified, both the man and his partner should undergo genetic testing.
- >1,500 gene mutations are known to cause CBAVD.

## Y-Chromosomal Micro-Deletions

- The Y-chromosome contains the contains the azoospermia factor (AZF) region.
- AZF contains the male phenotypic developmental pathway (Figure 22.1).

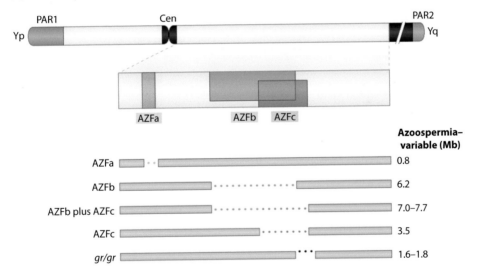

| Region | Frequency | Prognosis |
|---|---|---|
| AZFa | Rare (~5%) | Azoospermia<br>Sertoli cell only syndrome |
| AZFb | Rare (~30%) | Azoospermia<br>Maturation arrest |
| AZFb/c | Rare | Severe oligospermia |
| AZFc | Commonest site for microdeletion (~65%) | Severe Oligospermia (rarely azoospermia)<br>Micro-TESE occasionally successful |

Figure 22.1 Y Chromosome micro-deletions. Complete Azoospermia Factor (AZF) micro-deletions, a direct cause of impaired spermatogenesis, and the gr/gr deletion, a risk factor for spermatogenic impairment. Cen, centromere; PAR, pseudoautosomal region; SCOS, sertoli-cell-only syndrome; SGA, spermatogenic (maturation) arrest. (Reprinted by permission from Springer Nature [11])

**Table 22.4** Johnson Scoring System for Testicular Biopsy

| Score | Histology |
| --- | --- |
| 10 | Complete spermatogenesis |
| | Organised epithelium |
| 9 | Many spermatozoa |
| | Disorganised epithelium |
| 8 | <10 Spermatozoa |
| 7 | Many spermatids |
| 6 | <10 spermatids |
| 5 | Many spermatocytes |
| 4 | < Spermatocytes |
| 3 | Spermatogonia |
| 2 | Sertoli cells only |
| 1 | No cells, tubular fibrosis |

*Notes:* Isolated diagnostic testicular biopsies are now less readily performed for azoospermia as most will be undergoing sperm retrieval for Intracytoplasmic sperm insemination (ICSI). A biopsy can be performed if no sperm is found upon retrieval.

- Lies towards the distal end of the Y-chromosome long arm (Yq).
- Three regions where micro-deletions can result in male factor infertility:
  - AZFa, AZFb, and AZFc (from proximal to distal).
  - Where AZFb and AZFc regions overlap
  - AZFc region is the most common region for micro-deletion.
- This abnormality is associated with reduced spermatogenesis.

- Testicular biopsy demonstrates some sperm (Table 22.4).
- Micro-TESE is occasionally successful (Sperm found in 10–15%) – a Johnson score of 8 is required for assisted reproductive therapy.

# Recommended Reading

1. Eardley I. The incidence, prevalence and natural history of erectile dysfunction Sex Med Rev. 2013;1:3–16.
2. Hatsimouratidis K, Burnett AL, Hatzichristou D, McCullough AR, Montorsi F, Mulhall JP. Phosphodiesterase type 5 inhibitors in postprostatectomy erectile dysfunction: a critical analysis of basic science rationale and clinical applications. Eur Urol. 2009;55:334–347.
3. Saenz de Tejada I, Angulo J, Cellek S, Gonzalez-Cavadid N, Heaton J, Pickard R, Simonsen U. Pathophysiology of erectile dysfunction. J Sex Med. 2005;2:26–39.
4. Yafi FA, Jenkins L, Albersen M et al. Erectile dysfunction. Nat Rev Dos Primers. 2016:2:17003.
5. Sanchez E, Pastuscak AW, Khera M. Erectile dysfunction, metabolic syndrome and cardiovascular risks: facts and controversies. Transl Androl Urol. 2017;6:28–36.
6. Cellek S, Cameron NE, Cotter MA, Muneer A. Pathophysiology of diabetic erectile dysfunction: potential contribution of vasa nervoroum and advanced gycation end-products. Int J Imp Res. 2012;25:1–6.
7. Buvat J. Pathophysiology of premature ejaculation. J Sex Med. 2011;8 (Suppl 4):316–27.
8. Parham A, Serefoglu EC. Retrograde ejaculation, painful ejaculation and haematospermia. Trans Androl Urol. 2016;5:592–601.
9. Wu FCW, Tajar A, Beynon JM, Pye SR. Identification of late-onset hypogonadism in middle aged and elderly men. N Engl J Med. 2010;363:123–35.
10. Berookhim BM, Schlegel PN. Azoospermia due to spermatogenic failure. Urol Clin N Am. 2014;41:97–113.
11. Krausz C and Riera-Escamilla A. Genetics of male infertility. Nat Urol Rev. 2018;15(6):369–84.
12. Lotti F, Maggi M. Sexual dysfunction and male infertility. Nat Rev Urol. 2018;15(5):287–307.

# Section IV

## MALIGNANT PATHOLOGY

# 23 Renal Cancer

*Sabrina H. Rossi and Grant D. Stewart*

## Adult Malignant, Primary, Sporadic Renal Cancers

- The World Health Organization (WHO) Classification for renal tumours is based on histopathological, molecular, and genetic characteristics (Table 23.1).
- Renal cell carcinoma (RCC) comprises >90% of adult renal cancer.
  - Adenocarcinoma arises from renal tubular epithelial cells.
- Other much rarer renal cancers with alternative cells of origin include:
  - Metanephric, nephroblastic, mesenchymal, neuroendocrine, and haematological renal tumours.

## Renal Cell Carcinoma

- RCC was historically referred to as 'Grawitz tumour' or 'hypernephroma'.

## Epidemiology

- *Incidence (rising)*
  - 7th most common cancer in the UK (6th in men and 10th in women).
  - UK 2017: 13,000 new cases.
  - Highest in developed countries, particularly in Europe and North America.
  - Lower rates in Asia and Africa.
  - Increasing prevalence of RCC risk factors (e.g., ageing population, obesity).
  - Increased incidental detection due to the widespread use of abdominal imaging.
- 50% of renal cancers are detected incidentally.
- 25% have metastases at presentation.
- *Mortality*
  - 50% die from RCC.
  - Mortality rates have stabilised or decreased in most developed countries.
    - Continue to rise in certain parts of Eastern Europe.
  - *UK:*
    - Five-year survival: >80% in stage I disease.
    - <10% in stage IV.
  - 2017: 4,600 deaths.

## Aetiology

### Non-Modifiable Risk Factors (Table 23.2)

- *Gender:* incidence is higher in males for all subtypes, except in chromophobe RCC.
- *Age:* incidence increases with age, peaking during the 6th and 7th decade.
- *Genetics*
  - *Sporadic* in ~95% of cases.
    - *Unilateral* and *unifocal.*
    - Relative risk of RCC in individuals who have a history of an affected first-degree relative with sporadic RCC is ~2x compared to the general population.
  - Associated with *hereditary* syndromes in 5% of cases (Table 23.3).
    - *Earlier* age of onset.
    - *Bilateral* and *multifocal.*

### Modifiable Risk Factors (Table 23.2)

- Smoking, obesity, and hypertension.
- *Renal disease:*
  - Acquired renal cystic disease (ARCD).
    - ~43% of patients on dialysis → risk increases with duration of dialysis
    - Development of multiple, usually small, cysts in small/shrunken kidneys.
  - End-stage renal failure (ESRF) on dialysis.
  - Renal transplant.
  - Increases the risk of RCC, especially multifocal papillary RCC or acquired cystic disease-associated RCC.

## Pathology

*Histological* subtype – major predictor of survival:

- The best prognosis – chromophobe and type 1 papillary RCC.
- Progressively worsening survival outcomes in:
  - Type 2 papillary RCC
  - Clear cell RCC

**Table 23.1** World Health Organization (WHO) Classification of Tumours of the Kidney

| Renal cell tumours | Mesenchymal tumours occurring mainly in adults |
|---|---|
| Clear cell RCC | Leiomyosarcoma |
| Multilocular cystic renal neoplasm of low malignant potential | Angiosarcoma |
| Papillary RCC | Rhabdomyosarcoma |
| Hereditary leiomyomatosis and RCC-associated RCC | Osteosarcoma |
| Chromophobe RCC | Synovial sarcoma |
| Collecting duct carcinoma | Ewing sarcoma |
| MiT family translocation RCC | Angiomyolipoma |
| SDH renal carcinoma | Epithelioid angiomyolipoma |
| Mucinous tubular and spindle cell carcinoma | Leiomyoma |
| Tubulocystic RCC | Haemangioma |
| Acquired cystic disease-associated RCC | Lymphangioma |
| Clear cell papillary RCC | Haemangioblastoma |
| RCC, unclassified | Juxtaglomerular cell tumour |
| Papillary adenoma | Renomedullary interstitial cell tumour |
| Oncocytoma | Schwannoma |
| **Metanephric tumours** | Solitary fibrous tumour |
| Metanephric adenoma | **Mixed epithelial and stromal tumour family** |
| Metanephric adenofibroma | Cystic nephroma |
| Metanephric stromal tumour | Mixed epithelial and stromal tumour |
| **Nephroblastic and cystic tumours occurring mainly in children** | **Neuroendocrine tumours** |
| Nephrogenic rests | Well-differentiated |
| Nephroblastoma | Large cell |
| Cystic partially differentiated nephroblastoma | Small cell |
| Paediatric cystic nephroma | Phaeochromocytoma |
| **Mesenchymal tumours occurring mainly in children** | **Miscellaneous tumours** |
| Clear cell sarcoma | Renal haematopoietic neoplasms |
| Rhabdoid tumour | Germ cell tumours |
| Congenital mesoblastic nephroma | **Metastatic tumours** |
| Ossifying renal tumour of infancy | |

*Source:* Adapted from Moch et al. [1].
*Abbreviations:* RCC, renal cell carcinoma; SDH, Succinate dehydrogenase-deficient

- Subset of papillary RCC – CpG island methylator phenotype
- Cancer-specific five-year survival following surgical management:
  - Papillary RCC at 91%.
  - Chromophobe RCC at 88%.
  - Clear cell RCC at 71%.
- Histological slides of RCC subtypes are shown in Figure 23.1.

## Clear Cell RCC (ccRCC)

- Composes ~75% of cases.
- Derived from *proximal convoluted tubule* (PCT) in the renal cortex.
- *Genetics:*
- *Sporadic ccRCC:*
  - >90% have genetic or epigenetic aberrations in the Von Hippel Lindau (*VHL*) gene.

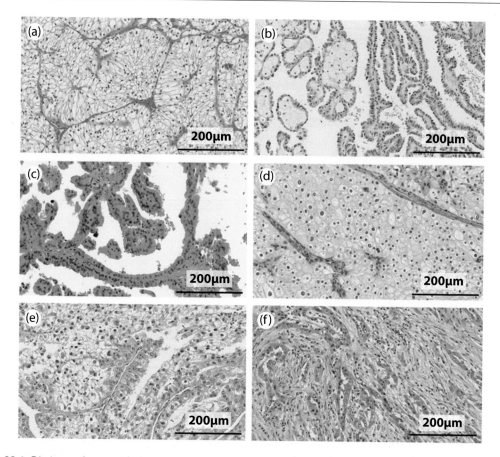

**Figure 23.1** Distinct subtypes of renal cell carcinoma. (a) Approximately 75% of renal cell carcinomas (RCCs) are clear cell RCC; (b) Papillary RCCs Make Up ~15% of all kidney cancers and are divided into two types based on staining features: Type 1 Basophilic and; (c) Type 2 Eosinophilic; (d) Chromophobe RCCs Make Up ~5% of Kidney tumours; (e) Other minor subtypes include MiT family translocation RCCs and; (f) Collecting duct RCCs. Additional minor subtypes include medullary RCC, clear cell papillary RCC, acquired cystic disease-associated RCC, tubulocystic RCC, Mucinous tubular and spindle RCC, succinate dehydrogenase-deficient RCC, hereditary leiomyomatosis, RCC-associated RCC and oncocytoma. Tumours not fitting into any of these categories are designated as unclassified RCC. (Reprinted by permission from Springer Nature [11])

- *VHL*: tumour suppressor gene. Chromosome 3 short arm (3p25).
- VHL protein is encoded by the gene and regulates oxygen sensing through interactions with hypoxia-inducible factors (HIF).
- *VHL mutations* – increased HIF (1-alpha)-mediated transcription of factors that increase angiogenesis (vascularised tumours), cell growth, and mitosis, including:
  - Vascular endothelial growth factor (VEGF)
  - Transforming growth factor α (TGF-α)
  - Platelet-derived growth factor β (PDGF-β)
    - Basis of targeted therapy.
- Other genes implicated in ccRCC:
  - Chromosome 3 (3p21): *PBRM1, BAP1,* and *SETD2* genes.
    - Responsible for chromatin remodelling.
  - *CDKN2A* (cell cycle).

- ~30% have mutations in genes (*MTOR, PTEN*) involving the PI(3)K/AKT/mammalian target of rapamycin (mTOR) pathway.
  - Leads to increased tumorigenesis, angiogenesis, cell growth, and tumour progression.
- *Hereditary ccRCC:*
  - Occurs in VHL disease.
  - Germline *mutation* in the *VHL* gene (Table 23.3).
- *Macroscopically:*
  - Unifocal, exophytic tumour.
  - Golden yellow (high fat content).
  - Well-circumscribed with a pseudocapsule.
  - Often have necrosis, haemorrhage, calcification, and/or cystic changes.
- *Microscopically:*
  - *Cytoplasm:* high lipid and glycogen content.
    - Dissolves upon histopathological processing.

**Table 23.2** Risk Factors for Renal Cell Carcinoma

| Risk Factor | Comment |
| --- | --- |
| **Established Risk Factors** | |
| Gender | Males to female ratio of approximately 2:1 |
| Age | Positive association |
| Race | Higher in African–Americans compared to Caucasians |
| Obesity | Positive association with a dose response |
| Smoking | Positive association with a dose response. |
| Hypertension | Positive association with a dose response. Effect of hypertensive medication, such as diuretics, on renal cancer risk, remains unclear. |
| Renal disease | Increased risk of renal cancer in patients with acquired cystic kidney disease, end-stage renal failure on dialysis and renal transplant (RCC affects the native kidney). |
| Alcohol | Moderate alcohol intake has a protective effect relative to abstinence. There is no additional benefit for higher consumption. |
| Family history | Affected first-degree relative confers a risk of renal cancer. A number of inherited rare genetic conditions also predispose to renal cancer, as summarised in Table 23.3. |
| **Risk factors that are less well characterised** | |
| Physical activity | High/strenuous physical activity is protective. |
| Type 2 Diabetes | Positive association |
| Renal stones | Increased risk in male patients with renal stones, but not females. |
| Occupational exposure | Trichloroethylene is considered a carcinogenic agent with sufficient evidence for the development of renal cancer according to the International Agency for Research on Cancer (IARC). Arsenic and inorganic arsenic compounds, cadmium and cadmium compounds, perfluorooctanoic acid printing processes and welding fumes have limited evidence according to the IARC. |
| Gamma radiation and X radiation | Carcinogenic agent with sufficient evidence in humans according to the IARC. |
| Analgesic use | Meta-analyses suggest acetaminophen is associated with a significant risk of developing kidney cancer. Conflicting results are available regarding non-aspirin NSAIDs. Aspirin did not demonstrate a significant association. |
| Parity and hormonal factors | Association noted in some studies, not others. |

*Source:* Adapted from Rossi et al. [2].
*Abbreviations:* NSAIDs, non-steroidal anti-inflammatory drugs, IARC, International Agency for Research on Cancer.

- Creates a distinctive, '*clear*' appearance; hence, its name.
- A minority demonstrate *eosinophilic*, granular cytoplasm.
- Cells surrounded by a large network of thin blood vessels (angiogenesis).
  - The high angiogenicity and immunogenicity of ccRCC have been harnessed in the management of metastatic disease (e.g., VEGF and T cell checkpoint inhibitors).

## Papillary RCC (pRCC)

- Comprises ~10–15% cases.
- Derived from *PCT*.
- Better prognosis than other subtypes.
- More often bilateral and multifocal (particularly in ESRF and ARCD).
- *Two subtypes:*
  - *Type 1:* More common and less aggressive.
  - *Type 2:* More aggressive.

**Table 23.3** Genetic Syndromes Which Predispose to Hereditary RCC

| Syndrome | Estimated Incidence | Genetics | Lifetime Risk of RCC | Renal Manifestations | Extrarenal Manifestations |
|---|---|---|---|---|---|
| Von Hippel Lindau (VHL) Disease | 1:30,000 to 1:35,000 | Autosomal dominant *VHL* gene on chromosome 3p25-26 | 50–70% | Clear cell RCC - Early age at onset. Bilateral, multifocal. Renal cysts | Retinal angioma. Haemangioblastoma of brainstem, cerebellum or spinal cord. Phaeochromocytoma. Renal, pancreatic and epididymal cysts. Inner ear tumours |
| Hereditary papillary RCC syndrome (HPRCC) | Unknown | Autosomal dominant *c-MET* gene on chromosome 7q31 | 90% | Type 1 papillary RCC. Bilateral, multifocal | No tumours in other organs |
| Hereditary leiomyomatosis and RCC (HLRCC) | 1:200,000 | Autosomal dominant *FH* gene on chromosome 1q42-43 | 15–20% | Most commonly type 2 papillary RCC, although collecting duct RCC has also been reported. Often very aggressive | Cutaneous and uterine leiomyomas |
| Succinate dehydrogenase RCC (SD RCC) | Unknown | Autosomal dominant SD genes: *SDHB* (most common), *SDHA, SDHC, SDHD* | 10–15% | Specific type of RCC | Paragangliomas, Gastrointestinal stromal tumours |
| Birt–Hogg–Dubé Syndrome | 1:200,000 | Autosomal dominant *FCLN* gene on chromosome 17p.11.2 | 10–30% | Chromophobe RCC, oncocytomas and hybrid oncocytic-chromophobe tumours. ccRCC and other subtypes have also been observed. | Cutaneous fibrofolliculomas, Lung cysts and spontaneous pneumothorax |
| Tuberous sclerosis | 1:6,000 to 1:10,000 | Autosomal dominant *TSC1* gene on chromosome 9p34 or *TSC2* gene on chromosome 16p13.3 | 1–5% | Renal cysts, angiomyolipoma (AML), ccRCC | Epilepsy, learning difficulties and adenoma sebaceum |

- *Genetics:*
  - Usually sporadic, but also includes familial syndromes associated with each type.
  - *Type 1*
    - *Sporadic* cases: gains (trisomy and tetrasomy) in chromosomes 7 and 17, and loss of chromosome Y in males.
    - *Hereditary* cases: *Hereditary papillary RCC syndrome* (HPRCC). Mutations in the *c-MET* (Chm 7q) proto-oncogene (Table 23.3).
  - *Type 2*
    - *Hereditary* cases: *Hereditary leiomyomatosis and RCC* (HLRCC) syndrome. Mutations in the *Fumurate Hydratase* gene (Chm 1q) (Table 23.3).
- *Macroscopically:*
  - Brown;
  - Well-circumscribed with a pseudocapsule; and
  - Often with the presence of haemorrhage and necrosis.
- *Microscopically:*
  - Arranged in a papillary or tubular architecture.
  - Type 1: *basophilic* with low cytoplasm.
  - Type 2: *eosinophilic* with abundant cytoplasm.

## Chromophobe RCC (chRCC)

- ~5% of cases.
- Derived from the *distal convoluted tubule* (DCT).
- *Incidence* is equal in both genders.
- *Genetics:*
  - Usually sporadic.
  - *Sporadic* cases: loss of whole chromosomes – 1, 2, 6, 10, 13, 17, and 21.
  - *Hereditary* cases: Hybrid oncocytic-chromophobe tumours, which have features of both oncocytomas and chRCC, are characteristic of the familial *Birt–Hogg–Dubé Syndrome* (Table 23.3).
- *Macroscopically:*
  - Light brown or pale *tan* in colour.
  - Well-circumscribed.
- *Microscopically:*
  - Large cells – wrinkled '*raisinoid*' nucleus.
  - Pale perinuclear cytoplasm and prominent cell membrane which causes a '*halo*' effect.
  - *Cytoplasmic microvesicles* – diagnostic on staining with *Hale colloidal iron stain*.
  - In contrast to ccRCC:
    - Network of *thick* blood vessels.
    - *Absence* of necrosis and calcifications.

## Collecting Duct Carcinoma

- Also referred to as *Bellini duct carcinoma*.
- Rare tumour with poor prognosis.
- Most commonly in males, with an earlier age of onset.
- Derived from *collecting ducts* in the medulla.
- *Macroscopically:*
  - Occupies the central location within the kidney due to its origin within the medulla.
  - Often cannot be distinguished from urothelial carcinoma of the renal pelvis invading the renal parenchyma.
- *Microscopically:*
  - Tubular and/or papillary architecture.
  - *Eosinophilic* cytoplasm.
  - Often high-grade.

## Renal Medullary Carcinoma

- Very rare.
- Almost exclusive to sickle cell disease and young African-American men.
- Derived from the epithelium of the renal papillae in the medulla.
- Similar features to collecting duct carcinoma and may be considered its variant.
- Very aggressive and often metastases are present at diagnosis.

## MiT Family Translocation RCC

- Gene translocations involving MiT family of transcription factor genes (e.g., genes *TFE3* and *TFEB*).
  - *Translocation:* gene rearrangement and fusion between non-homologous chromosomes.
  - Fluorescent in situ hybridisation (FISH) may be used to demonstrate chromosomal translocation and determine diagnosis.
- Most frequently in children and adolescents but may also occur in adults.
- Aggressive phenotype.

## Other RCC Subtypes (Table 23.1)

- Acquired cystic disease-associated RCC.
  - Separate subtype of RCC.
  - Exclusive to patients with acquired cystic disease.
  - May be multifocal.
  - Often partially cystic.
  - Microscopically, they have a characteristic 'sieve-like' appearance.
- *Unclassified RCC*
  - ~5% of RCCs either fit more than one category or cannot be classified due to poor differentiation – '*unclassified*'.
  - Variable prognosis as they represent different subtypes.

# Tumour Grading and Staging

- Grade and stage are important prognostic factors.

**Table 23.4** Comparison of Fuhrman Grading and WHO/ISUP Grading System

| Grade | Fuhrman | | | WHO/ISUP |
| | Nuclear Diameter | Nuclear Shape | Nucleoli | Nucleoli |
|---|---|---|---|---|
| 1 | 10 µm | Round, uniform | Absent, inconspicuous | Absent or inconspicuous and basophilic at 400x magnification. |
| 2 | 15 µm | Irregular outline | Visible at 400x | Conspicuous and eosinophilic at 400x magnification and visible but not prominent at 100x magnification. |
| 3 | 20 µm | Obvious irregular outline | Visible and prominent at 100x | Conspicuous and eosinophilic at 100x magnification. |
| 4 | As Grade 3 | As Grade 3 | Bizarre multilobed + spindles | Extremely unclear pleomorphism, multinucleate giant cells, and/or rhabdoid and/or sarcomatoid differentiation. |

- Pathological features associated with a worse prognosis include:
  - Histological coagulative necrosis
  - Rhabdoid morphology
  - Sarcomatoid morphology
    - High-grade spindle cells with very aggressive potential.
    - Previously considered a separate histological subtype.
    - Now recognised as a loss of differentiation, can occur in any other subtype, and most common in ccRCC and chRCC.

## Grading

- WHO/ISUP (International Society of Urological Pathology) grading system is currently recommended (superseded Fuhrman grading system).
- *Fuhrman* grading system (Table 23.4):
  - *Grades 1–4:* based on nuclear size, outline, and nucleolar prominence
  - High degree of inter and intra-observer variability is noted.
- *WHO/ISUP classification*
  - More reproducible.
  - *Grades 1–4* (Table 23.4):
    - Grades 1–3 are based on nuclear prominence.
    - Grade 4 is based on the presence of pronounced nuclear pleomorphism, giant cells, sarcomatoid, or rhabdoid features.
- The prognostic value of WHO/ISUP and Fuhrman grading systems has been validated in ccRCC and pRCC, but not in rarer (or more recently recognised) pathological subtypes.
- chRCC: nuclear atypia – recommended for those un-graded.

## Staging

- TNM 8th edition is the most up-to-date staging classification (Table 23.5).
- *Renal contrast CT:*
  - $\geq$15 Hounsfield unit (HU) change post-contrast = *enhancement*.
- Local tumour spread is into renal capsule, perirenal fat, and adrenal gland.
- RCC may spread into the renal vein, inferior vena cava, and right atrium.
- *Lymphatic spread* → to hilar and para-aortic lymph nodes
- *Haematogenous spread:*
  - Lung, bone, liver, and brain (listed in order of descending frequency).
  - Glandular metastases: rarely can metastasise to the pancreas, thyroid, breast, parotid gland, and contralateral adrenal (which should be differentiated from metastases to the ipsilateral adrenal via local invasion).
    - Tend to be solitary metastases.
    - Relatively indolent, with good overall survival.
- RCC subtypes determine metastatic spread:
  - ccRCC: lungs. Vena cava involvement is more common than other subtypes.
  - chRCC: commonly in the liver.
  - pRCC: commonly in lymph nodes.
- *Risk stratification:* Leibovich (Mayo) scoring system (0–11 points):
  - Pathological T stage (0–4)
    - T1a = 0; T1b = 2; T2 = 3; T3–4 = 4
  - Tumour size <10 cm = 0
  - Tumour size >10 cm = 1
  - Nodal status (0–2)
    - Nx/N0 = 0; N1–2 = 2

**Table 23.5** 2016 TNM Classification System for Renal Cell Carcinoma

| T – Primary Tumour | | |
|---|---|---|
| TX | Primary tumour cannot be assessed | |
| T0 | No evidence of primary tumour | |
| T1 | Tumour $\leq$7 cm or less in greatest dimension, limited to the kidney | |
| | T1a | Tumour $\leq$4 cm or less |
| | T1b | Tumour >4 cm but $\leq$7 cm |
| T2 | Tumour >7 cm in greatest dimension, limited to the kidney | |
| | T2a | Tumour >7 cm but $\leq$ 10 cm |
| | T2b | Tumours >10 cm, limited to the kidney |
| T3 | Tumour extends into major veins or perinephric tissues but not into the ipsilateral adrenal gland and not beyond Gerota fascia | |
| | T3a | Tumour grossly extends into the renal vein or its segmental (muscle-containing) branches, or tumour invades peri-renal and/or renal sinus fat (peripelvic fat), but not beyond Gerota fascia |
| | T3b | Tumour grossly extends into the vena cava below the diaphragm |
| | T3c | Tumour grossly extends into vena cava above the diaphragm or invades the wall of the vena cava |
| T4 | Tumour invades beyond Gerota fascia (including contiguous extension into the ipsilateral adrenal gland) | |
| **N – Regional Lymph Nodes** | | |
| NX | Regional lymph nodes cannot be assessed | |
| N0 | No regional lymph node metastasis | |
| N1 | Metastasis in regional lymph node(s) | |
| **M – Distant Metastasis** | | |
| M0 | No distant metastasis | |
| M1 | Distant metastasis | |

- Nuclear grade (0–3)
  - G1–2 = 0; G3 = 1; G4 = 3
- Tumour necrosis (0–1)
  - No = 0; yes = 1
- Low risk = 0–2, intermediate = 3–5, high risk = 6–11

# Pathophysiology of Signs and Symptoms

- ~50% are incidental.
- *Triad* (~10%):
  - Loin pain (clot colic or advanced disease)
  - Haematuria (involvement of nephrons/urinary tract)
  - Mass
- *Paraneoplastic* syndrome (20–30%):
  - *Hypercalcaemia* (20–30%).
    - PTH-related peptide
    - 1,25-dihydroxy vitamin D production
    - Osteolytic metastases

- *Hypertension* (~35%).
  - Renin production
  - Renal artery stenosis (encasement)
- *Polycythaemia* (3–5%).
  - EPO by tumour or adjacent parenchyma due to hypoxia.
- *Stauffer's syndrome* (~5%).
  - Non-metastatic hepatic dysfunction
  - Deranged liver function test
  - Often have discrete areas of hepatic necrosis

# Challenges in Pathology
## Small Renal Masses (SRM)

- *Definition:* solid or complex cystic mass of <4 cm.
- *Growth rate:* out of 209 SRM – 0.13 cm/year on imaging (63% grew – 0.26 cm/year).
- *Metastatic* rate: 1.1%
- Difficulty in pre-operative differentiation bet-

ween RCC, oncocytoma, and fat-poor angio-myolipoma (AML).
- ~20% solid SRM removed at surgery = benign.
- Benign SRM from surgical excision:
  - 34–58% oncocytomas; 10–38% AML
- There is a rising likelihood of malignancy and higher grade with increasing lesion size.
  - Proportion of benign histology by size:
    - <1 cm: 40%; 1–2 cm: 21%; 2–3 cm: 20%; 3–4 cm: 17%
    - 4–7 cm: 9%; >7 cm: 6%

### Renal Biopsy

- Helpful diagnostic tool but can be inconclusive.
  - Difficulties in assigning tumour type and differentiating benign oncocytomas from malignant chRCC and eosinophilic ccRCCs.
- Should not be performed for cystic renal masses.
- RCC is characterised by intratumoral heterogeneity, meaning renal biopsy is limited by the area of the tumour sampled.
  - Intratumoral heterogeneity = cells within the same tumour show different genotypic and phenotypic characteristics.
- *Indications* for renal biopsy:
  - Prior to active surveillance.
  - Prior to minimally invasive treatment, such as cryotherapy or radiofrequency ablation.
  - Prior to systemic treatment for metastatic disease.
  - Uncertainties (e.g., lymphoma, secondary).

## Adult Primary, Hereditary Renal Cell Carcinoma (Table 23.3)

### Hereditary RCC

- *Autosomal dominant* inheritance pattern.
- It is usually an early onset RCC.
- *Bilateral* and *multifocal*.
- Not aggressive in the majority, except in hereditary leiomyomatosis and RCC syndrome.
- *Annual surveillance* is recommended with MRI scanning.
- Treat when lesions grow to *>3 cm* (except for HLRCC).

### Von Hippel Lindau Disease

- Germline mutations in the *VHL* gene (3p25).
- Increased risk of ccRCC.
- Associated conditions:
  - Retinal angioma
  - Central nervous system haemangioblastoma
  - Pancreatic neuroendocrine tumour
  - Phaeochromocytoma

- Endolymphatic sac inner ear tumour
- Multiple visceral cysts
- Annual surveillance for RCC recommended.

## Hereditary Papillary RCC (HPRCC)

- Germline mutation in *c-MET* proto-oncogene (Chm 7q).
- *Gene function:*
  - *C-MET* protein encoded by the gene: tyrosine kinase receptor for hepatocyte growth factor (HGF).
  - Disruption of signalling pathway leads to:
    - Cell proliferation, invasion, and increased angiogenesis.
- Associated with development of type 1 pRCC.
  - RCC occurs to those in their mid-40s.
  - Often multifocal and bilateral.
  - Small and hypovascular tumours.
  - With good prognosis.
- No associated extrarenal manifestations.

## Hereditary Leiomyomatosis and RCC (HLRCC)

- Germline mutations in the *FH* gene (Chm 1q).
- *Gene function:*
  - *FH* gene encodes the fumarate hydratase enzyme.
  - Component of the Krebs cycle.
  - The absence of FH staining on immunohistochemistry may confirm the diagnosis.
- The *Warburg* effect:
  - Characteristic of RCC.
  - Cells make ATP through glycolysis rather than Krebs cycle, despite normoxic conditions.
- Increased risk of cutaneous and *uterine leiomyomas* and type 2 pRCC.
- Extrarenal manifestations occur earlier (during the 2nd and 3rd decade).
  - More common than RCC (which develops around the 4th decade).
- HLRCC often develops unifocal RCC, unlike other hereditary renal tumours.
  - Can be very aggressive and can metastasise early.
  - Annual surveillance is key.

## Succinate Dehydrogenase RCC (SDHRCC)

- Germline mutation in any of the four *SDH* genes.
- *Gene function:*
  - Succinate dehydrogenase (SDH): tetrameric enzyme in the Krebs cycle, upstream to fumarate hydratase.

- Each four SDH subunits are encoded by four genes:
  - *SDHA*, *SDHB*, *SDHC*, and *SDHD*
  - Mutations in the *SDHB gene* are the most common.
- Absence of SDH staining on immunohistochemistry may confirm the diagnosis.
- *Renal manifestations:*
  - Early onset RCC, often bilateral and multifocal.
  - RCC may be aggressive in a small subset.
- *Extrarenal manifestations:*
  - Paragangliomas
  - Gastrointestinal stromal tumours

## Birt–Hogg–Dubé Syndrome

- Germline mutations in the folliculin (*FLCN*) gene (Chm 17p).
- *Gene function:*
  - Tumour suppressor gene leads to the activation of the mTOR pathway.
- *Renal manifestations:*
  - Increased risk of *distal nephron* tumour:
    - chRCC, oncocytomas, and hybrid oncocytic-chromophobe tumours.
    - Other types of RCC (including ccRCC) have also been noted.
  - Age of onset at the ~5th decade.
  - Associated with fibrofolliculomas, lung cysts, and spontaneous pneumothorax.
  - Often has good prognosis.

## Tuberous Sclerosis

- Germline mutations in one of the two tuberous sclerosis genes:
  - *TSC1* on Chm 9
  - *TSC2* on Chm 16
- Proteins encoded by the two genes work as a complex.
  - Mutations in either gene gives rise to a similar phenotype.
- *Renal manifestations:*
  - AML: lifetime risk of ~80%.
  - Renal cysts: lifetime risk of ~50%.
  - ccRCC: lifetime risk of ~1–5%.
- *Extrarenal manifestations:*
  - *Classical triad:*
    - Epilepsy, learning difficulties, cutaneous adenoma sebaceum

## Other Hereditary Conditions Associated with RCC

### BAP1 Tumour Syndrome

- Germline mutations in the *BAP1* gene.

- Increased risk of ccRCC, mesothelioma, uveal, and cutaneous melanoma.

### Cowden's Syndrome

- Germline mutations in the *PTEN* tumour suppressor gene.
- Increased risk of papillary RCC, breast cancer, and epithelial thyroid cancer.

### Cowden-Like Syndrome

- Germline mutations in the *KILLIN* gene, a tumour suppressor gene adjacent to the *PTEN gene.*
- Similar phenotype to Cowden's syndrome.

### Familial Non-Syndromic RCC

- >2 relatives are affected by RCC, but no other features are present as part of a syndrome.

# Other Adult Primary Malignant Renal Tumours

## Sarcoma of the Kidney

- Derived from the mesenchyme of the kidney.
- Leiomyosarcoma is the most common, followed by liposarcoma.
  - *Leiomyosarcoma* originates from smooth muscle cells in the renal capsule or perinephric tissue.
  - *Liposarcoma* originates from fat.
- Characterised by:
  - Large size and a rapid growth rate.
  - Aggressive, frequent metastasis (especially in the lungs).
  - Very high recurrence rates and overall poor outcome.

## Lymphoma of the Kidney

- Frequently found in association with systemic evidence of lymphoma.
  - Examples: splenomegaly, generalised lymphadenopathy, and B symptoms.
- Primary renal lymphoma without systemic features is much rarer.
- *Risk factors* include:
  - Immunosuppression
  - Autoimmune disease
  - Graft versus host disease
  - History of radiotherapy
- Lymphoma is sensitive to chemo-radiotherapy, so correct diagnosis is key.

## Adult Secondary Renal Tumours

- On autopsy studies, renal metastases are found in 7–12% of patients with other primary malignancies.
  - Lung is the most common primary site.
  - Other sites via haematological spread:
    - Breast, gastrointestinal, melanoma, and haematological cancers
- Metastases are often multifocal.
- Evidence of metastases in other organs is common.
  - Solitary renal metastases without involvement of other organs are rare.

# Paediatric Tumours

## Wilms' Tumour

- Also known as *nephroblastoma*.
- Derived from nephrogenic rests = tissue which resembles embryonic developing kidneys that fail to involute.
- Most common abdominal malignancy in children.
- Peak incidence: age 2–4 years (may occur rarely in adults).
- Bilateral tumours in 5% of cases.
- *Macroscopically:*
  - Distinct pseudocapsule
  - Large, soft, and pale grey — appearing similar to brain tissue
- *Microscopically:*
  - Contains three components in varying proportions: blastema, epithelium, stroma.
  - Two histological subtypes:
    - *'Favourable histology'*
      - 85–90% of cases with well-differentiated cells.
    - *'Unfavourable histology'*
      - 5–10% of cases with anaplastic features.
- *Genetics*:
- *Sporadic* cases:
  - Composes ~90% of cases.
  - Mutations/deletions in the *WT1* gene noted in 10–30% of sporadic disease.
- *Hereditary* cases:
  - WAGR syndrome: Wilms' tumour, Aniridia, Genitourinary malformation, mental Retardation.
  - Associated with a deletion in Wilms' Tumour 1 gene (*WT1*), Chm 11p13.
  - *Gene function:* tumour suppression and a role in renal embryonic development.
- Treated with neoadjuvant chemotherapy and subsequent surgery.
- Excellent prognosis with >90% survival.

# Benign Renal Cysts and Tumours

## Renal Cysts

### Simple Renal Cysts

- Definition: fluid-filled sacs lined with epithelium.
- Most common benign renal lesion.
- *Risk factors:*
  - Age: ~60% in those >80 years of age.
  - Males
  - Hypertension
  - Renal impairment
- Simple cysts: negligible malignant potential – do not require follow-up.
- Acquired renal cystic disease associated with ESRF is associated with increased risks of malignancy.
- Majority of renal cysts are asymptomatic.
  - Increasing cyst size may be associated with:
    - Pain
    - Complications, such as spontaneous haemorrhage or cyst rupture
- Anatomical location:
  - *Parapelvic* cysts: originate in the renal parenchyma and extend into the renal sinus.
  - *Peripelvic* cysts: originate within the sinus. Believed to be lymphatic in origin.

### Complex Renal Cysts

- Classified radiologically according to the *Bosniak classification* (Table 23.6).
  - Assesses the appearance of:
    - Cyst wall
    - Number and thickness of septations
    - Calcifications
    - Enhancement
  - Management is based on the risk of malignancy.
- Malignancy rates >50% in Bosniak III, ~90% in Bosniak IV lesions.
- European Association of Urology (EAU) Guidelines recommend:
  - Surveillance for Bosniak IIF cysts.
  - Operative management for Bosniak III and IV cysts.

## Oncocytoma

- Benign tumours derived from intercalated cells of the collecting duct.
- 3–7% of all solid renal masses.
- *Epidemiology:*
  - Male: Female; 2:1.
  - Prevalence increases with age.
  - The majority is sporadic.
  - Associated with the familial *Birt–Hogg–Dubé Syndrome.*

**Table 23.6** Bosniak Classification of Renal Cysts, Observed Malignancy Rates, and EAU Management Guidelines

| Classification | Definition | Malignancy rate | Recommended Management |
|---|---|---|---|
| Bosniak I | Simple cyst<br>• Regular, smooth, thin wall<br>• No septations, calcifications or contrast enhancement | Benign | No follow up required |
| Bosniak II | Mildly complex cyst<br>• Regular, smooth, thin wall<br>• Few thin septations<br>• Fine calcifications<br>• High-attenuating lesions <3 cm<br>• No contrast enhancement | ~6–9% | No follow up required |
| Bosniak IIF | Moderately complex cyst<br>• Well demarcated<br>• Minimally thickened wall<br>• Multiple thin septations<br>• Minimal enhancement of septations and/or wall<br>• Thick calcifications<br>• High-attenuating lesions >3 cm<br>• No enhancing soft tissue | ~6–18% overall. 12% Bosniak IIF cysts reclassified to III/IV. In Bosniak IIF cysts that are not reclassified, malignancy rates are <1% | Follow up recommended for up to 5 years |
| Bosniak III | Indeterminate<br>• Irregular appearance, thick wall<br>• Thick septations (>1 mm)<br>• Increasing amount of thick calcifications<br>• Contrast enhancement | ~50% | Treat as RCC: Surgery or active surveillance |
| Bosniak IV | High risk malignancy<br>• Irregular appearance, thick wall<br>• Contrast enhancement<br>• Soft tissue | ~90% | Treat as RCC: Surgery |

- Commonly found incidentally during abdominal imaging.
- Less commonly present with symptoms of a renal mass.
- *Macroscopically:*
  - Round, well-circumscribed, brown masses.
  - Characteristic central stellate scar of fibrous connective tissue.
    - *'Spoke-and-wheel'* appearance on angiography/CT due to the hypervascular edges and central scar tissue.
    - Central scar may be absent in small oncocytomas.
    - RCCs with central necrosis may give a similar appearance.
- *Microscopically:*
  - *Eosinophilic* cytoplasm.

- Abundance of mitochondria.
- Diagnostic challenge: differentiating onco-cytoma from the eosinophilic variant of chRCC on renal biopsy because they have a similar microscopic appearance.

# Angiomyolipoma (AML)

- A benign tumour.
- Derived from perivascular epithelioid cells.
  - Mesenchymal in origin.
- *Three components, giving rise to the name:*
  - Thick-walled blood vessels, smooth muscle, and adipose tissue.
- *Epidemiology:*
  - Sporadic AMLs are more common in women.
  - Mean age of diagnosis is at 45 years.

- *Aetiology:*
  - In most cases, sporadic and solitary.
  - Familial AML is associated with tuberous sclerosis.
    - Often multifocal and smaller, with a younger age of onset.
- *Macroscopically:*
  - Well-circumscribed.
  - Yellow colour suggests high fat content.
  - Pale grey colour suggests high content of smooth muscle.
- Radiographically (ultrasound and CT):
  - Presence of fat is diagnostic (CT <20 HU).
  - Fat-poor AMLs – diagnostic challenge. Not easily differentiated from RCC (in particular, ccRCC containing fat).
- Small AMLs are usually asymptomatic.
- Larger tumours may present with classical symptoms of a renal mass.
- An uncommon complication is retroperitoneal haemorrhage.
  - Risk increases with tumour size.
  - *Wunderlich syndrome: Lenk's triad.*
    - Acute loin pain, loin mass, hypovolaemic shock
- Tumours <4 cm in size are usually managed conservatively.
- Symptomatic tumours/rapid growth – treated surgically or by embolisation.

# Recommended Reading

1. Moch H, Cubilla AL, Hunmphrey PA, et al. The 2016 WHO classification of tumours of the urinary system and male genital organs-part A: renal, penile, and testicular Tumours. Eur Urol. 2016;70(1):93–105.
2. Rossi SH, Klatte T, Usher-Smith J, Stewart GD. Epidemiology and screening for renal cancer. World J Urol. 2018;36(9): 1341–1353.
3. Cancer Research UK Kidney Cancer statistics. https://www.cancerresearchuk.org/health-professional/cancer-statistics/statistics-by-cancer-type/kidney-cancer.
4. Ljungberg B, Albiges L, Abu-Ghanem Y, Bensalah K, Dabestani S, Montes SF, et al. European Association of Urology Guidelines on Renal Cell Carcinoma: the 2019 update. Eur Urol. 2019.
5. Cancer Genome Atlas Research N. Comprehensive molecular characterization of clear cell renal cell carcinoma. Nature. 2013;499(7456):43–49.
6. Ricketts CJ, De Cubas AA, Fan H, Smith CC, Lang M, Reznik E, et al. The cancer genome atlas comprehensive molecular characterization of renal cell carcinoma. Cell Rep. 2018;23(1):313–326 e5.
7. Gospodarowicz MK, Brierley JD, Wittekind C. TNM classification of malignant tumours: John Wiley & Sons; 2017.
8. Rossi SH, Prezzi D, Kelly-Morland C, Goh V. Imaging for the diagnosis and response assessment of renal tumours. World J Urol. 2018;36(12):1927–1942.
9. Maher ER. Hereditary renal cell carcinoma syndromes: diagnosis, surveillance and management. World J Urol. 2018;36(12):1891–1898.
10. Verine J, Pluvinage A, Bousquet G, Lehmann-Che J, de Bazelaire C, Soufir N, et al. Hereditary renal cancer syndromes: an update of a systematic review. Eur Urol. 2010;58(5):701–710.
11. Hsieh JJ, Purdue MP, Signoretti S, et al. Renal cell carcinoma. Nat Rev Dis Primers. 2017;3:17009.
12. Bosniak MA. The current radiological approach to renal cysts. Radiology. 1986;158(1):1–10.
13. Schoots IG, Zaccai K, Hunink MG, Verhagen P. Bosniak classification for complex renal cysts reevaluated: a systematic review. J Urol. 2017;198(1):12–21.

# 24 Urothelial and Urethral Cancer

*Ibrahim Jubber, Karl H. Pang, and James W.F. Catto*

## Epidemiology of Urothelial Cancer

### Demographics

#### Bladder Cancer (BC)

- 90–95% of all urothelial cell carcinoma (UCC)
- Male to female – 3:1
- 7th most common cancer worldwide in men, 9th when both genders are considered.
- One of the most expensive to manage.
- Highest incidence rates – North America, Europe, and Western Asia.
- Trends vary and reflect patterns of smoking and occupational hygiene.
- *UK 2017:* 10,200 new cases and 5,600 deaths.

#### Upper Urinary Tract Urothelial Carcinoma (UTUC)

- 5–10% of UCC.
- Concurrent with BC in ~17%.

## Aetiology and Risk Factors

- Risks for UCC are summarised in Table 24.1
- Tobacco smoking is the most common risk factor.
- BC and UTUC share common risk factors.
- Risk factors associated with UTUC include:
  - Lynch syndrome
  - Arsenic in drinking water (Taiwan).
  - Aristolochic acid (nitrophenanthrene caroboxylic acid produced by Aristolochia plants):
    - Environmental contamination or ingestion of herbal remedies.
    - Reacts with genomic DNA forming aristolactam-deoxyadenosine.
  - Alcohol – odd ratio 1.23 in ever-drinkers versus never-drinkers.

## Genetic Risk Factors

### Inherited Gene Polymorphisms

- Inheritance of low-cancer risk gene polymorphisms.

- Polymorphisms may be of unknown function:
  - Such as those found in Chr. 19q12 by genome wide screens.
- Genes important in urothelial carcinogens metabolism are shown in Figure 24.1.
  a. *N-acetyltransferase 2 (NAT-2)*
  - Regulates the rate of detoxification of aromatic amines (e.g., nitrosamine, a known urothelial carcinogens) through acetylation.
  - Carriers of the '*slow*' variant (because of a DNA polymorphism on one amino acid) of this gene have an increased risk of BC. Relative risk (RR) 1.4-fold compared with the '*fast*' variant.
  - Risk in *slow* variants is greater in tobacco smokers.
  - 56% of Caucasians are *slow acetylators* compared to 11% Asians.
  b. *Glutathione S-transferase (GST)*
  - Encoded by the *GSTM1* gene.
  - Detoxifies polyaromatic hydrocarbons (PAHs).
  - Homozygous deletion of *GSTM1* gene (Null *GSTM1*) – BC RR 1.9 fold.

### Inherited Cancer Syndromes

- *Lynch Syndrome* (Hereditary Non-Polyposis Colon Cancer).
  - DNA mutant mismatch repair gene (*MLH1* and *MSH2*).
  - High-risk family syndrome – elevated risk of urothelial cell carcinoma (UCC).
    - Most urothelial carcinoma are in the upper urinary tract (UTUC)
    - BC – RR 4.2 for males and 2.2 for females.

## Acquired Risk Factors

### Tobacco Smoking

- Most common risk factor for UCC. Estimated to account for 50% of UCC.
- UTUC: RR increased from 2.5 to 7.0.

**Table 24.1** Risk Factors for Bladder Cancer

| Risk | Association |
|---|---|
| Tobacco smoking | 50–60% male cases, 20–30% female |
| Occupational exposures | Work-related cases 8–15% |
| | 10–30 years latency period |
| | Aromatic amines, polycyclic aromatic hydrocarbons, Dyes, rubbers, textiles, paints, leathers, chemicals |
| Medical | EBRT or brachytherapy |
| | EBRT for gynaecological cancer- RR 2-4 |
| | Diabetes (Pioglitazone) |
| Bladder schistosomiasis and inflammation | Bilharzia parasite – associated with SCC |
| | Urinary calculi and chronic inflammation |
| Gender | Male incidence higher |
| | Female worse survival outcome- HR 1.2 |
| Genetic factors | Family history – 2-fold with an affected relative |
| | Gene polymorphism – NAT, GST |
| | Lynch syndrome |

*Abbreviations:* EBRT, external beam radiation therapy; RR, relative risk; SCC, squamous cell carcinoma; HR, hazard ratio; NAT, N-acetyltransferase; GST, Glutathione S-transferase.

- Carcinogenic components are combustion products:
  - Arylamines (particularly 4-aminobiphenol).
  - Polycyclic aromatic hydrocarbons.
  - *N*-nitroso compounds.
  - Heterocyclic amines.
  - Various epoxides.
- These compounds result in DNA damage:
  - Double strand breaks.
  - Base modifications.
  - Bulky adduct formation.
- *Electronic cigarettes* do not use combustion and so may not cause UCC.
- *Current smokers:* ~3x the risk of never-smokers.
- *Ex-smokers:* ~2x the risk of never-smokers.
  - Therefore, smoking cessation may reduce the risk of developing BC.

## Occupational Exposures

- 2nd most common risk factor for BC. Estimated to account for 5–10% of UCC.
- Exposure through inhalation, ingestion, or skin contact.
- Carcinogens are classified with respect to carcinogenicity by the International Agency for Research on Cancer (IARC):

- *Aromatic amines*
  - *4-aminobiphenyl* (IARC Class 1: *'definitively' carcinogenic* to humans).
  - *2-napthylamine* (IARC Class 1):
    - Rubber, plastic, dye industries (hair dyes), painting materials.
- *Polycyclic aromatic hydrocarbons (PAH)*
  - Atmospheric pollutants or lubricants.
  - Fused aromatic ring structure.
  - *Naphthalene* (IARC class 2b: *'possibly'-carcinogenic* to humans).
  - *Benzo[a]pyrene* (IARC class 1).
    - Metal and aluminium manufacturing industries.
    - Workers in proximity to tobacco smoke and diesel fumes (recreational and bar staff and drivers).
- The latency period between exposure and cancer is 10–30 years.

## Environmental Factors

- Arsenic in drinking water and chlorination of drinking water (with subsequent levels of trihalomethanes).

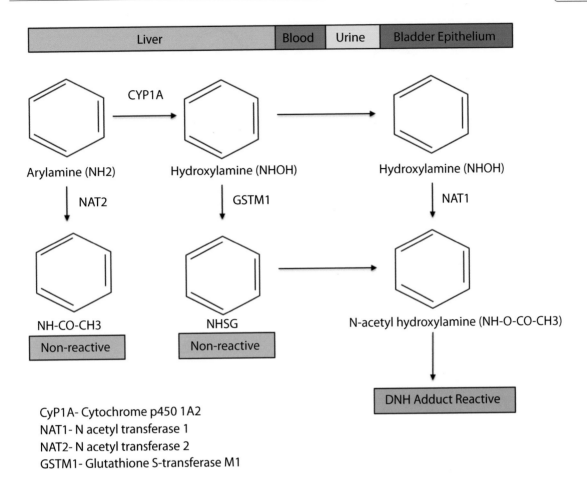

CyP1A- Cytochrome p450 1A2
NAT1- N acetyl transferase 1
NAT2- N acetyl transferase 2
GSTM1- Glutathione S-transferase M1

Figure 24.1 Metabolism of bladder cancer carcinogens arylamine and hydroxylamine. Arylamines are *N*-acetylated by NAT-2 in the liver to non-reactive compounds. *N*-hydroxylation by CYPIA leads to the production of hydroxylamine which is transported to the bladder and metabolised by NAT1 to a highly reactive species that can form DNA adducts.

## Iatrogenic Factors

- *Diabetic drugs:* the use of pioglitazone (a thiazolidinedione).
  - Increase the risk of BC by up to 1.6 fold.
- *Cyclophosphamide*
  - Increase the risk of BC by ~4.5 fold.
  - Dose-dependent.
- *Pelvic radiotherapy*
  - Examples: to treat ovarian, testicular, cervical, uterine, prostate cancer, lymphoma.
  - Radiotherapy for prostate cancer: ~2-fold increased risk of BC.
  - Radiotherapy for cervical cancer: 2–4-fold increased risk.

## Nutrition Factors

- Most nutrients or metabolites are excreted in the urine and have prolonged contact with the urothelium.
- *Fruits and vegetables:* contain active compounds important in detoxification.
- *Vitamins and antioxidants:* preventative effect on BC development.
- *Meats/animal protein:* nitroso compounds – increases risk of UC.

## Clinical Presentation of Urothelial Cancer

- Visible (VH) or non-visible haematuria (NVH).
- Haematuria: >3 red blood cell per high powered field (HPF).
- Malignancy found in ~3% NVH and 13.8% VH.
- Causes of haematuria are shown in Figure 24.2.
- Other signs and symptoms: lower urinary tract symptoms, palpable mass (advanced disease).

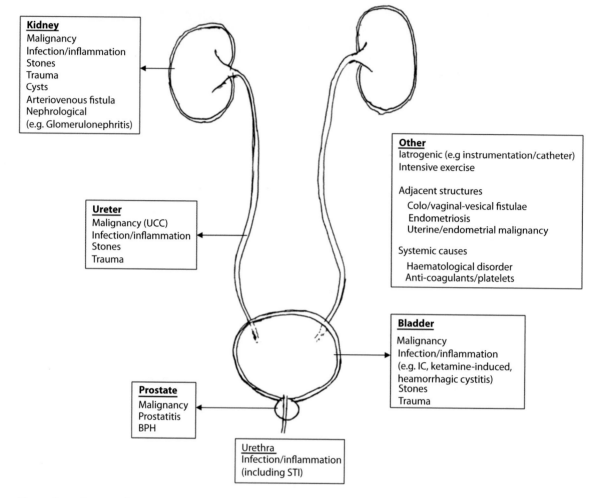

**Kidney**
Malignancy
Infection/inflammation
Stones
Trauma
Cysts
Arteriovenous fistula
Nephrological
(e.g. Glomerulonephritis)

**Other**
Iatrogenic (e.g instrumentation/catheter)
Intensive exercise

Adjacent structures
    Colo/vaginal-vesical fistulae
    Endometriosis
    Uterine/endometrial malignancy

Systemic causes
    Haematological disorder
    Anti-coagulants/platelets

**Ureter**
Malignancy (UCC)
Infection/inflammation
Stones
Trauma

**Bladder**
Malignancy
Infection/inflammation
(e.g. IC, ketamine-induced,
heamorrhagic cystitis)
Stones
Trauma

**Prostate**
Malignancy
Prostatitis
BPH

**Urethra**
Infection/inflammation
(including STI)

**Figure 24.2** Causes of haematuria. UCC, urothelial cell carcinoma; BPH, benign prostate hyperplasia; IC, interstitial cystitis; STI, sexually transmitted infection. (Reprinted by permission from Springer Nature [19])

# Pathology

- WHO Classification of urothelial tract tumours are summarised in Table 24.2.

## Benign Lesions

### Epithelial Metaplasia

- Focal areas of transformed urothelium.
- Normal nuclear and cellular architecture.
- Glandular or squamous in origin.
- Related to urinary catheter, infection, or trauma.
- Keratinising squamous metaplasia seen in exstrophy, chronic bladder inflammation and schistosomiasis = *premalignant*.

- Non-keratinising squamous metaplasia = *NOT* premalignant.

### Leukoplakia

- Squamous metaplasia with marked keratinisation.
- Whitish patches.
- Considered premalignant and may progress to squamous cell carcinoma in up to 20%.

### Malakoplakia

- Yellow patches.
- *Michaelis–Gutmann* bodies with distinctive basophilic inclusions.

**Table 24.2** World Health Organization (WHO) Classification of Urothelial Tumours

| Urothelial tumours | Neuroendocrine tumours |
|---|---|
| *Infiltrating UC* | Small cell |
| Nested | Large cell |
| Microcystic | Well-differentiated |
| Micropapillary | Paraganglioma |
| Lymphoepithelioma-like | **Melanocytic tumours** |
| Plasmacytoid/signet ring cell/diffuse sarcomatoid | Malignant melanoma |
| Giant cell | Naevus |
| Poorly differentiated | Melanosis |
| *Non-invasive urothelial neoplasms* | **Mesenchymal tumours** |
| UC in situ | Rhabdomyosarcoma |
| Non-invasive papillary UC low-grade | Leiomyosarcoma |
| Non-invasive papillary UC high-grade | Angiosarcoma |
| PUNLMP | Inflammatory myofibroblastic |
| Urothelial papilloma | Perivascular epithelioid cell |
| Inverted urothelial papilloma | Solitary fibrous |
| Urothelial proliferation of uncertain malignant potential | Leiomyoma |
| Urothelial dysplasia | Granular cell |
| **Squamous cell neoplasms** | Neurofibroma |
| Pure squamous cell carcinoma | **Urothelial tract haematopoietic and lymphoid tumours** |
| Verrucous carcinoma | **Miscellaneous tumours** |
| Squamous cell papilloma | Carcinoma of Skene, Cowper, and Littre glands |
| **Glandular neoplasms** | Metastatic tumours and tumours extending from other organs |
| Adenocarcinoma | Epithelial tumours of the upper urinary tract |
| Villous adenoma | Tumours arising in a bladder diverticulum |
| **Urachal carcinoma** | Urothelial tumours of the urethra |
| **Tumours of Mullerian type** | |
| Clear cell carcinoma | |
| Endometrioid carcinoma | |

*Source:* Adapted from Humphrey et al. [10]
*Abbreviations:* PUNLMP, papillary urothelial neoplasm of low malignant potential; UC, urothelial carcinoma.

## Inverted Papilloma

- Benign proliferative lesion.
- <1% of all bladder tumour.
- Most common on the trigone.
- No cytological or atypia.
- Invaginates lamina propria but not into muscularis.

## Papilloma

- Benign proliferative lesion on a delicate stalk. Normal urothelium.

## Nephrogenic Adenoma

- Benign lesion that resembles primitive renal collecting tubules.

- Involves mucosa and submucosa.
- Vascular, therefore may get haematuria.
- Associated/caused by inflammation.

## Cystitis Cystica

- Common finding in obstruction/inflammation. Not malignant.
- Cystic nests lined by columnar epithelium and proliferation of von Brunn's nests.

## Cystitis Glandularis

- Associated with adenocarcinoma.
- Transitional cells undergo glandular metaplasia.

## Bladder Cancer

- Most (>90%) BC are UCC in origin.
- Less common include:
  - Squamous cell carcinoma (5%)
    - Associated with Schistosoma haematobium (Figure 24.3) and chronic inflammation (bladder stones, long-term catheterisation).
  - Adenocarcinoma (1–2%)
    - Primary urachal or non-urachal, or secondary from prostate/bowel/ovarian cancer.
  - Small cell (<1%)
    - Neuroendocrine in origin
  - Sarcoma (<1%)
  - Melanoma (<1%)
  - Lymphoma (<1%)
- UCC may be:
  - Pure urothelial
  - Mixed (e.g., with squamous or glandular components)
  - UCCs have a variant growth pattern (e.g., micropapillary or nested patterns).
- Mixed, variant UCC and non-UCC may be more aggressive than pure UCC.
  - Present at a higher stage than pure UCC.
  - Have ominous features (e.g., solid growth, lymphovascular invasion (LVI), or metastases).
- Multiple growth patterns of UCC including:
  - Flat carcinoma in situ (CIS)
  - Papillary tumours that can be low (LG) or high grade (HG)
  - Sessile tumours (HG) with a solid growth pattern
  - Mixed papillary/solid
- Stage and grade are predictors of behaviour and survival.
  - Grade is indicative of the growth potential.
  - Stage describes the extent of the cancer.
- The ability of HG tumours to invade and metastasise is a result of micro-metastatic disease from LVI.

- Initial presentation: ~75% non-muscle invasive (NMIBC), ~20% MIBC.

## Upper Tract UCC

- Non-urothelial is uncommon.
- Variants in ~25%, squamous differentiation in ~15%, sarcomatoid (rare).
- Treated UTUC have recurrence in:
  - Bladder, 22–47% (UTUC recurrence following cystectomy for BC is ~2–4%).
  - Contralateral ureter, 2–5%
- ~60% present with invasive disease, 5% is bilateral.
- Location in the renal pelvis is more common than in the ureter.
- Within the ureter: distal ureteric UCC is more common.

## Schistosomiasis (Bilharzia)

- Parasitic infection
- Skin penetration and enter portal vasculature (Figure 24.3).
  - *Schistosoma haematobium* (terminal spines) – vesicular vessels (bladder).
  - *S. mansoni* and *S. japonicum* (lateral spines) – mesenteric vessels (intestine).
- Endemic in the Middle East (Egypt) and most of Africa.
- *S. haematobium* produces 200–500 eggs/day. Egg: 80–158 μm long.
- Acute infection (Katayama fever) occurs 3–9 weeks after infection.
- Chronic infection: urinary symptoms, urinary tract infection, squamous cell carcinoma.

## Immunohistochemistry (IHC)

- Cytokeratin: CK7, CK20
- GATA3
- p40, p63
- PDL-1
- Uroplakin

## Tumour Stage

- Stage is assessed by histopathological evaluation, bimanual examination and imaging (Tables 24.3 and 24.4).
- BC are subdivided into:
  - NMIBC (CIS, pTa, pT1).
  - MIBC (T2–4).

## Carcinoma In Situ (CIS)

- Flat and non-invasive.

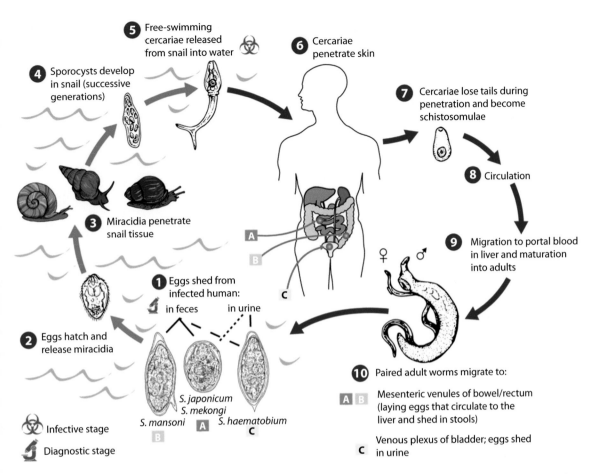

**Figure 24.3** Schistosoma life cycle. (1) *Schistosoma* eggs are eliminated with faeces or urine, depending on species; (2) Under appropriate conditions the eggs hatch and release miracidia; (3) Penetrate specific snail intermediate hosts; (4) The stages in the snail include two generations of sporocysts and; (5) The production of cercariae; 6) Upon release from the snail, the infective cercariae swim, penetrate the skin of the human host; (7) Forked tails, are shed becoming schistosomulae; (8-9) The schistosomulae migrate via venous circulation to lungs, then to the heart, and then develop in the liver, exiting the liver via the portal vein system when mature; (10) Male and female adult worms copulate and reside in the mesenteric venules, the location of which varies by species (with some exceptions). For instance, S. japonicum is more frequently found in the superior mesenteric veins draining the small intestine (A), and *S. mansoni* Occurs more often in the inferior mesenteric veins draining the large intestine (B). However, both species can occupy either location and are capable of moving between sites. S. intercalatum and S. guineensis also inhabit the inferior mesenteric plexus but lower in the bowel than S. mansoni. S. haematobium most often inhabits in the vesicular and pelvic venous plexus of the bladder (C), but it can also be found in the rectal venules. The females (size ranges from 7 to 28 mm, depending on species) deposit eggs in the small venules of the portal and perivesical systems. The eggs are moved progressively towards the lumen of the intestine (*S. mansoni, S. japonicum, S. mekongi, S. intercalatum/guineensis*) and of the bladder and ureters (*S. haematobium*), and are eliminated with faeces or urine, respectively. (Reused from da Silve Aj and Moser M. Centers for Disease Control and Prevention: Schistosomiasis. Aug 2019.)

- Confined to the epithelium and has an intact basement membrane.
- High-grade lesion → precursor to invasive cancer.
- Loss of umbrella cells is a characteristic that can distinguish CIS from dysplasia.

- Cells are poorly cohesive – CIS often results in positive urine cytology.
- Often multifocal – can occur in the bladder, upper urinary tract, prostatic ducts and urethra.
- Without treatment, 54% progress to MIBC.

**Table 24.3** 2016 TNM Classification of Bladder Cancer

**T – Primary tumour**

| | | |
|---|---|---|
| TX | Primary tumour cannot be assessed | |
| T0 | No evidence of primary tumour | |
| Ta | Non-invasive papillary carcinoma | |
| Tis | Carcinoma *in situ*: 'flat tumour' | |
| T1 | Tumour invades subepithelial connective tissue | |
| T2 | Tumour invades muscle | |
| | T2a | Tumour invades superficial muscle (inner half) |
| | T2b | Tumour invades deep muscle (outer half) |
| T3 | Tumour invades perivesical tissue | |
| | T3a | Microscopically |
| | T3b | Macroscopically (extravesical mass) |
| T4 | Tumour invades any of the following: prostate stroma, seminal vesicles, uterus, vagina, pelvic wall, abdominal wall | |
| | T4a | Tumour invades prostate stroma, seminal vesicles, uterus or vagina |
| | T4b | Tumour invades pelvic wall or abdominal wall |

**N – Regional lymph nodes**

| | | |
|---|---|---|
| NX | Regional lymph nodes cannot be assessed | |
| N0 | No regional lymph node metastasis | |
| N1 | Metastasis in a single lymph node in the true pelvis (hypogastric, obturator, external iliac, or presacral) | |
| N2 | Metastasis in multiple regional lymph nodes in the true pelvis (hypogastric, obturator, external iliac, or presacral) | |
| N3 | Metastasis in common iliac lymph node(s) | |

**M – Distant metastasis**

| | | |
|---|---|---|
| M0 | No distant metastasis | |
| | M1a | Non-regional lymph nodes |
| | M1b | Other distant metastases |

## Lamina Propria Invasion (pT1)

- Degree of pT1 invasion and LVI is prognostic.
- There is a risk of understaging patients with pT1 if:
  - There is no detrusor muscle in the transurethral resection specimen, if the initial resection was incomplete, or if the lesion is high grade.

## Muscle Invasion

- >50% with MIBC have occult/clinically inapparent metastatic disease at presentation.

- In cN0 MIBC pre-op staging, ~1/5 have positive nodes on radical cystectomy and lymphadenectomy specimen.

## Histological Grading

- *Two classifications* are used for grading UCC.
  1. *The World Health Organization (WHO) 1973 classification*:
     - Well (Grade 1), moderately (Grade 2) and poorly differentiated (Grade 3).
  2. *The WHO 2004 classification (papillary lesions)*:
     - Papillary Urothelial Neoplasm of Low Malignant Potential (PUNLMP).

**Table 24.4** 2016 TNM Classification of for Upper Tract Urothelial Carcinoma

| T – Primary tumour | | |
|---|---|---|
| TX | Primary tumour cannot be assessed | |
| T0 | No evidence of primary tumour | |
| | Ta | Non-invasive papillary carcinoma |
| | Tis | Carcinoma *in situ* |
| T1 | Tumour invades subepithelial connective tissue | |
| T2 | Tumour invades muscularis | |
| T3 | (Renal pelvis) Tumour invades beyond muscularis into peripelvic fat or renal parenchyma (Ureter) Tumour invades beyond muscularis into periureteric fat | |
| T4 | Tumour invades adjacent organs or through the kidney into perinephric fat | |
| **N – Regional lymph nodes** | | |
| NX | Regional lymph nodes cannot be assessed | |
| N0 | No regional lymph node metastasis | |
| N1 | Metastasis in a single lymph node 2 cm or less in the greatest dimension | |
| N2 | Metastasis in a single lymph node more than 2 cm, or multiple lymph nodes | |
| **M – Distant metastasis** | | |
| M0 | No distant metastasis | |
| M1 | Distant metastasis | |

- Low grade (LG).
- High grade (HG).
- G1 tumours split into PUNLMP and LG.
- G2 reassigned to LG and HG.
- G3 reassigned to HG.

## Precursor Lesions

- Normal bladder urothelium is multilayered (~7 cells thick).
- Cells mature from the basement membrane cells up to the surface cells.
- The mucosal lining has:
  - Large umbrella cells.
  - Membrane composed of uroplakin proteins.
  - The umbrella cells prevent urinary toxins from transforming urothelial cells.

- *Hyperplasia*
  - Thickening of the urothelium mucosa to >10 cells.
  - Often found adjacent to LG papillary tumours and may be a precursor to these.
  - There is no cytological atypia or mitoses.

- *Dysplasia*
  - Flat lesions with cytological and architectural abnormalities.

- Preneoplastic, but does not meet the criteria for CIS.
- It can occur de novo (primary) or with previous or concurrent UCC (secondary).
  - Secondary is more common than primary dysplasia.
- Progression rates – 15–19% for primary, 30–36% for secondary dysplasia.
- Aberrations in Chm 9 and TP53 are reported.

- Cystoscopic views and histological slides of BC and CIS are shown in Figure 24.4.

## Histological Variants

- Influence prognosis and management.
  - Incidence of variants ~20% (Figure 24.5).
- *Micropapillary*
  - Incidence of up to 6%.
  - Strong male preponderance.
  - Histologically resembles ovarian serous carcinoma.
  - Associated with advanced stage at presentation, poor prognosis
  - Poor response to intravesical treatment – early radical treatment recommended.

- *Nested*
  - Rare variant.

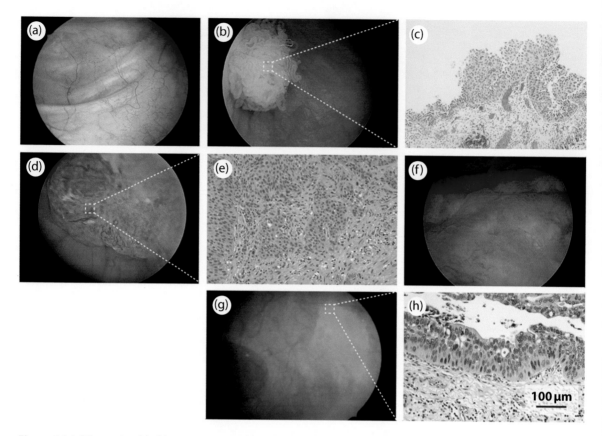

**Figure 24.4** Diagnosing bladder cancer. (a) Normal bladder appearance by cystoscopy; (b) Papillary bladder cancer by cystoscopy; (c) Histology slide (haematoxylin and eosin (H&E) staining of low-grade (pTa) non-muscle-invasive bladder cancer, magnification ×100; (d) Muscle-invasive bladder cancer by cystoscopy; (e) Histology slide (H&E) of high-grade (pT2) cancer, magnification ×200; (f) Cystoscopy image of the characteristic appearances of carcinoma in situ (CIS) as 'velvety' red patches at the base of the bladder; (g) Blue-light cystoscopy image of CIS visible at the anterosuperior portion of the bladder; (h) Histology slide (H&E) of CIS. (Reprinted by permission from Springer Nature [17])

- Male preponderance.
- Can be confused with benign lesions such as von Brunn's nests or cystitis cystica.
- Clinically aggressive and has a poor prognosis.

- *Sarcomatoid*
  - Rare variant.
  - Incidence of 0.2–4.3%.
  - Biphasic with epithelial and mesenchymal morphologies.
  - Mesenchymal features can include differentiation into tissues not usually found in the bladder (e.g., bone, cartilage, and skeletal muscles (heterologous differentiation)).
  - Advanced at presentation and associated with a poor prognosis.

- *Plasmacytoid*
  - Rare entity.
  - Encountered at an advanced stage and has a poor prognosis.

## Bladder Tumour Dissemination

- *Lymphovascular invasion:*
  - Can lead to metastases.
  - Present in ~25% of MIBC.
  - Poor prognostic sign – 40% risk of nodal disease.
  - Independent predictor of survival.

- *Pagetoid spread*:
  - Cancer cells grow underneath a layer of normal-looking surface urothelium.
  - Primarily seen in CIS.
  - Can occur in prostatic urethra or distal ureters.

- *Direct extension*:
  - Direct extension into the basal lamina, connective tissue and the lymphovascular system is caused by genetic and epigenetic changes.

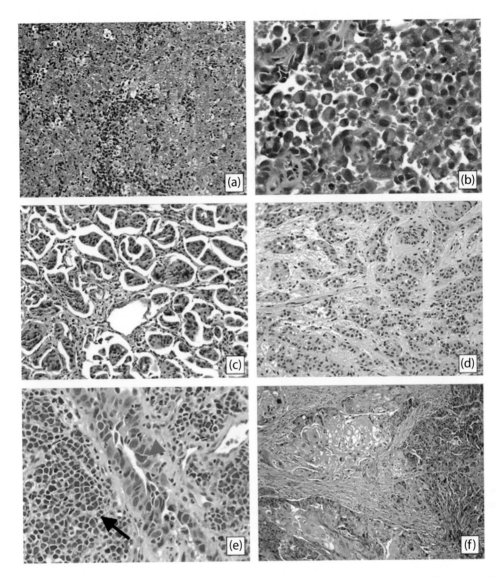

Figure 24.5 Histological variants of Urothelial Cancer (UC). Hematoxylin and eosin staining. (a) Lymphoepithelioma-like variant histologic differentiation; (b) Plasmacytoid differentiation in UC; (c) Micropapillary differentiation; (d) Nested urothelial carcinoma; (e) Small cell neuroendocrine differentiation (arrow) with conventional urothelial component (arrowhead); (f) Squamous differentiation. (Reprinted with permission from Elsevier [11])

- Facilitated by collagenases, motility and growth factors and cell adhesion molecules.

- *Lymphatic drainage* – important in the extent of pelvic lymph node dissection (PLND) (Figure 24.6).
  - External iliac.
  - Obturator.
  - Internal iliac (hypogastric).
  - Common iliac.
  - Presacral.
  - Abdominal (paracaval, iteraaortocaval, para-aortic).

## Multifocality and Tumour Recurrence

- BC may be multi or unifocal.
- ~5% will have a synchronous UTUC.
- BC has a high local recurrence rate (up to 80% in HG disease). Two main theories to explain this (32–34):
  *1. Oligoclonal disease (Field change)*
- Transformation of multiple unrelated urothelial cells (secondary to common carcinogen exposure).
- Leads to synchronous/metachronous non-related UC at different sites.
  *2. Monoclonal disease (Implantation)*

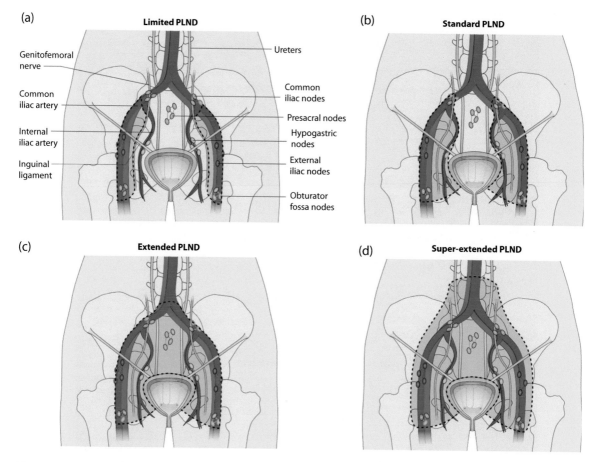

**Figure 24.6** Extent of lymphadenectomy. (a) Limited PLND: limited to obturator fossa; (b) Standard PLND: includes nodal dissection between the bifurcation of the common iliac artery proximally, the inguinal ligament distally, the genitofemoral nerve laterally, and the bladder wall medially and includes the distal common iliac, external iliac, obturator, and hypogastric nodes; (c) Extended PLND: removal of nodes between the aortic bifurcation and common iliac vessels proximally, the genitofemoral nerve laterally, the circumflex iliac vein distally, and the internal iliac vessels posteriorly; (d) super-extended plnd: dissection that is continued proximally to the root of the inferior mesenteric artery. (Reprinted by permission from Springer Nature [20])

- A single common genetically transformed cell that spreads by:
  - Intraepithelial migration or
  - Intraluminal seeding.
- *Intraluminal seeding:* tumour cells detaching from the primary lesion, seeding in the urine, and subsequently implanting at other sites in the urothelium.

## Recurrence and Progression in NMIBC

- NMIBC is a heterogeneous disease.
- 30–80% develop recurrent disease.
- Up to 45% progress to MIBC over 5 years. Very rare in low-grade BC.

- Prognostic factors for recurrence in NMIBC:
  - Grade and stage.
  - Number and size of the tumour(s).
  - Presence of CIS.
  - Previous recurrences.

- Important prognostic factors for progression in NMIBC:
  - Grade and stage.
  - Presence of CIS.
  - Variant histology.
  - Presence of LVI.

- Prognostic factors are based on the European Organisation for Research and Treatment of Cancer (EORTC) trials.

**Table 24.5** Weighting System Used to Calculate Recurrence and Progression Scores (EORTC 2006)

| Factor | Recurrence | Progression |
|---|---|---|
| **Number of tumours** | | |
| Single | 0 | 0 |
| 2–7 | 3 | 3 |
| ≥8 | 6 | 3 |
| **Tumour diameter** | | |
| <3 cm | 0 | 0 |
| ≥3 cm | 3 | 3 |
| **Prior recurrence rate** | | |
| Primary | 0 | 0 |
| <1 recurrence/year | 2 | 2 |
| >1 recurrence/year | 4 | 2 |
| **Category** | | |
| Ta | 0 | 0 |
| T1 | 1 | 4 |
| **Concurrent CIS** | | |
| No | 0 | 0 |
| Yes | 1 | 6 |
| **Grade** | | |
| G1 | 0 | 0 |
| G2 | 1 | 0 |
| G3 | 2 | 5 |
| **Total score** | 0–17 | 0–23 |

*Notes:* The new EAU 2021 NMIBC scoring model is based on data from 3,401 patients. There are slight changes to the parameters which include: • Number of tumours: single, multiple; • Maximum tumour diameter: <3 cm, >3 cm; • Stage: Ta, T1; • Concomitant CIS: no, yes; • WHO Grade 2004/2016: LMP-LR, HG OR WHO Grade 1973: G1, G2, G3.
*Source:* Reprinted with permission from Elsevier [13].

- Patient data available from 2596 patients diagnosed with Ta and T1 tumours.
- Scoring system is based on different prognostic factors can be used to calculate probabilities for recurrence and progression (Tables 24.5 and 24.6).
- The latest EAU 2021 guidelines include extra parameters – Age <70y or >70y; WHO Grade 2004/2017 LMP-LG or HG (www.nmibc.net).
- The EAU guidelines recommend stratifying

patients with NMIBC into four risk groups based on risks of recurrence or progression.
- Low, intermediate, high risk and very high risk (Table 24.7).
- This risk group stratification is used to guide treatment decisions.

# Risk Stratification of Non-Metastatic UTUC

- Risks are based on focality, tumour size, grade on cytology/biopsy and invasion (Table 24.8).
- *Prognostic factors* include:
  - Age, tobacco consumption, performance status, co-morbidity.
  - Tumour focality, location, grade.
  - Neutrophil to lymphocyte ratio, hydronephrosis.
  - CIS, LVI, tumour architecture, positive surgical margins, variant histology, tumour necrosis.

# Molecular Biology of Bladder Cancer

- There are multiple genetic and epigenetic alterations including genes that affect:
  - Signal transduction, cell cycle, invasion, angiogenesis, apoptosis.
- Papillary LG and HG BC arise via distinct pathways.
- HG BCs have high levels of genomic instability (in contrast to low grade) and share many similarities regardless of stage.

## Low-Grade BC

- LG papillary BCs are stable at the chromosomal level compared to HG.
- Deletions in regions of Chm 9 are the most common events.
- Common genetic events are mutations of:
  - *FGFR3* (79%), *Ras* (12%) and *PIK3CA* (54%).
  - *STAG 2* (37%), *KDM6A* (52%) and *TERT* (60–80%).
- *FGFR3* mutations
  - Activate the FGF growth pathway.
  - Associated with a favourable clinical phenotype (fewer progression and recurrence events).
  - FGF-targeting small molecules are now entering clinical practice (e.g., erdafitinib is FDA approved).
- *H-Ras* mutations
  - Activate a similar pathway to FGFR3 (RAS–MAPK and RAS–MEK–ERK pathways).
  - Mostly mutually exclusive.
- *PIK3CA* mutations

**Table 24.6a** EORTC Probability of Recurrence and Progression According to Total Score

| Recurrence Score | Probability of Recurrence at 1 Year | | Probability of Recurrence at 5 Years | |
|---|---|---|---|---|
| | % | 95% CI | % | 95% CI |
| 0 | 15 | 10–19 | 31 | 24–37 |
| 1–4 | 24 | 21–26 | 46 | 42–49 |
| 5–9 | 38 | 35–41 | 62 | 58–65 |
| 10–17 | 61 | 55–67 | 78 | 73–84 |
| Progression Score | Probability of Progression at 1 Year | | Probability of Progression at 5 Years | |
| | % | 95% CI | % | 95% CI |
| 0 | 0.2 | 0–0.7 | 0.8 | 0–1.7 |
| 2–6 | 1 | 0.4–1.6 | 6 | 5–8 |
| 7–13 | 5 | 4–7 | 17 | 14–20 |
| 14–23 | 17 | 10–24 | 45 | 35–55 |

*Abbreviation:* CI, confidence interval.
*Source:* Reprinted with permission from Elsevier [13].

**Table 24.6b** Probabilities of disease progression in 1, 5 and 10 year(s) for the new EAU NMIBC risk groups.

| Risk group | Probability of Progression and 95% Confidence Interval (CI) | | |
|---|---|---|---|
| | 1 Year | 5 Years | 10 Years |
| **New Risk Groups with WHO 2004/2016** | | | |
| Low | 0.06% (CI: 0.01%–0.43%) | 0.93% (CI: 0.49%–1.7%) | 3.7% (CI: 2.3%–5.9%) |
| Intermediate | 1.0% (CI: 0.50%–2.0%) | 4.9% (CI: 3.4%–7.0%) | 8.5% (CI: 5.6%–13%) |
| High | 3.5% (CI: 2.4%–5.2%) | 9.6% (CI: 7.4%–12%) | 14% (CI: 11%–18%) |
| Very High | 16% (CI: 10%–26%) | 40% (CI: 29%–54%) | 53% (CI: 36%–73%) |
| **New Risk Groups with WHO 1973** | | | |
| Low | 0.12% (CI: 0.02%–0.82%) | 0.57% (CI: 0.21%–1.5%) | 3.0% (CI: 1.5%–6.3%) |
| Intermediate | 0.65% (CI: 0.36%–1.2%) | 3.6% (CI: 2.7%–4.9%) | 7.4% (CI: 5.5%–10%) |
| High | 3.8% (CI: 2.6%–5.7%) | 11% (CI: 8.1%–14%) | 14% (CI: 10%–19%) |
| Very High | 20% (CI: 12%–32%) | 44% (CI: 30%–61%) | 59% (CI: 39%–79%) |

*This does not include patients with variant histologies, LVI, CIS in the prostatic urethra, primary CIS or recurrent patients.
*Abbreviation:* WHO, World Health Organization.

**Table 24.7** EAU 2021 Stratification of NMIBC

| Risk Group | Characteristics |
|---|---|
| Low-risk Tumours | • Primary, Solitary, Ta/Ta LG/G1 tumour <3cm, no CIS, <70 years<br>  Ta LG/G1 without CIS with at most ONE of the additional clinical risk factors* |
| Intermediate-risk Tumours | • Patients without CIS who are not included in either the low, high or very high-risk groups |
| High-risk Tumours | • All T1 HG/G3 without CIS, except those included in the very high-risk group<br>  All CIS patients, except those included in the very high-risk group |
| | **Stage, grade with additional clinical risk factors:**<br><br>• Ta LG/G2 or T1 G1, no CIS with all 3 risk factors<br>• Ta HG/G3 or T1 LG, no CIS with at least 2 risk factors<br>• T1 G2 no CIS with at least 1 risk factor |
| Very High-risk Tumours | **Stage, grade with additional clinical risk factors:**<br><br>• Ta HG/G3 and CIS with all 3 risk factors<br>• T1 G2 and CIS with at least 2 risk factors<br>• T1 HG/G3 and CIS with at least 1 risk factor<br>• T1 HG/G3 no CIS with all 3 risk factors |

* Additional clinical risk factors include age >70 y, multiple papillary tumours, tumour >3 cm.

**Table 24.8** Risk Stratification of Non-Metastatic UTUC

| | Low Risk<br>All Factors Need To Be Present | High Risk<br>Any Factor Can Be Present |
|---|---|---|
| **Focality** | Unifocal | Multifocal |
| **Tumour size** | <2 cm | >2 cm |
| **Urinary cytology** | Low grade | High grade |
| **Ureteric biopsy** | Low grade | High grade |
| **CT urogram** | No invasion | Invasion |
| **Others** | | Hydronephrosis |
| | | Previous radical cystectomy for HG BC Variant histology |

*Abbreviation:* HG BC, high-grade bladder cancer.

- Can lead to increased kinase activity, enhanced signalling and dysregulated pathway activation.
- *STAG 2* mutations
  - Affect chromosomal stability and are associated with poorer outcomes
- *KDM6A*
  - An epigenetic regulator.
  - Mutations may be more common in females (gene located on the X Chm).
  - Lead to epigenetically unstable cancers (often without chromosomal changes).
- *TERT* mutation
  - Leads to upregulation of telomerase, longer chromosomal telomeres (i.e. less cell death).
  - More aggressive cell phenotype (more deaths from BC).

# High-Grade BC

- Invasive BC appear to arise from regions of CIS.
- *Molecular pathways:*
  - Chromosomal aberrations (both gains and deletions).
    - Example: loss of regions of Chm. 17p (*P53* gene).
  - Epigenetic instability (changes to histone

modification, non-coding RNA expression and DNA methylation).
- Gene mutations.
- Common gene mutations include
  - *p53* (48% in TCGA survey):
    - Tumour suppressor gene – role in cell cycle regulation.
  - *Epigenetic regulators*:
    - *KMT2D* (28%), *KDM6A* (26%), *ARID1A* (25%), and *KMT2C* (18%).
    - Mutations affect the modelling of chromosomes (via histone modification) to allow up/downregulation of key cellular proteins (and subsequent carcinogenic traits).
  - *Cell kinases*:
    - *PIK3CA* (22%) and *ERBB2* (12%).
    - Lead to gain of function changes and enhanced signalling (leading to dysregulated pathway activation).
  - *Retinoblastoma* gene (*RB1*: 17%):
    - Mutation leads to loss of a cell cycle checkpoint and uncontrolled cell proliferation.
  - *DNA repair: ERCC2* (9%).
  - mRNA editing: *APOBEC 3A/B* (~80% in the TCGA have a mutation signature).
  - *Growth factors: FGFR3* (14%), *HER2*, *EGFR* family.
- Genetic and epigenetic alterations lead to modified gene expression:
  - Example: loss of tumour suppressor or gains in oncogenes.

## Molecular Classification of MIBC

- Various molecular classification systems for MIBC exist:
  - Lund in Sweden
  - MD Anderson and North Carolina in the USA
  - NIH's TCGA consortium
- Most recently, TCGA consortium identified 5 sub-classes of MIBC (Figure 24.7) which they termed:

1. *Luminal papillary*
   - Prominent *FGFR3* mutation.
   - Other highly expressed genes: *UPK2, UPK1A, FOXA1, GATA3, PPARG*.
   - Papillary architecture.
   - Low likelihood of response to neoadjuvant chemotherapy (NAC).
   - Tyrosine Kinase inhibitors of FGFR3 may be an effective treatment approach.

2. *Luminal infiltrated*
   - Rich immune infiltrate.
   - High expression of epithelial-mesenchymal transition (EMT) and myofibroblast markers.

- Increased expression of PD-L1, PD-1, MiR-200 family.
- Thought to be sensitive to immune checkpoint therapy.

3. *Luminal*
   - High expression of uroplakin and genes expressed in differentiated urothelial umbrella cells, e.g., *KRT20, UPK2, UPK1A, SNX31*
   - Optimal therapy remains to be elucidated.
   - Future trials may evaluate NAC or targeted treatments based on the cancer's mutational profile.

4. *Basal/squamous*
   - Female predominance.
   - Squamous differentiation and basal keratin expression.
   - Increased expression of *CD44, KRT5, KRT6A, KRT14, TGM1, DSC3, PI3, CIS* genes
   - High expression of PD-L1 and CTLA4 expressing T cells.
   - Both Cisplatin-based NAC and immune checkpoint therapy are options.

5. *Neuronal*
   - Neuroendocrine differentiation.
   - Increased expression of *MSI1, PLEKHG4B*, neuronal differentiation and development genes.
   - Aggressive cancers.
   - Thought to be sensitive to Etoposide-cisplatin therapy.

# Urine Cytology and Biomarkers in Urothelial Cancer

## Urine Cytology

- Analysis of urine for cancer cells.
- Ideally performed on a *mid-morning* urine sample:
  - *Early morning* urine samples can be degenerative.
  - Whole voided urine collected as the midstream urine is more acellular.
- Urine can also be collected via bladder washout (barbotage) or ureteric washings.
- Stain with Papanicolaou or haematoxylin and eosin dyes.
- High sensitivity in G3 and HG tumours (84%).
- Low sensitivity in G1/LG tumours (16%).
- Sensitivity for CIS: 28–100%.
- Useful as an adjunct to cystoscopy to detect HG tumours.
- Can be used in primary detection or follow up of high-risk NMIBC.
- Interpretation of cytology is variable and is experience dependant.
- Interpretation can be affected by low cellular yield, urinary tract infection, stones, intravesical instillations.

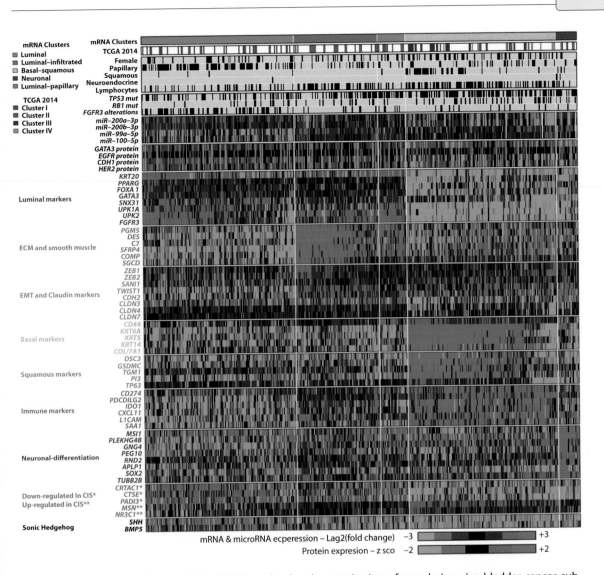

**mRNA Clusters**
- Luminal
- Luminal–infiltrated
- Basal–squamous
- Neuronal
- Luminal–papillary

**TCGA 2014**
- Cluster I
- Cluster II
- Cluster III
- Cluster IV

mRNA & microRNA ecperession – Lag2(fold change)   −3 [    ] +3
Protein expresion – z sco   −2 [    ] +2

**Figure 24.7** The Cancer Genome Atlas (TCGA) molecular characterisation of muscle invasive bladder cancer sub-types using 5 mRNA expression subtypes. Above is a heat map, a method which visualises gene expression data. Each small tile in one row represents a MIBC sample (412 Samples). Rows labelled KRT20 to BMP5 correspond to expression changes (mRNA Expression) for selected genes. red tiles represent MIBC samples with increased expression of the gene and green tiles represent MIBC samples with decreased expression. The shade of green or red corresponds to the degree of change in gene expression (see key bottom right). Black represents unchanged expression. The proposed gene expression subtypes based on the gene expression profiles are at the top (mRNA clusters). (Left to right): luminal- papillary, luminal-infiltrated, luminal, basal-squamous and neuronal. Also shown (below mRNA subtypes) are (top to bottom): four previously reported TCGA subtypes (2014), Selected clinical covariates, key genetic alterations and normalised expression for miRNAs and proteins. (Reprinted with permission from Elsevier [16])

## Urinary Biomarkers

- Numerous urine tests have been developed for use in the diagnosis or follow up of BC.
- FDA biomarkers include NMP22 (Nuclear Matrix Protein 22), ImmunoCyt, BTA (Bladder Tumour Antigen) test, UroVysion (FISH).

- *Others:* FGFR3/TERT
- Compared to urine cytology these tests often have a higher sensitivity but a lower specificity.
- No urinary biomarkers have been accepted for diagnosis or follow up in routine practice or clinical guidelines.

# Urethral Cancer

## Epidemiology

- Primary urethral cancer is rare.
- <1% of all genitourinary malignancies.
- Male ~3x more common than female.
- ~4.4% urethral recurrence rate following radical cystectomy for urothelial cancer.

## Aetiology

- *Male*:
  - Urethral stricture.
  - Chronic irritation (intermittent catheterisation, urethroplasty).
  - External beam radiation therapy.
  - Radioactive seed implantation (brachytherapy).
- Chronic inflammation/urethritis.
- *Female*:
  - Recurrent urinary tract infection.
  - Urethral diverticulum.

## Histopathology

- Urothelial cell carcinoma (UCC): 54–65%.
- Squamous cell carcinoma (SCC): 16–22%.
- Adenocarcinoma: 10–16%.

## Staging and Grading

- The World Health Organization (WHO) staging system is shown in Table 24.9.
- *Urothelial grading*

| Table 24.9 2016 TNM Classification of Urethral Cancer | |
|---|---|
| **T – Primary tumour** | |
| TX | Primary tumour cannot be assessed |
| T0 | No evidence of primary tumour |
| **Urethra (male and female)** | |
| Ta | Non-invasive papillary, polypoid, or verrucous carcinoma |
| Tis | Carcinoma *in situ* |
| T1 | Tumour invades subepithelial connective tissue |
| T2 | Tumour invades any of the following: corpus spongiosum, prostate, periurethral muscle |
| T3 | Tumour invades any of the following: corpus cavernosum, beyond prostatic capsule, anterior vagina, bladder neck (extraprostatic extension) |
| T4 | Tumour invades other adjacent organs (invasion of the bladder) |
| **Urothelial (transitional cell) carcinoma of the prostate** | |
| Tis pu | Carcinoma *in situ*, involvement of the prostatic urethra |
| Tis pd | Carcinoma *in situ*, involvement of prostatic ducts |
| T1 | Tumour invades subepithelial connective tissue (for tumours involving prostatic urethra only) |
| T2 | Tumour invades any of the following: prostatic stroma, corpus spongiosum, periurethral muscle |
| T3 | Tumour invades any of the following: corpus cavernosum, beyond prostatic capsule, bladder neck (extraprostatic extension) |
| T4 | Tumour invades other adjacent organs (invasion of the bladder or rectum) |
| **N – Regional lymph nodes** | |
| NX | Regional lymph nodes cannot be assessed |
| N0 | No regional lymph node metastasis |
| N1 | Metastasis in a single lymph node |
| N2 | Metastasis in multiple lymph nodes |
| **M – Distant metastasis** | |
| M0 | No distant metastasis |
| M1 | Distant metastasis |

- PUNLMP: papillary urothelial neoplasm of low malignant potential.
- Low grade: well-differentiated.
- High grade: poorly differentiated.
- *Non-urothelial grading*
  - Gx: grade not assessable, G1: well, G2: moderately, G3: poorly differentiated.

# Recommended Reading

1. Cumberbatch MGK, Jubber I, Black PC et al. Epidemiology of bladder cancer: a systematic review and contemporary update of risk factors in 2018. Eur Urol. 2018.
2. García-Closas M, Malats N, Silverman D et al. NAT2 slow acetylation and GSTM1 null genotypes increase bladder cancer risk: results from the Spanish Bladder Cancer Study and meta-analyses. Lancet. 2005;366(9486): 649–59.
3. Rothman N, Garcia-Closas M, Chatterjee N et al. A multi-stage genome-wide association study of bladder cancer identifies multiple susceptibility loci. Nat Genet. 2010;42(11): 978–84.
4. Cumberbatch MG, Rota M, Catto JWF, La Vecchia C. The role of tobacco smoke in bladder and kidney carcinogenesis: a comparison of exposures and meta-analysis of incidence and mortality risks. Eur Urol. 2016;70(3): 458–66.
5. Bourke L, Bauld L, Bullen C et al. E-cigarettes and Urologic Health: A Collaborative Review of Toxicology, Epidemiology, and Potential Risks. Eur Urol. 2017;71(6):915–23.
6. Cumberbatch MGK, Cox A, Teare D, Catto JWF. Contemporary occupational carcinogen exposure and bladder cancer: a systematic review and meta-analysis. JAMA Oncol. 2015;1(9):1282–90.
7. Brierley J, Gospodarowicz M, Wittekind C. TNM classification of malignant tumours, 8th Edition 2016.
8. Babjuk M, Burger M, Comperat EM et al. European Association of Urology Guidelines on Non-muscle-invasive Bladder Cancer (TaT1 and Carcinoma In Situ) - 2019 Update. Eur Urol. 2019;76(5):639–57.
9. Sylvester RJ et al. European Association of Urology (EAU) Prognostic Factor Risk Groups for Non-muscle-invasive Bladder Cancer (NMIBC) Incorporating the WHO 2004/2016 and WHO 1973 Classification Systems for Grade: An Update from the EAU NMIBC Guidelines Panel. Eur Urol. 2021 Apr;79(4):480–488.
10. Humphrey PA, Moch H, Cubilla AL et al. The 2016 WHO classification of tumours of the urinary system and male genital organs-Part B: prostate and bladder tumours. Eur Urol. 2016;70(1):106–19.
11. Shah RB, Montgomery JS, Montie JE, Kunju LP. Variant (divergent) histologic differentiation in urothelial carcinoma is under-recognized in community practice: impact of mandatory central pathology review at a large referral hospital. Urol Oncol. 2013;31(8):1650–5.
12. Chalasani V, Chin JL, Izawa JI. Histologic variants of urothelial bladder cancer and nonurothelial histology in bladder cancer. Can Urol Assoc J. 2009;3(6 Suppl 4):S193–8.
13. Sylvester RJ, van der Meijden AP, Oosterlinck W et al. Predicting recurrence and progression in individual patients with stage Ta T1 bladder cancer using EORTC risk tables: a combined analysis of 2596 patients from seven EORTC trials. Eur Urol. 2006;49(3):466-5; discussion 75-7.
14. Hurst CD, Knowles MA. Mutational landscape of non-muscle-invasive bladder cancer. Urol Oncol. 2018;S1078–439.
15. Knowles MA, Hurst CD. Molecular biology of bladder cancer: new insights into pathogenesis and clinical diversity. Nat Rev Cancer. 2015;15(1):25–41.
16. Robertson AG, Kim J, Al-Ahmadie H et al. Comprehensive Molecular Characterization of Muscle-Invasive Bladder Cancer. Cell. 2017;171(3):540–56.e25.
17. Sanli O, Dobruch J, Knowles MA et al. Bladder cancer. Nat Rev Dis Primers. 2017;3:17022.
18. Schneider AK, Chevalier MF, Derre L. The multifaceted immune regulation of bladder cancer. Nat Rev Urol. 2019;16(10)613–30.
19. Chapple, CR et al. Urologic principles and practice. Springer specialist surgery series, Second edition. Springer 2020 (figure 16.2).
20. Perera, M et al. Pelvic lymph node dissection during radical cystectomy for muscle-invasive bladder cancer. Nat Rev Urol. 2018;15(11): 686–692.

# 25 Prostate Cancer

*Karl H. Pang and James W.F. Catto*

## Epidemiology of Prostate Cancer

### Demographics

- Most common cancer in men.
- Second most common cause of cancer-related death in men.
- *UK 2017:* 48,600 new cases of prostate cancer (PCa) and 12,000 deaths.
- Incidence varies between different geographical areas:
  - Highest in Australia/New Zealand and Northern America.
  - Low in Eastern and South-Central Asia.
- Demographics often mirror the public health policy. In the USA, there has been a rise in the percentage of men with advanced disease following changes in the PSA screening advice.

## Aetiology and Risk Factors

- Family history and germline mutations (e.g., BRCA 2, see later):
  - ~9% men with PCa have a *'hereditary disease'*.
  - Defined as >3 affected relatives or ≥2 relatives with early-onset PCa (<55 years).
  - One first-degree relative with PCa: relative risk (RR) = 1.8.
  - Father and brother with PCa: RR = 5.5.
  - Two brothers with PCa: RR = 7.7.
- Increasing age
- Afro-Caribbean
- *Metabolic syndrome*
  - Hypertension
  - Waist circumference: >102 cm
  - Diabetes: metformin users
  - Obesity: increased risk of high-grade PCa
- *Dietary*
  - Alcohol
  - Dairy: weak association.
  - Tomatoes: favourable effect of tomato and lycopene.
  - Phytoestrogens: reduced risk.
  - Soy: reduced risk of PCa, but increased risk of advanced diseases.
  - Vitamin D: both low and high concentrations are associated with increased risk.
- Vitamin E/selenium: inverse relationship between serum selenium levels and PCa.
- Selenium or Vitamin E supplements have no beneficial effect in preventing PCa.
- Medications
  - 5-alpha-reductase inhibitors (5-ARI): not approved for chemoprevention.
    - Prostate Cancer Prevention Trial (PCPT):
      - Finasteride reduces the risk of PCa by 24.8%.
      - Increases the proportion of high-grade tumours.
    - Reduction by Dutasteride of Prostate Cancer Events (REDUCE):
      - Dutasteride reduces the risk of PCa by 22.8% over four years.
    - Theories to explain the increasing proportion of high-grade cancers:
      - Histological artefact resulting in incorrect grading.
      - More effective prevention in low Gleason grade 6 than with grades 7–10.
      - Reduction in gland volume may improve high-grade detection.
      - Affected PSA and digital rectal examination (DRE).
  - Hypogonadal men receiving testosterone supplements do not have an increased risk of PCa.
  - Aspirin, non-steroidal anti-inflammatories: conflicting data.
- Other high-risk factors
  - Balding
  - Gonorrhoea
  - Occupational (night-shift work, cadmium)
  - Cigarette smoking
  - HPV-16
- Potential protective factors
  - Higher ejaculation frequency (>21x per month)
  - Mediterranean diet
- The associations with PCa studied to date lack evidence for casualty. Therefore, no specific preventive or dietary measures are recommended to reduce the risk of developing PCa.

# Genetics and Pathophysiology
## Genes and Pathways

(Reference to Genome-Wide Association Studies [*GWAS*] and The Cancer Genome Atlas [*TCGA*] data).

- Transcription
  - HOXB13 – transcription factor
- DNA repair genes
  - 19% have alterations in DNA repair pathway.
  - *BRCA 1, BRCA 2, ATM, FANCD2, RAD51C, CDK12, CHEK2*
- Androgen receptor (AR) pathways
  - *AR* gene mutation and amplification.
- PI3K/AKT/mTOR pathway
  - *PTEN* (17%), *PIK3CA, PIK3CB, AKT1, AKT-E17K*
- MAPK pathway
  - Defects in genes found in 25%.
  - *BRAF, HRAS, RAC1, RRAS2*
- Cell cycle
  - CDK4, CDK6, *RB1*
- Single nucleotide polymorphism (SNP)
  - rs11568818, rs2735839, rs752822
- Neuroendocrine transdifferentiation
  - Loss of *RB1* and *TP53* (~50% in neuroendocrine tumours, but 14% adenocarcinoma).
  - *MYCN* amplification
- ETS family subtypes
  - Fusion genes involving ETS transcription factor family, like the following:
    - ERG (46%), ETV1 (8%), ETV4, FLI1
    - Transmembrane protease serine 2 – ETS-related gene (TMPRSS2-ERG) fusion is the most common alteration.
  - *SPOP* (11%), *FOXA1* (3%), and *IDH1* (1%) subtypes

## Epigenetic Events

- Inheritable changes that alter expression without changing the gene sequence or chromosomal structure.
- Often reversible.
- Known epigenetic mechanisms include:
  1. Modification of histone proteins.
  2. Modification of DNA.
  3. Expression of non-coding RNAs (ncRNA).

## Pathophysiology

- Charles Huggins discovered the relevance of androgen regulation in 1941.
  - Androgen deprivation therapy (ADT) by surgical castration for men with advanced metastatic PCa results in remarkable benefits.
- The synthesis of androgen involves the hypothalamic–pituitary–gonadal/testicular (HPG) axis and adrenal glands (Figure 25.1).
- The activation of AR by androgens results in gene expression of many genes that are involved in PCa development.
- ADT aims to lower/block androgen activity:
  - *Lowering testosterone*
    - Bilateral orchidectomy to remove testosterone-producing Leydig cells.
    - GHRH agonist: downregulates GnRH receptors.
    - GHRH antagonist: blocks GnRH receptors.
    - CYP17A1 inhibitor (*Abiraterone):* inhibits androgen synthesis.
  - *Blocking androgen effect*
    - Non-steroidal anti-androgens (Bicalutamide): block androgen receptors.

# Histopathology
## Histological Subtypes

- ~70% PCa occurs in the peripheral zone; 20% in the transition zone; 5–10% in the central zone; and rarely in the anterior fibromuscular area.
- Pathological subtypes are based on the 2016 WHO classification (Table 25.1).

### Malignant

- Acinar adenocarcinoma (+/– variants)- most common.
  - Cytological atypia and architectural changes (Gleason patterns – see later).
- Neuroendocrine
- Mesenchymal
- Haematolymphoid
- Metastatic (e.g., from colorectal, bladder cancer)

### Pre-Malignant

- Intraductal carcinoma (WHO 2016 *new entity*).
  - Intra-acinar and/or intraductal neoplastic epithelial proliferation that has some features of HGPIN but exhibits greater architectural and/or cytological atypia.
- Atypical small acinar proliferation (*ASAP*)
  - 31–40% risk of PCa on repeat prostate biopsy.
  - A focus of small acinar structures formed by atypical epithelial cells.
  - *Does not* appear to raise PSA.
- High-grade prostate intraepithelial neoplasia (*HGPIN*)
  - >3 positive biopsy sites = 30% risk of PCa.
  - A continuum of intraluminal proliferation of atypical secretory cells lining pre-existing ducts and acini in the prostate.
  - *Does not* appear to raise PSA.
- PIN with adjacent atypical gland (*PINATYP*)
  - ~50% risk of PCa.

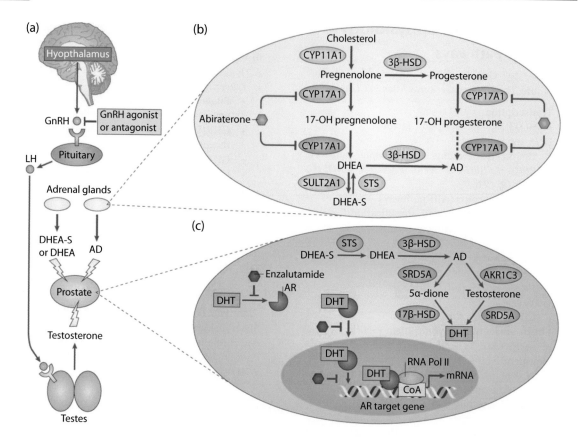

**Figure 25.1** Androgen receptor signalling is regulated by the hypothalamic–pituitary–testicular axis, adrenal gland steroidogenesis and prostate cell intrinsic factors. (a) The hormones gonadotropin-releasing hormone (GnRH) and luteinizing hormone (LH) bind to their cognate receptors, resulting in testosterone secretion from leydig cells. GnRH agonists leads to downregulation of the GnRH receptor (GnRH-R). GnRH antagonists provide immediate GnRH-R blockade. Both agents suppress LH production – decline in serum testosterone to castrate levels. The adrenal glands secrete dehydroepiandrosterone sulphate (DHEA-S; predominantly), DHEA and androstenedione (AD) into the circulation (b) Adrenal androgen de novo steroidogenesis (enzymes in ovals). CYP17A1 (cytochrome P450 family 17 subfamily a polypeptide 1 has 17α-Hydroxylation (Red) and 17, 20-lyase (Blue) activities; both are inhibited by abiraterone (dashed arrow: a weak effect); (c) Prostate conversion of adrenal androgens to dihydrotestosterone (DHT). DHT binds to the androgen receptor (AR) in the cytoplasm, triggering a conformational change that leads to nuclear translocation. DHT-bound AR Homodimerizes and, with Co-activators (CoAs) and RNA polymerase II (RNA Pol II) or Co-repressors, binds to DNA at cis androgen response elements to activate or repress AR target gene expression, respectively. Enzalutamide Inhibits AR by competing with DHT for binding, blocking nuclear translocation, and blocking DNA and cofactor binding. AKR1C3, aldo-keto reductase family 1 member C3; 3β-HSD, 3β-hydroxysteroid dehydrogenase/Δ5-4-isomerase; 17β-HSD, 17β-hydroxysteroid dehydrogenase; SRD5A, steroid 5α-reductase; STS, steryl-sulfatase; SULT2A1, bile salt sulfotransferase. (Reprinted by permission from Springer Nature [11])

- A few atypical glands immediately adjacent to HGPIN.

## Immunohistochemistry (IHC)

- Uses mono/polyclonal antibodies to check certain antigens (markers).
- Used to differentiate between different tissue and cancer types.

- PCa *stains* include:
  - Prostate-specific antigen (PSA)
  - PSA phosphatase (PAP)
  - High molecular weight cytokeratins – negative stain (stains prostatic basal cells, positive cytokeratin = rule out adenocarcinoma)
  - p63 (nuclear – negative stain)
  - Alpha-methylacyl-CoA racemase/P504S (mitochondrial enzyme, AMACR)

**Table 25.1** World Health Organization (WHO) Classification of Prostate Tumours

| Epithelial tumours | Haematolymphoid tumours |
|---|---|
| *Glandular neoplasms* | Diffuse large B-cell lymphoma |
| Acinar adenocarcinoma | Chronic lymphocytic leukaemia/small lymphocytic lymphoma |
| Atrophic | Follicular lymphoma |
| Pseudohyperplastic | Mantle cell lymphoma |
| Microcystic | Acute myeloid leukaemia |
| Foamy gland | B lymphoblastic leukaemia/lymphoma |
| Mucinous (colloid) | **Miscellaneous tumours** |
| Signet ring-like cell | Cystadenoma |
| Pleomorphic giant cell | Nephroblastoma |
| Sarcomatoid | Rhabdoid |
| Prostate intraepithelial neoplasia, high grade | Germ cell |
| Intraductal carcinoma | Clear cell adenocarcinoma |
| Ductal adenocarcinoma | Melanoma |
| Cribriform | Paraganglioma |
| Papillary | |
| Solid | |
| Urothelial carcinoma | |
| *Squamous neoplasms* | |
| Adenosquamous carcinoma | |
| Squamous cell carcinoma | |
| Basal cell carcinoma | |
| **Neuroendocrine tumours** | |
| Adenocarcinoma with neuroendocrine differentiation | |
| Well-differentiated | |
| Small cell | |
| Large cell | |
| **Mesenchymal tumours** | |
| Stromal tumour of uncertain malignant potential | |
| Stromal sarcoma | |
| Leiomyosarcoma | |
| Rhabdomyosarcoma | |
| Leiomyoma | |
| Angiosarcoma | |
| Synovial sarcoma | |
| Inflammatory myofibroblastic | |
| Osteosarcoma | |

(*Continued*)

**Table 25.1** (Continued)

| |
|---|
| Undifferentiated pleomorphic sarcoma |
| Solitary fibrous |
| Solitary fibrous, malignant |
| Haemangioma |
| Granular cell |

*Source:* Adapted from Humphrey et al. [6].

- Homeobox-containing transcription factor (NKX3.1)
- Prostate-specific membrane antigen (membrane glycoprotein, PSMA)
- PSA/PAP expression can be decreased after androgen deprivation therapy.
- AMACR and NKX immunostains are useful in these cases.

## Diagnosis and Investigations

- Clinical examination (digital rectal examination [DRE] and systemic).
- Serum PSA, PSA kinetics (see Chapter 11)
- Biomarkers (see below)
- Imaging (multi-parametric MRI, staging CT abdomen-pelvis)
- Prostate biopsy

### Risk Calculators

- Risk calculators may be used to help determine the potential risk of cancer. This may reduce the number of unnecessary biopsies. The calculators are developed from cohort studies.
- PCPT cohort http://myprostatecancerrisk.com/
- ERSPC cohort http://www.prostatecancer-riskcalculator.com/seven-prostate-cancer-risk-calculators

## Tumour Staging

- Staging is based on surgical pathology (pT1) or clinical assessment, DRE (T2+), and imaging (Table 25.2).

## Tumour Grading

- In *2005,* there were five Gleason patterns (1–5) described.
  - The Gleason score (GS) was used to grade PCa.
  - The GS is the most common Gleason pattern, plus the second most common pattern. GS ranged from 2–10.

- In *2014,* the International Society of Urological Pathology (ISUP) established a new grading system.
  - GS = Gleason grade of the most common pattern, plus the highest-grade pattern.
  - GS 2–5 are no longer assigned, therefore the GS now ranges from 6 to 10.
  - Gleason patterns were re-described (Figure 25.2).
  - Five grades are now used to classify PCa (Table 25.3).

## Tumour Risk Stratification

### D'amico

- PCa diagnosis is stratified into risk groups based on the initial risk tools developed by D'amico (Table 25.4).
- Management is based on risks, age/life-expectancy, performance status, co-morbidities, and the patient's preference.

### PREDICT

- The Cambridge *'PREDICT Prostate'* (www.prostate.predict.nhs.uk) is a prognostic model and decision-aid designed to inform treatment decision-making amongst men with newly diagnosed non-metastatic PCa. Parameters include:
  - Age, PSA, Gleason score, ISUP grade group, T-stage, number of biopsies taken/involved, BRCA status, previous hospital admissions in the last two years, co-morbidities, and metastasis.

## Tumour Dissemination

- Local invasion
  - Seminal vesicles, bladder, rectum (Denonvillier's fascia), base of penis
- Distant metastasis
  - Lymphatics (pelvic lymph nodes) and haematogenous (bones, lung, liver, brain)
  - Vascular spread to the pelvic organs and the vertebrae:

**Table 25.2** 2016 TNM Classification System for Prostate Cancer

| T – Primary Tumour (stage based on digital rectal examination [DRE] only) | | |
|---|---|---|
| TX | Primary tumour cannot be assessed | |
| T0 | No evidence of primary tumour | |
| T1 | Clinically inapparent tumour that is not palpable | |
| | T1a | Tumour incidental histological finding in 5% or less of tissue resected |
| | T1b | Tumour incidental histological finding in more than 5% of tissue resected |
| | T1c | Tumour identified by needle biopsy |
| T2 | Tumour that is palpable (DRE) and confined within the prostate | |
| | T2a | Tumour involves one half of one lobe or less |
| | T2b | Tumour involves more than half of one lobe, but not both lobes |
| | T2c | Tumour involves both lobes |
| T3 | Tumour extends through the prostatic capsule | |
| | T3a | Extracapsular extension (unilateral or bilateral) |
| | T3b | Tumour invades seminal vesicle(s) |
| T4 | Tumour is fixed or invades adjacent structures other than seminal vesicles: external sphincter, rectum, levator muscles, and/or pelvic wall | |
| **N – Regional (pelvic) Lymph Nodes**[1] | | |
| NX | Regional lymph nodes cannot be assessed | |
| N0 | No regional lymph node metastasis | |
| N1 | Regional lymph node metastasis | |
| **M – Distant Metastasis**[2] | | |
| M0 | No distant metastasis | |
| M1 | Distant metastasis | |
| | M1a Non-regional lymph node(s) | |
| | M1b Bone(s) | |
| | M1c Other site(s) | |

1 Metastasis that is no larger than 0.2 cm can be designated pNmi;
2 When more than one site of metastasis is present, the most advanced category is used. (p)M1c is the most advanced category.

- - Prostatic venous plexus
  - Batson venous plexus (valveless)
  - Internal vertebral venous plexus
- The anatomy of lymphatic drainage is important when deciding on the extent of lymphadenectomy (Figure 25.3).
- Bony metastasis
  - Sclerotic (osteoblastic activity):
    - Deposition of a new bone.
    - The transforming growth factor, bone morphogenic protein (BMP), and endothelin-1 are involved.
    - Stimulates secretion of RANK ligand → induces osteoclasts (Denosumab – a RANKL monoclonal antibody which may be used to reduce skeletal-related events)
  - Note: 'osteolytic' metastasis (e.g., renal cell carcinoma):
    - May result in bone destruction.
    - Associated with osteoclastic and PTH-related peptide activity.
- Diagnosed with technetium 99-methylene diphosphonate (MDP) bone scan.
  - MDP binds hydroxyapatite crystals.

**Discrete Well-formed Glands (Gleason Pattern 3)**

**Cribriform/Poorly-formed/Fused Glands (Gleason Pattern 4)**

**Sheets/Cords/Single Cells/Solid Nests/Necrosis (Gleason Pattern 5)**

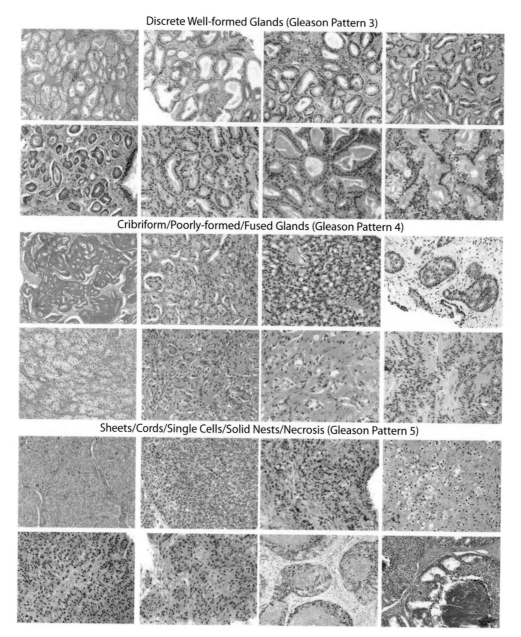

**Figure 25.2** Gleason patterns 3–5. From left to right. *1st Row*: Closely packed uniform-sized and -shaped large glands. Large variably sized and shaped glands, some with infolding. Uniform medium-sized glands. Variably sized glands. *2nd Row*: Occasional tangentially sectioned glands among well-formed small glands. Occasional tangentially sectioned glands among well-formed glands with open lumina. Back-to-back discrete glands. Branching glands. *3rd Row*: Large irregular cribriform glands with well-formed lumina. Irregular cribriform glands with slit-like lumina, glomeruloid structures, and fused glands. Irregular cribriform glands with small round lumina. Small round cribriform glands. 4th Row: Poorly formed glands with peripherally arranged nuclei. Small poorly formed glands. Small poorly formed glands. Fused poorly formed glands. 5th row: Sheets of cancer. Sheets of cancer with rosette formation. Small nests and cords of tumour with scattered clear vacuoles. Individual cells. 6th row: Nests and cords of cells with only vague attempt at lumina formation. Solid nests of cancer. Solid nests with comedonecrosis. Cribriform glands with central necrosis. (Reprinted by permission from Springer Nature [7])

**Table 25.3** The International Society of Urological Pathology 2014 Grading System

| ISUP Grade | Gleason Score | Histological Description |
|---|---|---|
| 1 | ≤6 | Only individual discrete well-formed glands. |
| 2 | 7 (3+4) | Predominantly well-formed glands with lesser component of poorly-formed/fused/cribriform glands. |
| 3 | 7 (4+3) | Predominantly poorly-formed/fused/cribriform glands with lesser component of well-formed glands. |
| 4 | 8 (4+4 or 3+5 or 5+3) | Only poorly-formed/fused/cribriform glands or Predominantly well-formed glands and lesser component lacking glands or Predominantly lacking glands and lesser component of well-formed glands. |
| 5 | 9–10 | Lacks gland formation (or with necrosis) with or without poorly formed/fused/cribriform glands. |

*Source:* Adapted from Epstein et al. [7].

**Table 25.4** EAU risk groups for biochemical recurrence of localised and locally advanced prostate cancer

| Low-risk | Intermediate-risk | High-risk | |
|---|---|---|---|
| PSA < 10 ng/mL | PSA 10–20 ng/mL | PSA > 20 ng/mL | Any PSA |
| and GS < 7 (ISUP grade 1) | or GS 7 (ISUP grade 2/3) | or GS > 7 (ISUP grade 4/5) | Any GS (any ISUP grade) |
| and cT1–2a | or cT2b | or cT2c | cT3–4 or cN+ |
| **Localised** | | | **Locally advanced** |

*Abbreviations:* GS, Gleason score; PSA, prostate-specific antigen; ISUP, International Society of Urological Pathology.

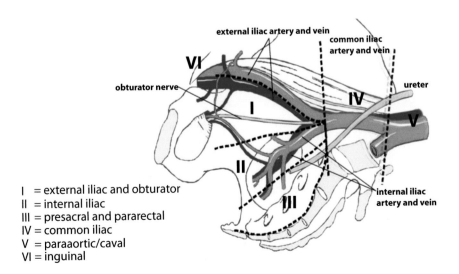

I = external iliac and obturator
II = internal iliac
III = presacral and pararectal
IV = common iliac
V = paraaortic/caval
VI = inguinal

**Figure 25.3** Regions of pelvic lymph node dissection (PLND). Limited PLND corresponds to region I; Extended PLND corresponds to regions I and II. (Reprinted with permission from Elsevier [10])

- May cause nerve root compression/cauda equina syndrome.

## Disease Progression

- Castration is defined as testosterone <50 ng/dL (20 ng/dL being used increasingly).
- Castration-resistance develops when PSA continues to rise despite a suppressed testosterone level.
- *EAU definition:* castrate serum testosterone of <50 ng/dL or 1.7 nmol/L plus either:
  a. *Biochemical* progression: three consecutive rises in PSA at least one week apart, resulting in two 50% increases over the nadir and a PSA of >2 ng/mL; or
  b. *Radiological* progression: the appearance of new lesions—either two or more new bone lesions on bone scan or a soft tissue lesion.
- The pathophysiology of castration-resistant PCa (CPRC) includes:

### Androgen Receptor Gene Mutation

- Occurs in 15–20% CRPC cases, >60% when *AR* gene amplification is included.
- *AR* gene: chromosome Xq11–12.
- AR: 920 amino acids, four functional domains.
- Four point mutations exist: T878A, L702H, W742C, H875Y.
- Anti-androgens may be converted into agonistic agents.
- Discontinuation of flutamide results in clinical improvement – *'anti-androgen withdrawal syndrome'*

### AR Splice Variants (ARV)

- Alternative splicing of the *AR* mRNA.
- AR-V1, AR-V7, AR$^{v567es}$

### Adrenal Androgens, Intraprostatic Testosterone, and Dihydrotestosterone (DHT)

- Medical/surgical castration reduces testosterone levels by >90%.
- Other adrenal androgens– dehydroepiandrosterone (DHEA) and androstenedione (AD) are converted into testosterone and DHT in the prostate (Figure 25.1c).
- Therefore, CRPC can be managed by inhibiting the synthesis of these androgens by a CYP17A1 inhibitor (abiraterone).

### Androgen Receptor Bypass Signalling

- Glucocorticoid receptor (GR)

- Glucocorticoids (GC) negatively regulates ACTH and adrenal androgens and are used in advanced/metastatic/CRPC.
- PCa with 'high' expressions of GR, with the androgen-lowering benefit of GC, is counteracted by GR activation.
- Androgen receptor independence
  - Loss of RB1, PTEN, and TP53 mutation.
  - MYCN and AURKA gain.

## Molecular Markers

- Serum, urine, tissue-based.
- *Uses:*
  - Guide initial and/or repeat prostate biopsies.
  - Assess risks.
  - Assess progression.

## Markers

- Serum *Prostate health index (PHI)*
  - ([2]proPSA / free PSA) √PSA
- Serum *4 Kallikreins (4K)*
  - Free PSA, total PSA, intact PSA + kallikrein-like peptidase 2 (hK2)
- Urine *PCA3*
  - mRNA (Chm 9)
  - PCA3:PSA mRNA score
- Urine *Mi Prostate score*
  - PCA3, TMPRSS2-ERG, KLK3, and serum PSA
- Urine *ExoDx Prostate (IntelliScore)*
  - Exosomes: PCA3, ERG, SPDEF
  - PSA, age, race, family history
- Urine *SelectMDx*
  - HOXC6, DLX1 (KLK3 as control)
  - Age, DRE, PSA, PSA density, prostate biopsy, and family history
- Tissue *Confirm MDx*
  - Methylation of RASSF1, GSTP1, APC
- *Polaris score*
  - RNA extracts from formalin-fixed paraffin-embedded (FFPE) tissue.
  - Expression of 31 cell cycle genes and 15 control genes.

## Recommended Reading

1. Andriole GL, Bostwick DG, Brawley OW et al. Effect of dutasteride on the risk of prostate cancer. N Engl J Med. 2010;362(13):1192–202.
2. Cancer Genome Atlas Research Network. The molecular taxonomy of primary prostate cancer. Cell. 2015;163(4):1011–25.
3. Light A, Ahmed A, Dasgupta P, Elhage O. The genetic landscapes of urological cancers and their clinical implications in the era of high-throughput genome analysis. BJU Int. 2020;126(1):26–54.
4. Ku S-Y, Gleave ME, Beltran H. Towards precision oncology in advanced prostate cancer. Nat Rev Urol. 2019; 16(11):645–54.

5. Huggins C, Stevens R, Hodges C. Studies on prostatic cancer II. The effects of castration on advanced carcinoma of the prostate gland. Arch Surg. 1941;43(2):209.

6. Humphrey PA, Moch H, Cubilla AL et al. The 2016 WHO classification of tumours of the urinary system and male genital organs-Part B: prostate and bladder tumours. Eur Urol. 2016;70(1):106–19.

7. Epstein JI. Prostate cancer grading: a decade after the 2005 modified system. Mod Pathol. 2018;31(S1):47–63.

8. Thurtle DR, Greenberg DC, Lee LS et al. Individual prognosis at diagnosis in nonmetastatic prostate cancer: Development and external validation of the PREDICT Prostate multivariable model. PLoS Med. 2019;16(3):e1002758.

9. Mottet N et al. Prostate cancer. EAU Guidelines 2020.

10. Mattei A, Fuechsel FG, Bhatta Dhar N et al. The template of the primary lymphatic landing sites of the prostate should be revisited: results of a multimodality mapping study. Eur Urol. 2008;53(1):118–25.

11. Watson PA, Arora VK, Sawyers CL. Emerging mechanisms of resistance to androgen receptor inhibitors in prostate cancer. Nat Rev Cancer. 2015;15(12):701–11.

12. Attard G, Parker C, Eeles RA et al. Prostate cancer. Lancet. 2016;387(10013):70–82.

13. Cucchiara V, Cooperberg MR, Dall'Era M et al. Genomic markers in prostate cancer decision making. Eur Urol. 2018;73(4):572–82.

# 26 Testicular Cancer

*Selma Masic, Abhishek Srivastava, and Alexander Kutikov*

## Epidemiology and Classification

- Rare malignancy, ~1% of cancers in UK men.
- *UK 2017:* 2,200 new cases and 65 deaths.
- UK mortality rates decreased by 29% (ongoing decline is projected).
- Most common solid malignancy in men ages 15–34 years.
- *Three age peaks:*
  - Infancy, 30–34 years, 60 years.
- Incidence of bilateral GCT: 2.5%.
  - 0.6% risk of synchronous tumours.
  - 1.9% risk of metachronous contralateral tumours.
- More common in Caucasian men than in Asian or African/African-American men.
- Incidence rates increased by 27% since the early 1990s due to increased awareness.
- *Stage migration:* less advanced disease, but more cases of seminoma.
  - 10–30% present with distant metastases.
  - 50% present with pure seminoma.
- 95% are germ cell tumours (GCT).
  - 50% pure seminoma.
  - 50% non-seminomatous germ cell tumours (NSGCT), including tumours containing seminoma.
- 95% arise in the testis, 5% are extragonadal.
- Highly curable with the advent of cisplatin-based chemotherapy in combination with surgery.
  - Five-year survival rate of >95%.
  - Long-term survival rate for patients with metastatic GCT is 80–90%.
- *Non-GCTs* are rare:
  - Sex cord-stromal tumours.
  - Tumours of collecting duct and rete testis.
  - Lymphoid and haematopoietic tumours.
  - Adnexa and tumours metastatic to the testes.
- The classification of testicular tumours is shown in Table 26.1.

## Risk Factors

- Cryptorchidism
- Race (3x more common in Caucasians and in Northern Europeans)
- Personal or family history of testicular cancer (TC)
- Germ cell neoplasia in situ (GCNIS) – formerly known as intratubular germ cell neoplasia (ITGCN)
- Testicular dysgenesis syndrome (TDS)
- HIV: increased risk of seminoma (cause unclear).

## Cryptorchidism

- ~10% have a history of undescended testis (UDT).
- 1–3% of those with UDT develop seminoma.
- 4–6x at risk of TC in the affected gonad.
- Relative risk (RR) decreases by half if orchiopexy is performed before puberty.
  - The contralateral descended testis is also at a slightly increased risk.

## Personal or Family History

- Personal history: 12-fold increased risk of GCT in the contralateral testis.
- Family history:
  - RR: 8–12x higher for men with an affected brother.
  - RR: 2–4x higher for men with an affected father.

## Microlithiasis

- ~2–6% incidence; ~80% bilateral.
- >5 calcifications in testicular parenchyma per image field on USS.
- Associated with an increased risk of ITGCN when found on USS of the contralateral testis in men with a history of GCT.
  - Malignancy in 1.6% from a five-year follow-up study of asymptomatic microlithiasis.
  - The significance in the general population is debated.
  - Follow up is not usually required but self-examination is advised.

**Table 26.1** World Health Organization (WHO) Classification of Testicular Tumours

| GCT derived from GCNIS | Tumour containing both germ cell and sex-cord-stromal elements |
|---|---|
| *Non-invasive germ cell neoplasia* | Gonadoblastoma |
| GCNIS | **Miscellaneous tumours of the testis** |
| Specific forms of intratubular germ cell neoplasia | Ovarian epithelial-type tumours |
| *Tumours of a single histological type (pure form)* | Serous cystadenoma |
| Seminoma | Serous tumour of borderline malignancy |
| Seminoma with syncytiotrophoblast cells | Serous cystadenocarcinoma |
| *Non-seminomatous GCT* | Mucinous cystadenoma |
| Embryonal carcinoma | Mucinous borderline tumour |
| Yolk sac tumour, postpubertal-type | Mucinous cystadenocarcinoma |
| Trophoblastic tumours | Endometrioid adenocarcinoma |
| Choriocarcinoma | Clear cell adenocarcinoma |
| Non-choriocarcinomatous | Brenner tumour |
| Placental site trophoblastic | Juvenile xanthogranuloma |
| Epithelioid trophoblastic | Haemangioma |
| Cystic trophoblastic | **Haematolymphoid tumours** |
| Teratoma, postpubertal-type | Diffuse large B-cell lymphoma |
| Teratoma with somatic-type malignancy | Follicular lymphoma |
| *Non-seminomatous GCT of more than one histological type* | Extranodal NK/T-cell lymphoma, nasal-type |
| Mixed GCT | Plasmacytoma |
| *GCT of unknown type* | Myeloid sarcoma |
| Regressed GCT | Rosai-Dorfman disease |
| **GCT unrelated to GCNIS** | **Tumours of collecting duct and rete testis** |
| Spermatocytic tumour | Adenoma |
| Teratoma, prepubertal type | Adenocarcinoma |
| Dermoid cyst | |
| Epidermoid cyst | |
| Well-differentiated neuroendocrine tumour | |
| Mixed teratoma and yolk sac tumour, prepubertal type | |
| Yolk sac tumour, prepubertal-type | |
| **Sex cord-stromal tumours** | |
| *Pure tumours* | |
| Leydig cell tumour | |
| Malignant Leydig cell | |
| Sertoli cell tumour | |
| Malignant Sertoli cell | |
| Large cell calcifying Sertoli cell | |

*(Continued)*

**Table 26.1** (Continued)

| |
|---|
| Intratubular large cell hyalinizing Sertoli cell |
| Granulosa cell tumour |
| Adult granulosa cell |
| Juvenile granulosa cell |
| Tumours in the fibroma-thecoma group |
| *Mixed and unclassified sex cord-stromal tumours* |
| Mixed sex cord-stromal |
| Unclassified sec-cord stroma, |

*Source:* Adapted from Moch et al. [2].
*Abbreviations:* GCNIS, germ cell neoplasia in situ; GCT, germ cell tumour.

## Testicular Dysgenesis Syndrome

- Result of the disruption of embryonal programming and gonadal development during foetal life due to environmental influences.
- *Associated with:*
  - Hypospadias, UDT
  - Infertility/impaired spermatogenesis

## Pathogenesis

- All GCTs (except spermatocytic seminoma) arise from GCNIS.
- Orchidectomy specimen placed in Bouin's solution (not formalin).

## GCNIS

- Present in 0.8% of the population, 80–90% of GCTs, and ~2.8% in UDT.
- 50% risk of carcinoma within five years.
- Not associated with worse prognoses when found in orchidectomy specimens.
- In confirmed TC:
  - 5–10% of GCNIS may be present in the *contralateral* testis and ~36% if:
    - Testis volume is <12 mL, <40 years of age, previous history of UDT.
- Develops from the transformation of normal gonocytes in utero.
  - Heterogeneity of expression of embryonic and germ-cell markers implies pluripotency and plasticity of this cell type.
  - Maintains the ability to develop into germinal and somatic tissues due to failure to differentiate.
  - Potential to develop into a diverse and distinct set of tumours.
- *Does not* elevate tumour markers.

- Diagnosed with placental alkaline phosphatase (PLAP) and OCT3/4 stains.

## Different Tumours Have Different Origins

- Seminomas resemble gonocytes with arrested differentiation.
- Embryonal carcinomas resemble undifferentiated stem cells.
- Choriocarcinomas and yolk sac tumours express extraembryonic differentiation.
- Teratomas express somatic differentiation.

## Genetics

- Environmental and genetic factors.
- *Genetic factors*
  - Epidemiological studies: low risk in African and Asian population.
  - Retention of risk from the country of origin in first-generation immigrants.
  - Retained low-risk of GCT in black Americans living in the USA for multiple generations.
  - Higher risk in patients with family history (brother > father).
  - Genome studies imply multiple involved genetic loci:
    - Seminomas and NSGCT overexpress sequences on Chm 12p.
      - 80% are due to increased number of isochromosome 12p (i12p).
  - Gain of Chm 7, 8, 21, X.
  - Loss of Chm 1p, 11, 13, 18.
  - Spermatocytic seminomas: gain in Chm 9.
  - Yolk sac tumours: loss of Chm 1p, 4, 6q and gain of 1q, 12(p13), and 20q.
  - Bilateral GCTs: activating *KIT* mutation.

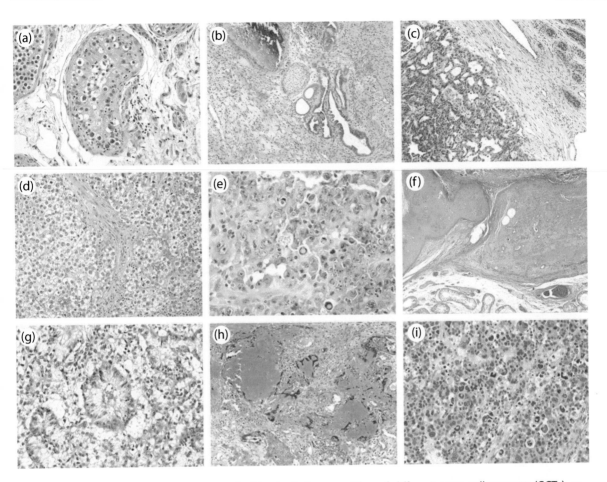

Figure 26.1 Testicular germ cell tumours. The histological composition of different germ cell tumours (GCTs), as assessed by haematoxylin and eosin staining under light microscopy, is shown. (a) Germ cell neoplasia in situ (GCNIS) (magnification ×400) Is the precursor lesion to most testicular cancers; (b) Prepubertal teratomas do not derive from GCNIS (magnification ×100); (c) Pepubertal yolk sac tumours (magnification ×100); (d) Seminomas (magnification ×200); (e) Embryonal carcinoma (magnification ×400); (f) Teratomas (magnification ×100); (g) Yolk sac tumours (magnification ×200); (h) Choriocarcinomas (magnification ×100); (i) Spermatocytic tumours (Magnification ×20). (Reprinted by permission from Springer Nature [10])

- GCNIS: OCT3/4 – marker for seminomas and NSGCTs.
- *Genetic/epigentic alterations:*
  - *KIT*
  - PI3K pathway (*KIT, KRAS, NRAS, PIK3CA, PIK3CD*)
  - Hypermethylation (*BRCA1, MGMT, RAD51C, RASSF1A*)
  - miR: 371a-3p, 367-3p, 373-3p
  - PD-L1
  - Seminomas: higher rates of demethylated DNA compared to NSGCTs.

## Histological Types

- Histological slides of GCTs are shown in Figure 26.1, and their clinical and pathological summary is shown in Table 26.2.

## Seminoma

- Most common and comprises 50% of all GCTs.
- Arises from GCNIS.
- Common precursor for other NSGCTs.
- *Presentation:*
  - Age ~40 years (later than NSGCTs).
  - 80% with localised disease.
  - 15% with retroperitoneal lymph nodes.
  - <5% with distant metastases.
- Originate in germinal epithelium of seminiferous tubules.
- Cells have abundant cytoplasm and on low power, a '*fried-egg*' appearance.
- A lymphocytic infiltrate is usually present.
- 15% of cases have syncytiotrophoblasts.
  - 15% of seminomas have elevated human chorionic gonadotropin (hCG).

**Table 26.2** Summary of Clinical and Histopathologic Features of Testicular Neoplasms

| | Seminomatous | | Non-seminomatous | | | | Stromal | | |
| --- | --- | --- | --- | --- | --- | --- | --- | --- | --- |
| | Seminoma | Spermatocytic seminoma | Embryonal | Yolk Sac | Choriocarcinoma | Teratoma | Leydig | Sertoli | Granulosa |
| **Age (years)** | 40 | Any age | 30 | <10 | 20–25 | 30 | | | 1 month |
| **Markers** | HCG 10% | None | ±AFP, HCG | AFP | HCG | None | T, 17-KS | E, T | E |
| **Histology** | Fried egg, lymphocytes | Similar to seminoma, no lymphocytes | Cohesive sheets | Schiller-Duval bodies, hyaline globules | Syncytiotrophoblast Cytotrophoblast | Endoderm, mesoderm, ectoderm layers | Reinke crystals | | |
| **Spread** | Lymph | Rare | Lymph | Lymph | Haem | Local | Rare | Rare | Rare |
| **Radiation** | Sensitive | - | Resistant | Resistant | Resistant | Resistant | - | - | - |
| **Chemo** | Sensitive | - | Sensitive | Sensitive | Sensitive | Resistant | - | - | - |
| **Misc** | 80% present with localised disease | Do not arise from GCNIS, no increased copies i12p | | | Haemorrhage | 50% of mixed GCT contain teratoma | | | |

Extragonadal 5% — Mediastinum Retroperitoneum

Gonadal 95%

*Abbreviations:* Lymph, lymphatic; Haem, haematogenous; Misc, miscellaneous; T, testosterone; E, oestrogen; KS, ketosteroid; AFP, alpha-feto protein; HCG, human chorionic gonadotropin; GCT, germ cell tumour.

- *Never* express alpha-feto protein (AFP).
  - If AFP is elevated in a pure seminoma during orchidectomy, a mixed GCT is assumed.
  - Tumour is classified and clinically managed as a NSGCT.
- Very radiosensitive unlike other NSGCTs.
- Chemosensitive.

## Spermatocytic Seminoma (Spermatocytic Tumour)

- Rare (makes up <1% of GCTs).
- Histologically and clinically distinct from seminomas.
- *Does not arise* from GCNIS.
- *Does not* have increased copies of i12p.
- Can occur at any age. Most commonly found in men >60 years old.
- Morphologically similar to seminomas. Can be distinguished through immunohistochemistry:
  - *Positive* staining for SSX, XPA, synaptonemal complex protein 1, CHK2, melanoma antigen family A4, and neuron-specific enolase.
  - *Negative* staining for KIT, PLAP, and OCT3/4.
  - Lack of lymphocytic infiltrate is seen with seminomas.
- Usually benign and treated with orchidectomy alone.

## Embryonal Carcinoma

- Pure embryonal carcinoma is rare (<2% of GCTs).
- Composes 85% of mixed GCTs.
- Presentation at ~30 years.
- Histologically appear as cohesive sheets of cells.
- Stain for cytokeratin and CD30.
- Syncytiotrophoblasts are occasionally seen.
- Usually not associated with tumour marker elevations.
- Elevated AFP and HCG in rare cases.

## Yolk Sac Tumour

- Pure yolk sac tumours are the most common prepubertal malignant GCT - rare in adults and compose 40% of mixed GCTs.
- Histologically show the most variability with many recognised patterns.
- Distinguished from embryonal carcinomas with:
  - High background AFP
  - Glypican 3
  - SALL4
  - Absence of OCT3/4, NANOG, and Sox-2
- *Schiller–Duval bodies* (pathognomonic):
  - Cellular structures resembling a glomerulus.

- Contain AFP and alpha 1-antitrypsin.
- Identified in 50% of the tumours.
- Hyaline (eosinophilic) globules can be found.
- Nearly all have *high AFP* of >100 ng/mL – AFP levels correlate with disease extent.
- HCG secretion is rare but possible.

## Choriocarcinoma

- Very rare in pure form.
- Composes 10% of GCTs.
- Presentation at ~30 years.
- Highly aggressive.
- Spread haematogeneously – usually widely disseminated at presentation.
  - Lungs, liver, brain (brain imaging at diagnosis recommended)
- Histologically characterised by syncytiotrophoblasts and cytotrophoblast cells together.
  - Vascular invasion, haemorrhage
- High propensity to bleed and gross areas of haemorrhage are common.
  - Bleeding complications – catastrophic when the lungs or the brain are involved.
- Large concentrations of syncytiotrophoblasts – *high hCG levels*, often >1000 IU/L.
- *No AFP production.*
- Worst prognosis.

## Teratoma ('Monster Tumour' in Greek)

- Contain at least two of three germ cell layers in different stages of maturation.
  - Endoderm, mesoderm, ectoderm
- Histologically comprised of solid and cystic areas.
- Depending on the germ cell layer components and stages of maturation, it may contain cartilage, bone, and teeth.
- Typically without tumour marker elevation.
- Benign in pre-pubescent boys.
- *Adults:*
  - Composes 50% of mixed GCTs.
  - Can be found in metastatic sites of NSGCTs.
- Potential for massive growth and invasion of surrounding structures.
- Potential for malignant transformation → poor prognosis
- *Resistant* to chemotherapy and radiation.

## Stromal Tumours

- Arise from surrounding tissue supporting gonadal cells:
  - Leydig cell tumours
  - Sertoli cell tumours

- Granulosa cell tumours
- Paratesticular rhabdomyosarcoma
- Very rarely adenocarcinoma of the rete testis and mesothelioma of tunica vaginalis
- Composes overall 5% of all testicular tumours.

## Leydig Cell Tumours

- Most common and composes 3% of testicular tumours.
- Benign in 90% of cases.
- Produce testosterone or 17-ketosteroid.
- Associated with Klinefelter's syndrome (47XXY).
- 20% express clinical manifestations including:
  - Gynaecomastia, poor libido, erectile dysfunction, or infertility.
  - Can be associated with precocious puberty in childhood tumours.
- *Microscopically:*
  - Eosinophilic cells.
  - Extracellular *Reinke crystals*: dark pink, cigar-shaped.
  - Stain negative for PLAP, AFP, hCG.
  - Stain positive for inhibin, calretinin.
- Usually cured by orchidectomy alone.

## Sertoli Cell Tumours

- 1% of testicular tumours.
- May secrete oestrogen or testosterone – gynaecomastia or virilisation.
  - Stain negative for PLAP, AFP, hCG.
  - Stain positive for inhibin and calretinin.
- Usually cured by orchidectomy alone.

## Granulosa Cell Tumours

- Extremely rare in adults.
- Most common tumours of infancy.
  - 75% are diagnosed during the neonatal period.
- Produce oestrogen.
- Adults – 50% are associated with gynaecomastia.
- Infants – may be associated with ambiguous genitalia and/or cryptorchidism.
- Usually cured by orchidectomy alone.

# Gonadoblastoma

- Arise in dysgenetic gonads.
  - Mixed gonadal dysgenesis
  - Ambiguous genitalia
  - Hypospadias
- 46XY karyotype is the most common.
- 45X/46/XY mosaicism compose a small fraction.
- Phenotypic females usually display virilisation.
- Phenotypic males usually display gynaecomastia.

# Haematopoietic Tumours

- Lymphoma with testicular involvement is the most common cause of testicular masses in men >60 years.
- Often bilateral.
- Large B-cell lymphoma is the most common.
- Acute lymphoblastic leukaemia (ALL) in young boys can involve the testes in a small percent of cases.
- Primary testicular plasmacytoma extremely rare.

# Tumour Markers

- ~50% of new TC have raised markers.
- ~90% of NSGCTs have raised markers.
- Measured at diagnosis, after orchidectomy, and during follow up.
- Diagnostic and prognostic.

# Alpha-Feto Protein (AFP)

- Produced by yolk sac elements.
- Half-life of 5–7 days.
- Not raised in pure seminoma or choriocarcinoma.
- Raised in ~50–70% NSGCTs.
- *Also raised in:*
  - Stomach, pancreatic, liver, and lung cancers
  - Benign hepatic dysfunction

# Beta Human Chorionic Gonadotrophin (beta-hCG)

- Produced by syncytiotrophoblast elements.
- Half-life of 24–36 hours.
- *Raised in:*
  - *All* choriocarcinoma
  - 40–60% embryonal carcinomas
  - 5–10% pure seminomas
- *Also raised in:*
  - Stomach, pancreatic, liver, lung, breast, kidney, bladder cancers
  - Marijuana smokers

# Lactate Dehydrogenase (LDH)

- Five isoenzymes, but LDH-1 is the most overexpressed.
- Main use: assessment of prognosis at diagnosis.
- Surrogate marker for tumour volume and cell necrosis.
- Half-life of ~24 hours.

# Staging

- The 2016 TNM classification of the International Union Against Cancer (UICC) is used to assess the anatomical extent of the disease (Table 26.3).

**Table 26.3** 2016 TNM Classification for Testicular Cancer

**T – Primary Tumour[1]**

| | |
|---|---|
| pTX | Primary tumour cannot be assessed (see note 1) |
| pT0 | No evidence of primary tumour (e.g., histological scar in testis) |
| pTis | Intratubular germ cell neoplasia (carcinoma *in situ*)* |
| pT1 | Tumour limited to testis and epididymis without vascular/lymphatic invasion; tumour may invade tunica albuginea but not tunica vaginalis* |
| pT2 | Tumour limited to testis and epididymis with vascular/lymphatic invasion, or tumour extending through tunica albuginea with involvement of tunica vaginalis** |
| pT3 | Tumour invades spermatic cord with or without vascular/lymphatic invasion** |
| pT4 | Tumour invades scrotum with or without vascular/lymphatic invasion |

**N – Regional Lymph Nodes – Clinical**

| | |
|---|---|
| NX | Regional lymph nodes cannot be assessed |
| N0 | No regional lymph node metastasis |
| N1 | Metastasis with one or more lymph node mass 2 cm or less in greatest dimension |
| N2 | Metastasis with a lymph node mass more than 2 cm but not more than 5 cm in greatest dimension |
| N3 | Metastasis with a lymph node mass more than 5 cm in greatest dimension |

**pN -- Regional Lymph Nodes – Pathological**

| | |
|---|---|
| pNX | Regional lymph nodes cannot be assessed |
| pN0 | No regional lymph node metastasis |
| pN1 | Metastasis with 5 or fewer lymph node mass 2 cm or less in greatest dimension |
| pN2 | Metastasis with a lymph node mass more than 2 cm but not more than 5 cm in greatest dimension; or more than 5 nodes positive, none more than 5 cm; or evidence or extranodal extension of tumour |
| pN3 | Metastasis with a lymph node mass more than 5 cm in greatest dimension |

**M – Distant Metastasis**

| | |
|---|---|
| MX | Distant metastasis cannot be assessed |
| M0 | No distant metastasis |
| M1 | Distant metastasis** |
| | M1a Non-regional lymph node(s) or lung metastasis |
| | M1b Distant metastasis other than non-regional lymph nodes and lung |

**S – Serum Tumour Markers (Pre chemotherapy)**

| | LDH (U/L) | hCG (mIU/mL) | AFP (ng/mL) |
|---|---|---|---|
| SX | Serum marker studies not available or not performed | | |
| S0 | Serum marker study levels within normal limits | | |
| S1 | < 1.5 x N and | < 5,000 and | < 1,000 |
| S2 | 1.5–10 x N or | 5,000–50,000 or | 1,000–10,000 |
| S3 | > 10 x N or | > 50,000 or | > 10,000 |

1  Except for pTis and pT4, where radical orchidectomy is not always necessary for classification purposes, the extent of the primary tumour is classified after radical orchidectomy; see pT. In other circumstances, TX is used if no radical orchidectomy has been performed.

# Prognostic Factors

## Seminomas

- Higher risk of relapse in Stage 1 if the tumour is >4 cm, or if the retes testis is involved.
- Both factors present yields a relapse rate of 32%.
- If only one factor is present, the relapse rate is at 16%.
- When both are absent, the relapse rate is at 12%.
- Consider contralateral testicular biopsy (two-pole, upper/lower technique).

## NSGCT

- Higher risk of relapse in Stage I with the following:
  - Lymphatic vascular invasion (LVI)
  - Embryonal cancer content >50%
  - Proliferate rare >70%
  - Absence of yolk sac components

## Patterns of Lymphatic Spread

- Based on the drainage of lymph nodes to the retroperitoneum.

- Common for right-sided tumours to have left-sided nodes.
- Rare for left-sided tumours to have positive right-sided nodes; ~1%.
- *Right-sided tumours:*
  - First landing site: inter-aortocaval area; followed by
  - Pre-caval and pre-aortic nodes.
  - Right common iliac and external iliac.
- *Left-sided tumours:*
  - First landing site: para-aortic and pre-aortic nodes; followed by
  - Inter-aortocaval nodes.
  - Left common iliac and external iliac nodes.
- The anatomy is important when planning retroperitoneal lymph node dissection (RPLND).
  - Indication includes residual mass post-chemotherapy for NSGCT.
  - *Templates:* bilateral or modified unilateral (Figure 26.2).
  - Modified unilateral is less morbid and reduces the rate of retrograde ejaculation.
- *Bilateral template:*
  - Cranial: superior aspect of renal vein.

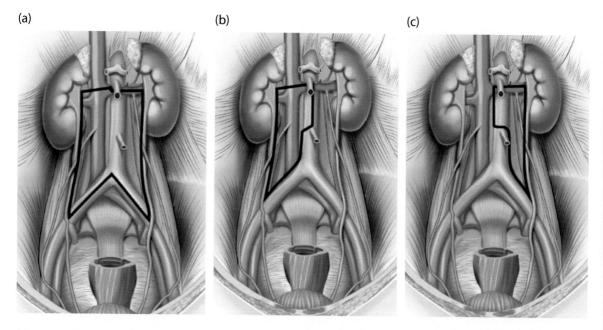

(a)  (b)  (c)

**Figure 26.2** Retroperitoneal lymph node dissection templates. (a) Bilateral; (b) Unilateral right; (c) Unilateral left. (Reprinted by permission from Springer Nature [11])

- Caudal: common iliac and proximal 1/3 external iliac and aortic bifucation.
- Lateral: medial margin of ureters.
- *Unilateral template* (typically for primary RPLND):
  - Inferior mesenteric artery is spared.
  - Right-side: lateral margins are the ureter and aorta.
  - Left-side: lateral margins are the ureter and vena cava.

# Recommended Reading

1. Einhorn LH. Treatment of testicular cancer: a new and improved model. J Clin Oncol. 1990;8(11):1777–81.
2. Moch H, Cubilla AL, Humphrey PA, Reuter VE, Ulbright TM. The 2016 WHO classification of tumours of the urinary system and male genital organs-part A: renal, penile, and testicular tumours. Eur Urol. 2016;70(1):93–105.
3. Akre O, Pettersson A, Richiardi L. Risk of contralateral testicular cancer among men with unilaterally undescended testis: a meta analysis. Int J Cancer. 2009;124(3):687–89.
4. DeCastro BJ, Peterson AC, Costabile RA. A 5-year followup study of asymptomatic men with testicular microlithiasis. J Urol. 2008;179(4):1420–23; discussion 3.
5. Skakkebaek NE, Berthelsen JG, Giwercman A, Muller J. Carcinoma-in-situ of the testis: possible origin from gonocytes and precursor of all types of germ cell tumours except spermatocytoma. Int J Androl. 1987;10(1):19–28.
6. Hanna NH, Einhorn LH. Testicular cancer--discoveries and updates. N Engl J Med. 2014;371(21):2005–16.
7. Oosterhuis JW, Looijenga LH. Testicular germ-cell tumours in a broader perspective. Nat Rev Cancer. 2005;5(3):210–22.
8. Krausz C, Looijenga LHJ. Genetic aspects of testicular germ cell tumors. Cell Cycle. 2008;7(22):3519–24.
9. Krag Jacobsen G, Barlebo H, Olsen J, Schultz HP, Starklint H, Sogaard H, et al. Testicular germ cell tumours in Denmark 1976-1980. Pathology of 1058 consecutive cases. Acta Radiol Oncol. 1984;23(4):239–47.
10. Cheng L, ALbers P, Berney DM et al. Testicular cancer. Nat Rev Primers. 2018;4(1):29.
11. Katz, MH, Eggener, SE. The evolution, controversies, and potential pitfalls of modified retroperitoneal lymph node dissection templates. World J Urol. 2009;27(4):477–483.

# 27 Penile Cancer

*Eleni Anastasiadis and Nicholas A. Watkin*

## Epidemiology

- The epidemiology of penile cancer varies by geographical region, race, ethnicity and age.
- Penile cancer is an uncommon malignancy in developed countries.
- Europe and USA: Overall incidence, one per 100,000 males.
- Some African, Asian, South American countries: rates are higher, can be up to 10% of male malignancies.
- Rare in cultures that perform ritual neonatal/childhood circumcisions
  - Lowest incidence for Israeli Jews — 0.3 per 100,000 men per year.
- In the United Kingdom (UK):
  - The incident rate is 2.3 per 100,000 men. Accounts for less than 1% of all new cancers in males.
  - The lifetime risk of being diagnosed is ~0.2%
  - There is an increased incidence in older men (~1/3 new diagnoses in age >75 years, highest rates in those >90 years of age)
  - Median age of diagnosis is 63 years.
- Penile cancer is usually a squamous cell carcinoma (SCC) with various subtypes.
- Typically arises from the epithelium of the inner prepuce or glans.
- ~ 45–63% linked to the Human Papilloma Virus (HPV) infection.
  - Type 16 is the most common, followed by 18 and 6.

## Risk Factors

- 30–50% caused by HPV infection.
- Associated with:
  - Multiple sexual partners (3–5x increased risk)
  - History of genital warts
  - HPV virus interaction with oncogenes and tumour suppressor (TS) genes (*p16, P53, Rb* genes)
- Tobacco use in any form is strongly associated (5-fold increase)
- Rural areas, low socioeconomic status (geographic variation)

- Chronic inflammation of the prepuce or glans – can increase odds by >10.
  - *Phimosis* (odds ratio 11–16 vs. no phimosis)
    - Present in 44–85% of newly diagnosed cancers.
    - In some studies men with phimosis had an increased risk (~65 fold) of developing penile cancer.
    - Poor penile hygiene and retention of smegma (desquamated epidermal cells and urinary products) underlying mechanisms of chronic inflammation.
    - Neonatal/childhood circumcision appears protective (~3x reduced risk).
    - Adulthood circumcision not thought to be protective.
  - *Recurrent balanoposthitis*
  - *Lichen sclerosis* (LS) et atrophicus (male genital LS)
- Treatment with psoralen and ultraviolet photochemotherapy (PUVA) in psoriasis.
  - Strongly dose-dependent.
  - High levels of PUVA causes ~286x increased incidence compared to the general population.
- *Others:* chronic rashes, tears, urethral strictures, obesity, poor penile hygiene, immunosuppresive drugs.

## Histological Classification of Penile Cancer

- 95% SCC (Table 27.1 and Figure 27.1), with different subtypes.
- Subtypes have different growth patterns and aggressiveness, HPV associations, and precursor lesions (Table 27.2).
- Keratinising type (usual type) is the most common.
- Multiple mixed forms present: warty-basaloid is the most common (50–60% of the mixed forms).
- Other epithelial tumours – small cell, Merkel Cell, clear cell, sebaceous cell, or basal cell carcinomas.
- Non-epithelial tumours such as melanoma or sarcoma are very rare.

**Table 27.1** World Health Organization (WHO) Classification of Penile Tumours

| Malignant epithelial tumours | Malignant tumours |
|---|---|
| Squamous cell carcinoma | Angiosarcoma |
| Non-HPV-related SCC | Clear cell sarcoma |
| SCC, usual type | Dermatofibrosarcoma protuberans |
| Pseudohyperplastic carcinoma | Epithelioid haemangioendothelioma |
| Pseudoglandular carcinoma | Epithelioid sarcoma |
| Verrucous carcinoma | Ewing sarcoma |
| Carcinoma cuniculatum | Giant cell fibroblastoma |
| Papillary SCC | Kaposi sarcoma |
| Adenosquamous carcinoma | Leiomyosarcoma |
| Sarcomatoid (spindle cell) carcinoma | Malignant peripheral nerve sheath tumour |
| Mixed SCC | Myxofibrosarcoma |
| HPV-related SCC | Undifferentiated pleomorphic sarcoma |
| Basaloid SCC | Osteosarcoma, extraskeletal |
| Papillary-basaloid carcinoma | Rhabdomyosarcoma |
| Warty carcinoma | Synovial sarcoma |
| Warty-basaloid carcinoma | **Lymphomas** |
| Clear cell SCC | **Metastatic tumours** |
| Lymphoepithelioma-like carcinoma | |
| Other rare carcinomas | |
| **Precursor lesions** | |
| Penile intraepithelial neoplasia | |
| Warty/basaloid/warty-basaloid | |
| Differentiated PeIN | |
| Paget disease | |
| **Melanocytic lesions** | |
| **Mesenchymal tumours** | |
| Benign tumours | |
| Benign fibrous histiocytoma | |
| Glomus tumour | |
| Granular cell tumour | |
| Haemangioma | |
| Juvenile xanthogranuloma | |
| Leiomyoma | |
| Lymphangioma | |
| Myointimoma | |
| Neurofibroma | |
| Schwannoma | |

*Source:* Adapted from Moch et al. [6]
*Abbreviations:* PeIN, Penile intraepithelial neoplasia; SCC, Squamous cell carcinoma.

## Immunohistochemistry (IHC)

- p16 and p53: for HPV-related PeIN/SCC
- Ki-67: differentiated PeIN from squamous hyperplasia
- Precursor/Premalignant penile lesions
- SCC may develop from the progression of premalignant lesions.
- Penile intraepithelial neoplasia (PeIN) = SCC pre-cancerous lesions.
  - Classified into differentiated and undifferentiated (Table 27.3 and Figure 27.1).
  - Depends on the degree of epithelial atypia.
- *Undifferentiated PeIN*
  - Full-thickness cytological atypia.
  - Lack of differentiation and abnormal mitotic activity throughout the epithelium.
  - Related to HPV-associated penile cancer.
  - Further subdivided into basaloid, warty, and warty-basaloid subtypes.
- Other rare patterns (pleomorphic, spindle, clear cell, pagetoid).
- *Differentiated PeIN*
  - Atypia is confined to the lower third of the epithelium.
  - Architectural atypia, elongated rete ridges and aberrant intraepithelial keratinisation.
  - Linked to chronic inflammation (e.g., LS).
  - Precursor lesions to well-differentiated and keratinising SCC.

## Clinical Manifestations of Pre-malignant Lesions

### Undifferentiated PeIN (HPV-related)

- Giant condylomata (Buschke-Löwenstein), Bowen's disease (BD), and Erythroplasia of Queyrat (EQ).
- Up to 33% may transform to invasive SCC.

**Table 27.2** Classification of Penile Cancer SCC Subtypes, Their Frequencies, Prognosis, Precursors Lesions and HPV Associations

| Histological SCC Subtype | Frequency (% of Cases) | HPV positivity (%) | Prognosis | Precursor Lesions (PeIN) |
|---|---|---|---|---|
| Keratinising type/ 'not otherwise specified' (NOS)/ usual type | 48–75% | 24–59 | Poor (30% DOD) | Differentiated PeIN |
| **Mixed warty-basaloid** | 9–17% | **82** | Poor (30% DOD) | Warty-basaloid PeIN |
| **Verrucous** | 3–8% | 0–23 | Good | Differentiated PeIN/LS |
| **Papillary** | 5–15% | 8-15 | Good | Differentiated PeIN |
| **Warty** | 6–10% | **22–100** | Good | Warty PeIN |
| **Basaloid** | 4–10% | **70–100** | Very Poor (>50% DOD) | Basaloid PeIN |
| **Sarcomatoid carcinoma** | 1–3% | 0–17 | Very poor (75% DOD) | |
| **Another SCC mixed** | 9–10% | +/– | Heterogenous group | |
| Pseudohyperplastic | <1% | 0 | Good | Differentiated PeIN/LS |
| Ca cuniculatum | <1% | 0 | Good | |
| Pseudoglandular ca | <1% | 0 | Poor | |
| Adenosquamous ca | <1% | – | Intermediate | |
| Mucoepidermoid ca | <1% | – | Poor | |
| Clear cell variant | 1–2% | 100 | Poor (20% DOD) | |

Those highlighted in bold are main types.
*Abbreviations:* Ca, carcinoma; DOD, die of disease; LS, lichen sclerosis; SCC, squamous cell carcinoma, PeIN, penile

**Table 27.3** Classification of Penile Intraepithelial Neoplasia (PeIN)

| | *Undifferentiated (HPV-related)* | *Differentiated (Non-HPV-related)* |
|---|---|---|
| **Histology** | Full-thickness cytological atypia with lack of differentiation and abnormal mitotic activity throughout the epithelium.<br> | Atypia confined to lower third of epithelium. Architectural atypia, elongated rete ridges and aberrant intraepithelial keratinisation.<br> |
| **Subtypes** | Basaloid PeIN, Warty PeIN, Warty-basaloid PeIN, Other rare patterns: (pleomorphic, spindle, clear cell, pagetoid) | Differentiated PeIN |
| **Associations** | HPV-associated penile cancer | Chronic inflammation (e.g., LS) Precursor lesions to well-differentiated and keratinising SCC |

*Source:* Table modified and Adapted from Hakenberg et al. [1]. Histology slides reprinted with permissions from A. Kaul et al, "Diagnosis and Management of Premalignant Penile Lesions" In: Culkin D. (eds) Management of Penile Cancer. Springer, New York, NY (2014)

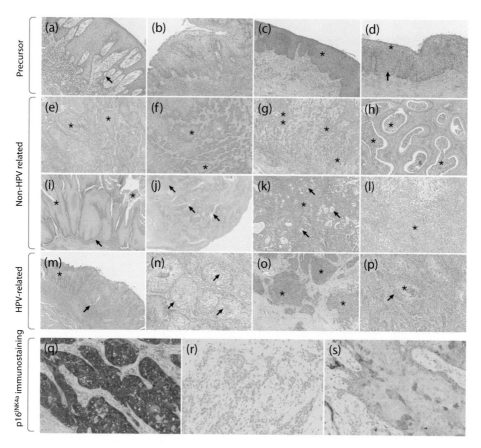

**Figure 27.1** Histology of penile carcinomas. Histopathological appearance of precursor lesions, non-HPV related invasive penile squamous cell carcinoma (PSCC) and HPV-related invasive PSCC in haematoxylin and eosin stains (upper panel) and different p16INK4a immunostaining patterns (lower panel). (a) Differentiated penile intraepithelial neoplasia (PeIN) with elongated and anastomosing rete ridges (arrow) and atypical basal layer cells (magnification x10); (b) Warty PeIN with squamous maturation, atypical parakeratosis, pleomorphism and koilocytosis (magnification x10); (c) Basaloid PeIN with a full- thickness presence of immature, small, monotonous basophilic cells in the epithelium (asterisk) (magnification x10); (d) Warty–basaloid PeIN with koilocytic changes in the upper epithelial cell layer (asterisk) and basaloid cells in the lower half of the epithelium (arrow) (magnification x10); (e) Usual PSCC, well-differentiated, grade I with well-delineated tumour nests with minimal atypia and central keratinization (asterisks) (magnification x5); (f) Usual PSCC, moderately differentiated, grade II with irregular tumour nests with more atypia, but maintained squamous maturation (asterisks) (magnification x5); (g) Usual PSCC, poorly differentiated, grade III with infiltrating tumour nests with minimal squamous maturation (asterisks) (magnification x5); (h) Pseudoglandular carcinoma with honeycomb appearance and acantholytic pseudolumina (asterisks) (magnification x5); (i) Verrucous carcinoma with papillomatosis, hyperorthokeratosis (asterisks) and broad- based pushing tumour front (arrow) (magnification x20); (j) Carcinoma cuniculatum with burrowing labyrinthine growth pattern (arrows) (magnification x0.5); (k) Adenosquamous carcinoma with squamous nests (asterisk) intermixed with a glandular component (arrows) (magnification x10); (l) Sarcomatoid carcinoma with atypical spindle cells (asterisk) (magnification x5). (m) Warty PeIN (asterisk) with microinvasion (arrow) (magnification x10); (n) Warty carcinoma with clear cells and pleomorphic koilocytes (arrows) (magnification x10); (o) Basaloid carcinoma with irregular nests of small uniform basaloid cells (asterisks) (magnification x10); (p) Warty–basaloid carcinoma with tumour nests with clear and koilocytic cell warty features in the centre (asterisk) and basaloid features in the periphery (arrow) (magnification x10); (q) Example of strong and diffuse p16INK4a immunostaining in a HPV- related carcinoma (magnification x20); (r) Negative p16INK4a immunostaining in a non-HPV-related carcinoma (magnification x20); (s) Patchy and focal staining is considered negative for p16INK4a overexpression and indicative for a non- HPV- related carcinoma (magnification x20). (Reprinted by permissions from Springer Nature [15])

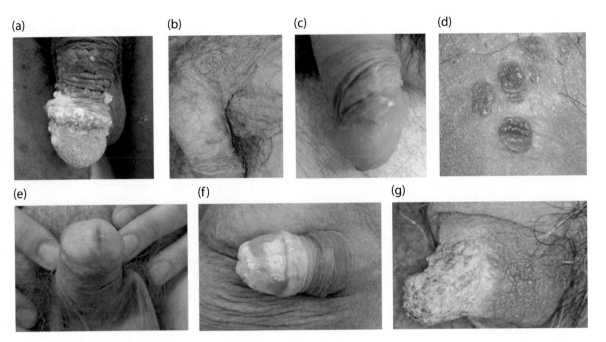

Figure 27.2 Premalignant lesions. (a) Giant condyloma acuminatum (Buschke-Löwenstein); (b) Bowen's Disease; (c) Erythroplasia of Queyrat (PeIN); (d) Bowenoid Papulosis; (e) Lichen Sclerosis; (f) Verrucous Hyperplasia; (g) Penile Cutaneous Horn. ([a,b,c,e,f] Reprinted by permission from Springer Nature [7]; (d) Reprinted with permission from Elsevier [13]; (g) Reprinted with permission from Elsevier [14].)

## Giant condylomata (Buschke-Löwenstein)

- May become invasive SCC in >50%.
- Large cauliflower-like growth due to a confluence of condyloma acuminate (smaller warty growths).
- Can grow on any part of the anogenital region.
- On penis, often appear on the frenulum and coronal sulcus (Figure 27.2a).
- Strong association with HPV-6 and 11.

## Bowen's Disease (BD) and Erythroplasia of Queyrat (EQ)

- The term Penile intraepithelial neoplasia (PeIN) is now used in preference to BD or EQ.
- *BD* - usually presents on the follicle bearing or keratinizing external genital skin and may appear as a single, scaly plaque (Figure 27.2b).
  - 5% risk of invasive SCC
- *EQ* - similar disease entity to BD
  - Typically on the mucosal surfaces of the glans, which may spread to the inner prepuce (Figure 27.2c)
  - One or more red, moist plaques Figure 27.2c
  - 10–30% risk of invasive SCC
- Prevalence of HPV in these conditions – 43–100%.

## Bowenoid Papulosis

- Self-limiting condition, typically in younger men.
- Mean duration of disease – 2–3 months.
- Related to HPV (usually HPV-16).
- Presentation (Figure 27.2d):
  - Multiple, small, well-demarcated brown/red/pink papillomatous papules or small patches on the penile shaft or mons pubis.
  - Less frequently on the glans or prepuce.
- <1% progress to an invasive SCC, those immuno-suppressed are most at risk.

## Differentiated PeIN (non-HPV-related)

### Lichen Sclerosis (LS)

- Chronic inflammatory, atrophic condition with unknown aetiology, commonly affects the anogenital area.
- Atrophic or sclerotic patches on the prepuce and/or glans (Figure 27.2e).
- *Histology:*
  - Hyperplastic or atrophic epithelium without cellular atypia.
  - Homogenisation of underlying stroma.
  - Mild vasocongestion.
- May Precede up to 30% of penile cancers.
- ~5% men with LS may progress to penile SCC.

## *Verrucous hyperplasia*

- Leads to verrucous carcinoma.
- Thickened, pale, fluffy area of mucosa without nodularity (Figure 27.2f).

## *Penile Cutaneous Horn*

- Conical, protruding, hyperkeratotic mass arising from the glans or coronal sulcus (Figure 27.2g).
- Associated with chronic inflammation and phimosis.
- The base of the lesion may show changes amounting to differentiated PeIN.

# Molecular Pathways in the Pathogenesis of Penile Cancer

- *Two distinct pathways*:
  1. HPV-dependent pathways
  2. HPV infection-independent pathways (due to inflammation)

## HPV-dependent Pathways

- Human papilloma virus.
  - Small, non-enveloped virus.
  - Contains double-stranded DNA within 55 nm diameter icosahedral capsids.
  - Member of the papovaviruses.
  - There are >200 types of HPV.
  - Can infect the epidermis (cutaneous types) and epithelial linings (mucosotropic).
  - Low- and high-risk types are based on its ability for malignant transformation.
  - *Low-risk:* HPV-6 and HPV-11 (most prevalent).
    - Localised benign genital warts (condyloma acuminata).
    - Do not typically progress to malignancy even if left untreated.
  - *High-risk:* most prevalent is HPV-16, followed by HPV-18 and HPV-31.
    - Can cause PeIN and invasive SCC.
- HPV infection alone is not sufficient for malignant transformation.
- Further genetic alterations are required.

a. *HPV oncogenes E5, E6, and E7.*
- Alter growth regulation by host proteins and induce genomic instability.
- HPV infects cells in the basal layer of the stratified squamous epithelium that becomes exposed from micro-trauma.
- Rely on host cell replication proteins to mediate viral DNA synthesis.

- Viral Oncoprotein *E6 and E7* binds and inactivates p53 and Rb tumour suppresor (TS) gene products, respectively, leading to the disturbance of the:
  1. $p14^{ARF}$/MDM2/p53 pathway (disrupting pathways that normally lead to cell-cycle arrest and apoptotic cell death)
  2. $p16^{INK4a}$/cyclin D/Rb pathway (disrupting pathways that normally results in cell-cycle arrest).
     - Inactivation of Rb protein results in an overexpression of $p16^{INK4a}$.
     - Overexpressed $p16^{INK4a}$ can be used as a marker of viral involvement.
     - This pathway is associated with basaloid and warty subtypes.
- HPV oncoproteins thus interfere with the control of cell division cycle and apoptosis.

b. *Amplification of MYC proto-oncogene.*
- Located on the chromosome 8q24.
- Insertion of the HPV-16 DNA within this region causes overexpression of *MYC oncogene*.

c. *Increased telomerase activity.*
- Telomerase adds telomere (repeated sequence of nucleotide) to chromosome ends → protect ends from deterioration or fusion to other chromosomes during cell division
- Telomeres shorten with each cell division.
- When the telomere length reaches critical limit → cell undergoes senescence and/or apoptosis
- HPV E6 oncoproteins increase telomerase activity, inducing immortalisation.

## HPV-independent Pathways

- Chronic inflammation is an important risk factor
- *Reactive oxygen/nitrogen species (ROS/RNS):*
  - Produced by inflammatory cells in an attempt to fight infectious agents.
  - May cause DNA damage.
  - *p16* TS gene inhibits cyclin D/E2F pathway, which causes cell arrest of damaged cells.
  - Chromosomal instability is frequently found in *p16* gene, thus, it is thought to be one of the critical pathways in penile carcinogenesis in the context of chronic inflammation
- *Cyclooxygenase-2 (COX-2) and prostaglandin E2 (PGE2):*
  - COX-2 is strongly expressed in penile cancer.
  - Causes an overproduction of PGs and thromboxanes.
  - PGE2 is involved in proliferation, angiogenesis, and activation of the epidermal growth factor (EGF).

# Tumour Progression and Metastatic Spread

a. *Proliferation*
- Overexpression of the epidermal growth factor receptor (EGFR) is strongly expressed in penile cancer.
- EGFR is an ERBB receptor tyrosine kinase.
- The activation of EGFR by EGF or transforming growth factor-α (TGF-α) → activation of intracellular tyrosine kinase unit → induces proliferative pathways
  - KRAS-BRAF pathway (EGFR-dependent pathway)
  - EGFR-RAS pathway
  - HER3 and HER4 receptor pathways

b. *Invasion*
- Breakdown of cell-to-cell adhesions.
- *E-cadherin* is an adhesion molecule.
- Low levels of E-cadherin → increased risk of lymph node metastases
- Matrix metalloproteinases → breakdown of type IV collagen found in the basement membrane → penetration of basement membrane → metastasis
- Tumour cells interact with their microenvironment (stromal-epithelial interactions).

c. *Neoangiogenesis*
- Vascular endothelial growth factor (VEGF) important in neoangiogenesis.
- Independent prognostic factor for metastatic progression.

## Tumour Grading and Staging

- Grade 1, well; G2, moderately; G3 poorly differentiated; G4, undifferentiated.
- The TNM classification system is used to stage penile cancer (Table 27.4).

# Lymph Node Metastasis and Inguinal Lymph Node Anatomy

- Spread and extent of inguinal node metastasis is considered the most important prognostic factor for survival.
- The first draining lymph nodes (or *'sentinel' nodes*) are invariably within the inguinal lymphatic basin.
- Cancer then spread to pelvic nodes and/or distant sites
- Penile SCC tends to have a prolonged locoregional phase.
- Lymphadenectomy is thus potentially curative.

## Lymphatic Drainage

- The prepuce and skin of the penile shaft:
  - Lymphatics converge dorsally.
  - Divide at the base of the penis.
  - Drain into the right and left superficial inguinal nodes.
- Glans penis
  - Drainage towards the frenulum.
  - Encircles the corona and unites with the dorsal lymphatic vessel.
  - Traverses through Buck's fascia to the base of the penis.
  - Drains into the superficial and deep inguinal lymph nodes via the presymphyseal lymphatics.
- Spread can occur bilaterally due to this lymphatic interconnectivity.
- Inguinal lymphatics drain into the ipsilateral pelvic nodes (external iliac nodes).
  - Crossover metastatic spread from one groin to contralateral pelvic nodes has never been reported.
- Spread from the pelvic nodes to the retroperitoneal nodes → systemic disease
- *Superficial* inguinal nodes are superior to the fascia lata within the femoral triangle.
- *Femoral triangle:*
  - Superior border – inguinal ligament
  - Medial border – lateral border of the adductor longus muscle
  - Lateral border – medial border of the sartorius muscle
  - Roof – fascia lata
  - Floor – iliopsoas and pectineus muscles, contains neurovascular structures
- *Deep* inguinal nodes are deep to the fascia lata, medial to the femoral vein.
  - *Cloquet's* (or Rosenmuller's) node is the most proximal node, considered to be between the inguinal and external iliac basins
- *Daseler's five zones* (Figure 27.3).
  - Vertical and horizontal line over the saphenofemoral junction creating five zones:
    - 1) Medial superior and 2) lateral superior zone
    - 3) Medial inferior and 4) lateral inferior zone
    - 5) Central zone which overlies the junction
- Sentinel inguinal nodes are located in the medial superior and central zone.
- No solitary lymphatic spread is reported from the penis to the inferior zones and no direct drainage to the pelvic nodes.

## Clinical assessment and management of lymph nodes

- Groin examination for enlarged lymph nodes
- Palpable lymph nodes are highly suggestive of lymph node metastatic involvement

**Table 27.4** 2016 TNM Classification of Penile Cancer

**T – Primary tumour**

| | | |
|---|---|---|
| TX | Primary tumour cannot be assessed | |
| T0 | No evidence of primary tumour | |
| Tis | Carcinoma *in situ* | |
| Ta | Non-invasive verrucous carcinoma[*] | |
| T1 | Tumour invades subepithelial connective tissue | |
| | T1a | Tumour invades subepithelial connective tissue *without* lymphovascular invasion and is not poorly differentiated |
| | T1b | Tumour invades subepithelial connective tissue *with* lymphovascular invasion or is poorly differentiated |
| T2 | Tumour invades corpus spongiosum with or without invasion of the urethra | |
| T3 | Tumour invades corpus cavernosum with or without invasion of the urethra | |
| T4 | Tumour invades other adjacent structures | |

**N – Regional lymph nodes**

| | |
|---|---|
| NX | Regional lymph nodes cannot be assessed |
| N0 | No palpable or visibly enlarged inguinal lymph nodes |
| N1 | Palpable mobile unilateral inguinal lymph node |
| N2 | Palpable mobile multiple or bilateral inguinal lymph nodes |
| N3 | Fixed inguinal nodal mass *or* pelvic lymphadenopathy, unilateral or bilateral |

**M – Distant metastasis**

| | |
|---|---|
| M0 | No distant metastasis |
| M1 | Distant metastasis |

**Pathological classification**

The pT categories correspond to the clinical T categories. The pN categories are based upon biopsy or surgical excision

**pN – Regional lymph nodes**

| | |
|---|---|
| pNX | Regional lymph nodes cannot be assessed |
| pN0 | No regional lymph node metastasis |
| pN1 | Metastasis in one or two inguinal lymph nodes |
| pN2 | Metastasis in more than two unilateral inguinal nodes or bilateral inguinal lymph nodes |
| pN3 | Metastasis in pelvic lymph node(s), unilateral *or* bilateral extranodal or extension of regional lymph node metastasis |

**pM – Distant metastasis**

| | |
|---|---|
| pM1 | Distant metastasis microscopically confirmed |

[*]Verrucous carcinoma is not associated with destructive invasion.

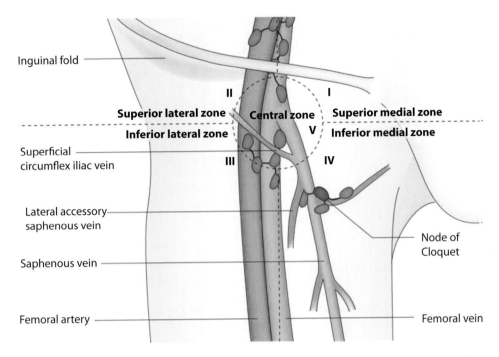

Figure 27.3 Illustration of Daseler's five zones and other lymph nodes. (Reprinted by permission from Springer Nature [12])

- Imaging of groins in this context will not alter management
- Pelvic CT or PET/CT scan can be used for further staging
- There is no reliable imaging modality that can assess for micro-metastatic disease in clinically non-palpable inguinal lymph nodes (cN0).
- In obese patients in which inguinal lymph node palpation may be difficult, the most reliable imaging modality is USS.
  - USS (+/– fine needle aspiration for cytology [FNAC]) involvement
    - Features that suggest metastatic disease involvement
      - absence of lymph node hilum
      - short-/long-axis ratio of <2
      - an enlarged lymph node
      - abnormal shape
      - cortical hypertrophy
      - hypoechogenicity due to a necrotic zone
- [18]FDG-PET/CT: high sensitivity (88–100%) and specificity (98–100%) for confirming metastatic disease in palpable inguinal nodes.
  - Does not detect disease if nodes are <10 mm
- Pathologically confirmed enlarged inguinal lymph node(s) (after FNAC or core biopsy confirmation) necessitates radical inguinal lymphadenectomy of the groin on that side.
- Ipsilateral pelvic lymphadenectomy if ≥2 inguinal nodes are involved on one side or if there is an extracapsular nodal extension (pN3).

## Clinically normal inguinal lymph nodes (cN0)

- The risk of micro-metastatic disease if no nodes are palpable or radiologically abnormal is 20-25%.
- In this group, adequate staging and management of the inguinal lymph nodes has important survival implications.
- Patients treated pre-emptively with bilateral lymphadenectomy, have a higher chance of survival compared to those who are managed expectantly with surveillance.
- Invasive surgical staging techniques are required
- Risk stratification is based on pathological findings in the primary tumour.
- Factors include: 1) stage, 2) grade, and 3) presence of lymphovascular invasion.
- In general, T1 grade 2 or higher disease: need invasive nodal staging.
- Each groin is managed independently i.e. if the right groin in cN0, and the left groin has a pathologically enlarged lymph node(s), the right groin will undergo Dynamic Sentinel Lymph node biopsy (DSLNB) or modified inguinal lymphadenectomy (MILND) and the left groin will undergo radical lymphadenectomy.

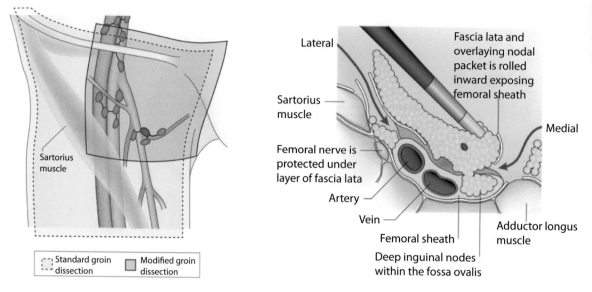

**Figure 27.4** Boundaries of standard/radical versus Modified Inguinal Lymphadenectomy and Fascial Layers in lymph node dissection. (Reprinted by permission from Springer Nature [12])

## Dynamic Sentinel Lymph Node Biopsy (DSLNB)

- Sentinel nodes are identified intraoperatively by patent blue dye and gamma emissions using a hand-held gamma probe.
- 2–12 hours before surgery: intradermal injection of radioactive tracer technetium 99m-labelled nano-colloid ($^{99m}$Tc) around the shaft of the penis proximal to the primary tumour.
- Dynamic and static images are collected using a dual-head gamma camera to locate the nodes.
- On the operating table – 1 mL *Patent Blue* dye is injected intradermally in the same location as the radionuclide injection.
- Locate nodes using a gamma probe to aid incision.
- Both gamma probe and blue dye are used to guide the dissection of sentinel nodes.
- Nodes are sent for histological examination.
- A pre-operative USS and FNAC of any abnormal nodes, is used in addition to pick up any pathological nodes. Pathological nodes may disrupt the typical lymphatic drainage system, and thus may fail to pick up the radioactivity.
- False-negative rates: 4–7%.

## The modified inguinal lymphadenectomy (MILND) (Figure 27.4)

- Same staging and therapeutic benefits as the standard (extended) radical lymphadenectomy (ELND), but less morbid.
- *ELND:*
  - Removes lymph nodes superficial and deep to the fascia lata.
  - Involves excision of the great saphenous vein.
- *MILND:*
  - Excision of lymph nodes superficial to the fascia lata.
    - Medial superficial and central zone inguinal nodes.
    - Preservation of the great saphenous vein.
  - Rationale for modified technique: deep nodes are *not* involved unless the superficial nodes are.
    - Negative superficial nodes exclude deeper node involvement.
- Complication rates are shown in Table 27.5.

**Table 27.5** Risks of Complications Following the Different Inguinal Nodal Dissection Techniques

| Complications | DSLNB (% Risk) | MILND (% Risk) | ELND (% Risk) |
|---|---|---|---|
| Seroma/lymphocele | 3.4 | 2.5–25 | 20–25 |
| Wound infection/haematoma/bleeding | 3.4 | 0.8–10 | 7 |
| Skin flap necrosis/dehiscence | <1% | 2.5 –10 | 12–40 |
| Genital/Lower limb oedema | 0.8 | 20 | 20–25 |
| Persistent oedema | 0.8 | 3 | 20 |
| DVT | 0 | 0 | 14 |
| Overall | 5–7 | 12–35 | 40–54 |

*Abbreviations:* DSLND, dynamic sentinel lymph node dissection; MILND, modified inguinal lymph node dissection; ELND, extended/radical lymph node dissection; DVT, deep vein thrombosis.

# Recommended Reading

1. Hakenberg OW, Comperat E, Minhas S, Necchi A, Protzel C, Watkin N et al. EAU guidelines on Penile cancer [Internet]. EAU Guidelines Office. 2018 [cited 2019 Aug 7]. Available from: https://uroweb.org/guideline/penile-cancer/ guidelin.
2. Cancer Research UK. Penile Cancer Statistics [Internet]. 2019 [cited 2019 Aug 7]. Available from: https://www.cancerresearchuk.org/health-professional/cancer-statistics/statistics-by-cancer-type/penile-cancer#heading-Zero
3. Yap T, Watkin N, Minhas S. Infections of the genital tract: human papillomavirus related infections. Eur Urol Suppl. 2017;16(4):149–62.
4. Bleeker MCG, Heideman DAM, Snijders PJF et al. Penile cancer: epidemiology, pathogenesis and prevention. World J Urol. 2008;27(2):141–50.
5. Stern RS. Genital tumors among men with psoriasis exposed to psoralens and ultraviolet a radiation (PUVA) and ultraviolet B radiation. N Engl J Med. 1990;322(16):1093–97.
6. Moch H, Cubilla AL, Humphrey PA, Reuter VE, Ulbright TM. The 2016 WHO classification of tumours of the urinary system and male genital organs-part A: renal, penile, and testicular tumours. Eur Urol. 2016;70(1):93–105.
7. Kaul, Asheesh, Corbishley et al. Diagnosis and management of premalignant penile lesions. In: Culkin D, editor. Management of Penile Cancer. New York: Springer Science+Business Media; 2014. pp. 107–22.
8. Protzel C, Spiess PE. Molecular research in penile cancer-lessons learned from the past and bright horizons of the future? Int J Mol Sci. 2013;14(10):19494–19505.
9. Bouchot O, Rigaud J, Maillet F, Hetet JF, Karam G. Morbidity of inguinal lymphadenectomy for invasive penile carcinoma. Eur Urol. 2004;45(6):761–766.
10. Schlenker B, Scher B, Tiling R et al. Detection of inguinal lymph node involvement in penile squamous cell carcinoma by 18F-fluorodeoxyglucose PET/CT: a prospective single-center study. Urol Oncol Semin Orig Investig. 2012;30(1):55–59.
11. Lam W, Alnajjar HM, La-Touche S et al. Dynamic sentinel lymph node biopsy in patients with invasive squamous cell carcinoma of the penis: a prospective study of the long-term outcome of 500 inguinal basins assessed at a single institution. Eur Urol. 2013;63(4):657–63.
12. Leone. A, Diorio GJ, Pettaway C et al. Contemporary management of patients with penile cancer and lymph node metastasis. Nat Rev Urol. 2017;14(6):335–347.
13. Bunker et al. Skin conditions of the male genitalia. Medicine. 2010;38(6):294–299.
14. Micali et al. Penile cancer. J Am Acad Dermatol. 2006;54(3):369–391.
15. Thomas A, Necchi A, Muneer A, Tobias-Machado M, Tran ATH, Van Rompuy AS et al. Penile cancer. Nat Rev Dis Primers. 2021;7(11):1–24.
16. Canete-Portillo S, Velazquez EF, Kristiansen G, Egevad L, Grignon D, Chaux A et al. Report From the International Society of Urological Pathology (ISUP) Consultation Conference on Molecular Pathology of Urogenital Cancers V : Recommendations on the Use of Immunohistochemical and Molecular Biomarkers in Penile Cancer. The American Journal of Surgical Pathology. 2020; 44(7):e80–e86.

# Section V

## THERAPEUTICS

# 28 Reconstruction

*Nadir I. Osman, Karl H. Pang, and Christopher R. Chapple*

## Wound Healing

### Primary Healing (By First Intention)

- The wound is closed within 12–24 hours of its creation.
- Focal disruption of the basement membrane.
- Death of a few epithelial and connective tissue cells.
- Epithelial regeneration is greater than fibrosis.
- *Delayed primary healing:*
  - The contaminated wound is left open for a period before closure.
  - Achieve through loose sutures or leaving the wound open to allow host defences to debride the wound.
- *Healing of superficial (partial thickness wound):*
  - Wounds such as superficial burns, abrasions, and split-thickness graft sites.
  - Injury involves the epithelium and superficial dermis. The basal layer is preserved.
  - Heal by re-epithelialisation → epithelial cells at the wound edge migrate to close the wound.

### Secondary Healing (By Secondary Intention)

- Wounds with extensive tissue loss or those left open after surgery.
- Re-epithelialisation alone cannot close the wound.
- Ingrowth granulation tissue from the wound margin → accumulation of extracellular matrix (ECM, including collagen) → wound contraction and epithelialisation.
- Myofibroblasts play a key role.

### Process of Wound Healing (Figure 28.1)

- Cells and growth factors involved in wound healing are summarised in Tables 28.1 and 28.2.
  1. *Haemostasis (immediate)*
     - Vascular constriction, platelet aggregation, degranulation, and fibrin formation (thrombus)
  2. *Inflammation (Days 1–3)*
     - Neutrophil / monocyte / lymphocyte infiltration, and monocyte differentiation to macrophage.
  3. *Proliferation (Day three to week two)*
     - Re-epithelialisation, angiogenesis, collagen synthesis, ECM formation
  4. *Maturation (Week two to several weeks)*
     - Collagen remodelling, vascular maturation, and regression

### Causes of Delayed Wound Healing

- Any disruption in the four phases of wound healing may cause a delay in healing.
- Healing requires good nutrition, blood supply, and a functioning immune/inflammatory response.
- *Local factors:*
  - Infection, ischaemia
  - Foreign body
  - Haematoma
  - Malignancy
  - Denervation
- *Systemic factors:*
  - Poor nutrition, vitamin A and C deficiency, and zinc and manganese deficiency
  - Obesity, diabetes mellitus, peripheral vascular disease, immunodeficiency
  - Malignant disease, irradiation
  - Age

## Tissue Transfer

- *Definition:* movement of tissue for the purposes of reconstruction.
- Tissue can be transferred either as a *graft* or *flap*.

## Grafts

- Tissue excised and transferred to a new host bed.
- *Examples:* split skin graft, full-thickness skin graft (e.g., postauricular skin prepuce), oral mucosa, bladder mucosa.

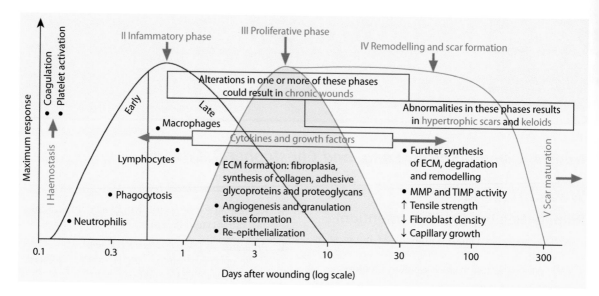

**Figure 28.1** Phases of wound healing. ECM, Extracellular Matrix; MMP, Metalloproteinases; TIMP, Tissue Inhibitors and Metalloproteinases. (Reprinted with permission from Elsevier [1])

**Table 28.1** Cells Involved in Wound Healing

| Cell Type | Function Related to Wound Healing |
|---|---|
| Platelets | - Involved in thrombus formation |
| | - α granules are a rich source of inflammatory mediators including cytokines (e.g., TGF-β, PDGF, β-thromboglobulin, platelet factor-4) |
| | - Major initial stimulus for inflammation |
| Neutrophils | - First cells to infiltrate the site of injury |
| | - Phagocytosis and intracellular killing of invading bacteria |
| Monocytes (macrophages) | - Phagocytose and destroy invading bacteria |
| | - Clear debris and necrotic tissue |
| | - Rich source of inflammatory mediators including cytokines |
| | - Stimulate fibroblast division, collagen synthesis and angiogenesis |
| Lymphocytes | - Not clearly defined |
| | - May produce cytokines in certain types of wound |
| Fibroblasts | - Produce various components of the ECM, including collagen, fibronectin, hyaluronic acid, proteoglycans |
| | - Synthesise granulation tissue |
| | - Help to reorganize the 'provisional' ECM |

*Source:* Reprinted with permission from Elsevier [1].
*Abbreviations:* ECM, extracellular matrix; TGF-β, Transforming growth factor-β; PDGF, Platelet-derived growth factor.

**Table 28.2** Growth Factors Involved in Wound Healing

| Growth Factor | Major Source | Function Related to Wound Healing |
|---|---|---|
| VEGF | Platelets, neutrophils | - Stimulates angiogenesis in granulation tissue |
| | | - Stimulates formation of collateral blood vessels in peripheral vascular disease |
| FGFs | Fibroblasts, endothelial cells, smooth muscle cells, macrophages; also brain, pituitary | - Proliferation of fibroblasts and epithelial cells, matrix deposition, wound contraction, angiogenesis |
| | | - Accelerates formation of granulation tissue |
| KGFs | Fibroblasts | - Proliferation and migration of keratinocytes |
| EGF | Platelets, macrophages, keratinocytes; also saliva, urine, milk, plasma | - Differentiation, proliferation, migration and adhesion of keratinocytes |
| | | - Formation of granulation tissue |
| PDGF | Platelets, fibroblasts, macrophages, endothelial cells | - Mitogenic for smooth muscle cells, endothelial cells and fibroblasts |
| | | - Chemoattractant for neutrophils and fibroblasts |
| | | - Fibroblast proliferation and collagen metabolism |
| G-CSF | Monocytes, fibroblasts, lymphocytes | - Stimulates production of neutrophils |
| | | - Enhances function of neutrophils and monocytes |
| | | - Promotes proliferation of keratinocytes |
| GM-CSF | Keratinocytes, macrophages, lymphocytes, fibroblasts | - Mediates proliferation of epidermal cells |
| TGF-α | Activated macrophages, platelets, epithelial cells | - Stimulates proliferation of epithelial cells and fibroblast |
| | | - Formation of granulation tissue |
| TGF-β | Platelets, macrophages, fibroblasts, neutrophils, keratinocytes | - Mitogenic for fibroblasts and smooth muscle cells |
| | | - Chemotactic for macrophages |
| | | - Stimulates angiogenesis (indirect) and collagen metabolism |
| IL-1 | Macrophages, lymphocytes, many other tissues and cells | - Neutrophil chemotaxis |
| | | - Fibroblast proliferation |
| TNF | Macrophages, mast cells, T-lymphocytes | - Fibroblast proliferation |
| IGF-1 | Fibroblasts, plasma, liver | - Fibroblast proliferation |
| | | - Stimulates synthesis of sulphated proteoglycans and collagen |
| HGF | Fibroblasts, keratinocytes, endothelial cells, tumour cells | - Re-epithelialisation, neovascularisation |
| | | - Formation of granulation tissue |

*Source:* Adapted from Enoch et al. [1].
*Abbreviations:* VEGF, vascular endothelial growth factor; FGFs, fibroblast growth factors; EGF, epidermal growth factor; KGFs, keratinocyte growth factors; TGF-β, transforming growth factor-β; TGF-α, transforming growth factor-α; IL-1, interleukin-1; TNF, tumour necrosis factor; HGF, hepatocyte growth factor; IGF-1, insulin-like growth factor-1; G-CSF, granulocyte-colony stimulating factor; GM-CSF, granulocyte macrophage-colony stimulating factor; PDGF, platelet-derived growth factor.

## Skin Grafts

- *Skin structure:*
  - *Epidermis* – superficial layer (stratified squamous keratinised).
  - *Intradermal plexus* (superficial plexus) – small numerous vessels.
  - *Dermis* – two layers
    - *Superficial:* adventitial dermis (or papillary/periadnexal).
    - *Deep:* reticular dermis – determines the mechanical properties.
  - *Subdermal plexus* (deep plexus) – large vessels, sparse distribution, lymphatics.
- *Full-thickness skin grafts (FTSG) features:*
  - Include entire epidermis and dermis.
  - Less prone to secondary contraction (contraction that occurs after graft transferred to recipient site).
  - Based on subdermal plexus – tenuous vascularity.
  - Include the reticular dermis – favourable mechanical properties.
- *Split thickness skin grafts (STSG) features:*
  - Epidermis
  - More prone to secondary contraction.
  - Based on intradermal plexus – favourable vascular characteristics.
  - Decreased metabolic rate vs FTSG.
  - No reticular dermis – less favourable mechanical characteristics.

## Oral Mucosa Grafts

- *Oral mucosa structure*
  - Epithelium (stratified squamous non-keratinised)
  - Lamina propria – superficial and deep layer
  - Panlaminar vascular plexus
- *Oral mucosa graft features:*
  - 'Wet' epithelium – closely resembles the urethral epithelium.
  - Rich panlaminar vascular plexus.
  - Good handling properties.
  - Resists infection (increased IgA levels).
- Grafts blood supply develops by a process called 'take':
  - *Imbibition:* graft absorbs (imbibe = drinks) nutrients from the underlying recipient bed (0–48 hours). Nutrients + waste are passed between the graft + recipient bed through passive diffusion. Graft temperature is *lower* than body temperature.
  - *Inosculation:* blood vessels in the graft grow to meet the vessels (inosculate = kiss) of the recipient bed (48–96 hours). Graft temperature = body temperature.

- *Neovascularisation:* new blood vessels form between the graft and recipient tissues.

## Graft Failure

- Fluid accumulation in the graft bed (e.g., haematoma, seroma – grafts fenestrated to allow fluid to escape).
- Shearing of the graft – grafts sutured to the recipient bed to prevent movement.

# Flaps

- Tissue is raised with its blood supply intact or are re-established surgically at the recipient site.
- *Examples:* small bowel, penile skin, fat pad (Martius flap).
- Classified based on:
  - Blood supply
  - Elevation method
  - Method of transfer
- Blood supply is *random or axial:*
  - *Random flaps:* no defined blood supply and depend on the dermal and subdermal plexus.
  - *Axial flaps:* depend on specific blood vessel with a known distribution. Subdivided by the structure carrying the blood supply.
    - *Musculocutaneous flaps* – the underlying muscle carries the blood supply.
    - *Fasciocutaneous flaps* – the fascia carries the blood supply.
- *Flaps elevation and methods of transfer:*
  - *Peninsular flap:* vascular and cutaneous connections are left intact.
    - *Advancement flaps* – the graft is moved parallel to the pedicle.
    - *Rotational flaps* – the graft is moved at a right angle to the long axis of pedicle.
  - *Island flap:* skin is divided, but the vascular connections are maintained.
  - *Free flap:* tissue + vessels are detached from the donor site and anastomosed to the vessels at the recipient site.

# Biomaterials

- *Definition:* any substance or combination of substances other than drugs — synthetic or natural in origin — which augments or replaces either partially or totally any tissue, organ, or function of the body for a period.
- Classified into *synthetic and biological grafts:*
- *Synthetic mesh*
  - Non-absorbable thermoplastic polymers.
  - Classified into four *groups* (amid classification):
    - Type 1: Macroporous monofilament >75 μm (polypropylene)

- Type 2: Microporous monofilament <10 μm (expanded PTFE)
  - Type 3: Macroporous multifilament
  - Type 4: Submicron porous (silicon)
- Macroporous monofilament polypropylene (Type 1) are commonly used in pelvic floor mesh to allow ingress of fibroblasts, collagen, and blood vessels.
- *Non-autologous biological grafts:*
  - Can either be allogenous (donor tissue banks) or xenogenous (e.g., porcine, bovine).
  - Decellularised predominately collagen extracellular matrices.
  - Processed to remove the cellular components.
  - Chemical cross-linked to resist enzymatic degradation in the body.
  - Sterilised using gamma or electron beam irradiation.
- *Host response to synthetic material:*
  - *Initial blood–material interactions* → adsorption of proteins to surface
  - *Provisional matrix formation (biofilm).*
    - Mitogens, chemo-attractants, cytokines, growth factors → activate/modulate inflammatory response
  - *Acute inflammation*
    - Neutrophil polymorphs predominate.
    - Mast cells degranulate and release histamine.
    - Interleukins 3 and 4.
  - *Chronic inflammation*
    - Mononuclear cells (monocytes and lymphocytes) predominate.
    - Usually lasts no longer than two weeks.
  - *Granulation tissue development*
    - Macrophages and fibroblasts predominate → neovascularisation
  - *Foreign body reaction*
    - 1–2 cell layers of macrophages, monocytes, and foreign body giant cells between the granulation tissue and the implant.
  - *Fibrosis*
    - The granulation tissue is replaced by collagen deposited by fibroblasts.
    - The implant is surrounded by scar tissue.

# Urinary Tract Reconstruction Using Bowel (Table 28.3)

## Cutaneous Urinary Diversion

- Non-continent.
- Urine drains into a collection bag.
- *Examples:* ileal conduit, cutaneous ureterostomy.

## Catheterisable Urinary Diversion

- Continent.
- Creation of a reservoir using the stomach, jejunum, ileum, colon, or sigmoid.
- Bowel segment is detubularised and constructed into a pouch.

## Bowel Wall Structure and Function

- Outer longitudinal muscle (condenses to form the taenia coli).
- Inner circular muscle.
- Autonomic innervation in between two layers (vagus nerve).

## Principles of Bowel Urinary Reservoirs

- *Aim:*
  - Large volume – adequate storage function.
  - Low surface area – limit electrolyte exchange and metabolic problems.
  - Low pressure – prevent upper tract deterioration/leakage.
- *Detubularisation:* opening along the antimesenteric border.
  - Prevents coordinated peristaltic contractions, which reduces pressure.
  - Allows re-configuration into spheroidal shape.
- *Spheroidal shape:*
  - Maximises volume for surface area:
    - Volume of cylinder proportional to the square of a radius $(v = \Pi\, r^2 \times L)$.
    - Volume of sphere proportional to the cube of a radius $(v = 4/3\Pi\, r^3 \times L)$.
  - Reduces pressure by increasing its radius (by virtue of the law of Laplace).
  - Excessive high radius will result in increased wall tension and increased risk of rupture.
- Motor activity usually returns after three months and may be pathological if it causes symptoms.

## Metabolic and Functional Consequences

### Renal Deterioration

- Anatomical obstruction
  - Stoma (e.g., stenosis, parastomal hernia), conduit/reservoir related.
  - Uretero-ileal anastomotic stricture.
- Functional obstruction
  - High reservoir pressures.
- Obstruction → upper tract dilatation (renal injury) → urinary stasis → infection/stone formation

**Table 28.3** Characteristics of urinary tract reconstruction using bowel

| Type | Features | Contraindications | Complications |
|---|---|---|---|
| Ileal conduit | - Ileum reservoir<br>- 10-15cm segment<br>- 10-15cm from the ileocaecal valve<br>- Refluxing uretero-ileal anastomoses<br>    (Bricker, Wallace). | - Pelvic irradiation<br>- Inflammatory bowel disease<br>- Short bowel syndrome | Early<br>- Urine/bowel leak<br>- Ileus<br>Late<br>- Parastomal hernia<br>- Stomal stenosis/retraction<br>- Uretero-ileal anastomotic stricture<br>- Stone formation<br>- Upper tract dilatation and renal failure<br>- Urinary tract infection<br>- Hyperchloraemic metabolic acidosis |
| Ureterosigmoidosto-my | - Sigmoid reservoir<br>Mansoura rectal bladder<br>- Sigmoid intussusception to prevent urine refluxing into colon.<br>- Ileal augmentation of the sigmoid to reduce intraluminal pressure.<br>- Uretero-sigmoid anastomosis-Kock nipple.<br>Mainz II<br>- Continent reconstruction using the anal sphincter.<br>- Sigmoid opened longitudinally and closed transversely.<br>- Tunnelled (non-refluxing) anastomosis.<br>- Modified Mainz<br>- incorporates ileal chimney. | - Pelvic irradiation<br>- Severe sigmoid diverticulosis<br>- Poorly functioning anal sphincter | Early<br>- Urine/bowel leak<br>- Ileus<br>Late<br>- Hyperchloraemic metabolic acidosis<br>- Ureterosigmoid cancer<br>- Renal deterioration |
| Cutaneous continent urinary diversion | - Mainz I<br>- Kock pouch<br>- Indiana pouch | - Renal impairment<br>- Hepatic impairment<br>- Pelvic irradiation-Inflammatory bowel disease<br>- Short bowel syndrome<br>- Cannot self-catheterise | Late<br>- Urinary tract infection<br>- Stone formation<br>- Upper tract dilatation and renal failure<br>- Hyperchloraemic metabolic acidosis<br>- Malignancy<br>- bowel mucosa exposed to urine |
| Orthotopic bladder substitution | - Retained functioning urethra and sphincter.<br>- Types: Hautmann W, Studer<br>- Require intermittent self-catheterisation through urethra.<br>- Empty bladder to completion by valsalva and relaxation of the pelvic floor. | - Urethral/sphincter impairment<br>- Cannot self-catheterise | - Similar to continent urinary diversions. |

## Electrolyte and Acid–Base (More Common with Reservoirs Compared with Conduits)

- Complications depend on:
  - The segment of bowel used.
  - The length of the segment.
  - The duration of urine in contact with the segment (conduit vs reservoir).
- *Stomach*
  - Usually uses greater curvature for reconstruction.
  - Contains gastric secretions (potassium and hydrochloric acid) into the urine.
  - Hypokalaemic, hypochloraemic metabolic alkalosis.
  - Acidic urine can cause dysuria.
- *Jejunum*
  - Secretes sodium and chloride into the urine.
  - Absorbs potassium and hydrogen.
  - Hyponatraemia, hyperkalaemia, hypochloraemic metabolic acidosis.
  - Alkaline urine.
  - Sodium loss results in water loss.
    - Dehydration increases aldosterone secretion → water reabsorption in kidney with sodium conservation and potassium secretion
- *Ileum/colon*
  - Absorption of ammonium chloride and excretion of bicarbonate.
  - Ammonium chloride $NH_4Cl$ → ammonia $NH_3$ + hydrochloric acid $HCl$
    - $NH_3$ → urea and $H^+$ ions
    - $HCl$ → $H^+$ and $Cl^-$
  - Results in hypokalaemic, hyperchloraemic metabolic acidosis.
  - Reconstruction is contraindicated in those with hepatic failure (reduced ability to metabolise ammonia) and renal failure (reduced compensation for acidosis).
  - Increased ammonia may induce encephalopathy.

## Bone Disease

- Osteomalacia – bone demineralisation.
- Chronic metabolic acidosis:
  - Hydrogen ions are buffered in exchange for calcium.
  - Demineralisation of bones (calcium lost in the urine).
- Impaired bowel absorption of calcium and vitamin D → demineralisation
- May retard bone growth in children and increase the risk of osteoporosis (especially in steroid use in postmenopausal women).

## Urinary Tract Infection (UTI)

- Colonisation with intestinal flora.
- Majority will have asymptomatic bacteriuria.
- Risk of infection increases with obstruction/ urinary stasis.
- Recurrent UTI may cause struvite stone formation.

## Mucus Production

- 35–40 g per day.
- Most abundant: colon > ileum > stomach.
- May cause blockage, UTI, and stone formation.

## Urolithiasis

- Increased risk occurs with:
  - Alkaline urine – struvite, calcium, phosphate.
  - Acidic urine (gastric segment) – uric acid stones.
  - Bacteriuria – urease producing bacteria (urea → ammonia and bicarbonate).
  - Abnormal anatomy – urinary stasis and enteric hyperoxaluria following ileal resection.
  - Acidosis – increases urine calcium/phosphate and decreases urine citrate.
  - Mucus – nidus for stone formation.
  - Foreign bodies (staples).
- Usually infection stones – ammonium magnesium phosphate (struvite).
- Hyperoxaluria – calcium oxalate stones.

## Spontaneous Perforation

- Rare at <1%.
- Occurs with high-pressure reservoirs.

## Bowel Function

- Ileal resection results in:
  - Malabsorption of bile salts (diarrhoea and reduced absorption of vitamins A, D, E, K), fat, vitamin B12.
  - Vitamin B12 deficiency takes >5 years to manifest:
    - Increased risk if >50 cm of terminal ileum is resected.
    - Macrocytic anaemia.
    - Demyelination – neurological complications.
    - Hyperpigmentation.
    - Tongue/mouth inflammation.
    - Gastrointestinal symptoms.
  - Cholesterol gallstones.

## Abnormal Drug Kinetics

- Reabsorption of drugs is excreted in the urine.
- Toxicity seen with phenytoin and methotrexate.

- When administrating toxic medications (e.g., chemotherapy), drain the conduit/diversion with a catheter to reduce reabsorption.

## Malignancy

- Ureterosigmoidostomy (~2.5%)
  - Latency period of >20 years.
  - Mixing of urine and faeces → carcinogenesis
  - 90% at anastomosis, 95% adenomatous.
- Ileal reservoirs (~1–2%)
  - Latent period of >10 years.
  - Associated with chronic inflammation/ recurrent UTI, urinary stasis.
  - Usually adenocarcinoma at the anastomosis region.

- Reduction of urinary nitrates to nitrites by colonic bacteria → reacts with urinary amines → N-nitrosamines → carcinogenic

# Recommended Reading

1. Enoch S and Leaper DJ. Basic science of wound healing. Surgery. 2008;26(2):31–37.
2. Hautmann RE, Hautmann SH, Hautmann O. Complications associated with urinary diversion. Nat Rev Urol. 2011;8(12) 667–77.
3. Pearce SM and Daneshmand S. Continent cutaneous diversion. Urol Clin North Am. 2018;45(1):55–65.
4. Roth JD and Koch MO. Metabolic and nutritional consequences of urinary diversion using intestinal segments to reconstruct the urinary tract. Urol Clin North Am. 2018;45(1):19–24.

# Pharmacology of the Lower Urinary Tract

*Pedro Abreu-Mendes, João Silva, and Francisco Cruz*

## Introduction

- The function of the lower urinary tract (LUT) is dependent upon the following:
  - Bladder smooth muscle (SM) activity.
  - Striated muscle in the urethral sphincter.
  - Pelvic floor.
    - These structures are a functional unit controlled by a complex interplay between the central and peripheral nervous system (PNS) and local regulatory factors.
- Three types of receptor control detrusor and bladder outlet activity:
  - Muscarinic (M) receptors
  - Beta-3 (β) adrenoceptors (AR)
  - Alpha-1A adrenoceptors

## A) Muscarinic Receptors and Anti-Muscarinic Drugs

### Muscarinic Receptors

- Five subtypes: M1-5.
- M receptors can be grouped into two clusters, based on chemical properties and preferred signal transduction pathways:
  1. M1, M3, and M5
  2. M2 and M4 subtypes
- M receptors have a widespread distribution throughout the body:
  - Urinary bladder
  - The central nervous system (CNS)
  - Eyes, salivary glands, heart, and the digestive tract
- Receptors are activated by the neurotransmitter acetylcholine (ACh), released from the intramural post-ganglionic parasympathetic nerve endings.
- Two muscarinic receptor subtypes are identified in the bladder SM:
  - *M2* and *M3* (also present in sensory fibres and urothelium, but their role in bladder function is unclear)
- *M2 receptors:*
  - Most abundant in the detrusor.
  - Act via a $G_i$ type receptor → decrease intracellular cyclic adenosine monophosphate (cAMP) → decrease intracellular calcium, inhibiting voltage-gated $Ca^{2+}$ channels + increase efflux of $K^+$ ions → promote SM *relaxation*
- *M3 receptors:*
  - Less expressed, but more functional than M2.
  - $G_q$-coupled receptors.
  - Upregulate phospholipase C (PLC) and inositol trisphosphate ($IP_3$) cascade → increase intracellular calcium → SM *contraction*
- The widespread distribution of M receptor subtypes is responsible for the systemic adverse effects (AEs) associated with the administration of anti-muscarinic drugs.
  - Somnolence, impaired memory and cognition, blurred vision, tachycardia, dry mouth, and constipation.
  - The latter two are the most common and have an incidence that increases with age.

## Anti-Muscarinic Drugs (Anticholinergic Drugs)

- All drugs of this class listed in Table 29.1 are recommended as first-line pharmacological treatment of patients with overactive bladder (OAB) symptoms refractory to conservative measures.
- Reduce voiding frequency and urge incontinence.
- Competitive antagonists which block M receptors.
- Divided by their selectivity to M receptors:
  - *Darifenacin* is the only M3-selective (moderately) drug.
  - The other drugs are *non-selective.*
- Drug activity is based on selectivity and affinity to the receptor.

### *Molecular Characteristics:*

- *Tertiary* (darifenacin, fesoterodine and its active metabolite 5-hydroxymethyl-tolterodine, oxybutynin, propiverine, solifenacin, and tolterodine)
  - Generally well absorbed from the gastrointestinal (GI) tract.

Table 29.1 Anti-Muscarinic Drugs 60 OD

| Drug | Administration | Structure | Daily Dose (mg) | ER Tablets (mg) | Half-life (h) | Ability to Cross BBB |
|---|---|---|---|---|---|---|
| Darifenacin* | Oral | Tertiary | 7.5 OD/BD, 15 OD | No | 13–19 h | Low |
| Fesoterodine | Oral | Tertiary | 4 OD/BD, 8 OD | No | 7 h | Low |
| Oxybutynin | Oral | | 5 BD/TDS (IR) | Yes 5 OD/BD | 2–3 h ER: 13 h | High |
| | Transdermal | Tertiary | Patch 3,9 mg OD, 2–3 times a week | | | |
| | | | Gel 3%: three pumps (84 mg/ day) OD | | | |
| | | | Gel 10% : one pump OD | | | |
| | Intravesical | | 1 mg/mL: recommended | | | |
| | | - | 0.2–0.4 mg/kg OD | | | |
| Propiverine | Oral | Tertiary | 30–45 OD (MR) | Yes | | |
| Solifenacin | Oral | Tertiary | 5–10 OD | No | 45–86 h | Moderate |
| Tolterodine | Oral | Tertiary | 1–2 BD (IR) | Yes 2–4 OD | 2–4 ER: 8.5 h | Moderate |
| Trospium | Oral | Quaternary | 20 BD | Yes | 20 | Low |

* Darifenacin is M3-selective.
*Abbreviations:* BBB, blood brain barrier; IR, immediate release; MR, modified release; ER, extended release; UI, urinary incontinence; NA, not available; OD, once daily; BD, twice daily; TDS, three times daily.

- Able to pass into the CNS due to high lipophilicity, small molecular size, and less charge.
- Some tertiary amines (e.g., darifenacin) are actively transported out of the CNS.

- *Quaternary* (trospium chloride, propantheline)
  - Generally not well absorbed.
  - Pass into the CNS to a limited extent, due to large molecular size and low lipophilicity – lower incidence of CNS side effects (better for the elderly).

## Route of Delivery

- *Oral*: extended (ER) or immediate release (IR). Some drugs have a longer half-life, reducing its posology and AE (Table 29.1).

- *Transdermal as patch/gel*: have the potential to improve patient compliance and tolerability by reducing AEs due to reduction of hepatic metabolites. Locally, they might cause skin reactions with pruritus and erythema.

- *Intravesical*: oxybutynin and trospium chloride increase bladder capacity and produce clinical improvement with few side effects in neurogenic and non-neurogenic detrusor overactivity patients. However, unless a delivery system is developed to allow a continuous release of the drug, intravesical delivery is limited to patients doing intermittent self-catheterisation.

- The majority of anti-muscarinic drugs are metabolised by the *P450 enzyme system*.
  - Carries risk of drug interactions causing enzyme inhibition/induction.
- Anti-muscarinics and their metabolites are not extensively excreted through urine.
  - Therefore, there is no need to adjust the therapeutic dose in renal insufficiency.
  - Exception for trospium, which is a quaternary amine not metabolised by P450 enzymes and is eliminated by the kidney.
- All anti-muscarinics are contraindicated in untreated *narrow-angle glaucoma*.

- AEs are related to the widespread distribution of M receptors.
  - Dry mouth – most common (one third).
  - Constipation.
  - Blurred vision and fatigue.
  - Cognitive dysfunction among elderly patients during long-term use.
  - Incidence of AEs may increase with age.
  - Cumulative anti-muscarinic effect can be expected in patients receiving multiple drugs with anticholinergic effect. In elderly patients, it is recommended to estimate the anticholinergic load.

## Treatment Outcome

- Most patients stop treatment within three months.
- 92% discontinue the first anti-muscarinic at 24 months.
- Most patients stop the medication due to lack of efficacy or side effects.
- Options for failure include:
  1. Switching to a second anti-muscarinic. The rate of failure with a 2nd anti-muscarinic is above 80%.
  2. Dose escalation of the anti-muscarinic if it is available in more than one dose. Increasing efficacy is accompanied by an intensification of AEs.
  3. Switching to another class of drugs.

# B) Beta-3 Adrenoceptors and Beta-3 Agonist

## Beta-3 Adrenoceptors (β3-AR)

- Three subtypes of β AR – β1-3.
- All are present in the detrusor muscle, although their activities are different.
- Predominate both normal and pathological/neurogenic bladders.
- β3 agonists activate adenyl cyclase (AC) → converts ATP to cAMP → detrusor relaxation
- β3-AR are also expressed in cholinergic nerve endings, suggesting a role (inhibitory) in the release of ACh.
- The role of β3-AR in sensory fibres is unclear.
- Expressed in the:
  - Urinary bladder
  - GI tract, gall bladder, uterus, and adipose tissue
  - Brain (although its function is unclear)
- Not expressed in the heart or in blood vessels.

- This distribution may explain why selective β3 agonist have a safe profile with AEs in RCT that are comparable to placebo in all age groups.

## β3-AR Agonists (Mirabegron)

- Mirabegron is the only licensed β3-AR agonist.
- It is the first-line pharmacologic treatment option in OAB symptoms refractory to conservative measures.
- 55% is excreted in urine, while the remaining 35% is excreted in faeces.
- Half-life of 50 hours.
- Highly lipophilic.
- Metabolised in the liver via multiple pathways, mainly by cytochrome P450 3A4 and 2D6 (CYP2D6).
- Improve urinary frequency and urgency incontinence, and its efficacy is not inferior to anti-muscarinics.
- Effective in patients refractory to anti-muscarinic drugs.
- No effect on bladder voiding function in men with urodynamically proven bladder outlet obstruction (BOO).
- *Adverse effects:*
  - Better profile than anti-muscarinics – no dry mouth or constipation.
  - Contraindicated in severe uncontrolled hypertension (systolic ≥180 mmHg or diastolic ≥110 mmHg).
  - Safe in elderly patients, with no CNS-related AEs.

## Antimuscarinics and β3 Agonists Combination

- More effective in reducing urinary frequency and urgency urinary incontinence than monotherapy (BESIDE and SYNERGY study).

# C) Alpha-1A Adrenoceptors and Alpha-Blockers

- Four Alpha1 ARs subtypes: Alpha-1A, 1B, 1D, 1L.
- Structurally and pharmacologically distinct and have different tissue distributions:
  - *Alpha-1A*: predominant subtype in the human prostate and bladder neck. Mediates smooth muscle contraction.
  - *Alpha-1B*: present in small arteries. Density increases in the vascular beds with the ageing process.

- *Alpha-1D*: predominates human detrusor muscle, spinal cord afferent nerves, and conduit arteries (aorta).
- *Alpha-1L*: present in the human prostate. Encoded by the same gene as Alpha-1A-AR.
- Selectivity for Alpha-1A AR does not translate into a clear clinical superiority, although it might change the side effect profile.
- Transmembrane glycoproteins.
- Activated by norepinephrine – heterotrimeric G protein, $G_q$, activates PLC.
- Increases $IP_3$ and calcium, resulting in the activation of protein Kinase C.
- *Key AE is associated with Alpha-1 AR:*
  - Selectivity for Alpha-1B AR has been considered disadvantageous from a cardiovascular (CV) point of view.
  - High selectivity for Alpha-1A, although decreases the risk of CV AEs, increases the risk of ejaculatory dysfunction.

## Alpha-Blockers

- *Examples:* oral alfuzosin, doxazosin, silodosin, tamsulosin, naftopidil (Japan only), and terazosin (Table 29.2).
- Only two of the drugs are considered selective:
  - Silodosin: alpha-1A.

- Naftopidil: moderate alpha-1D selectivity.
- Main indication – lower urinary tract symptoms (LUTS)/benign prostate hyperplasia (BPH):
  - Reduces the International Prostate Symptom Score (IPSS) by 35–40%.
  - Increases Qmax by 20–25%.
  - Decreases bladder outlet obstruction index (BOOI) in men with urodynamically proven BOO.
- *Adverse effects:*
  - Dizziness, rhinitis, headache, asthenia, postural hypotension are AEs related to the alpha-1B AR. More common in non-selective alpha-blockers.
  - Silodosin (Alpha-A1 selective) – better CV profile but higher rate of ejaculatory dysfunction.
  - Tamsulosin (and possibly silodosin also) is associated with a high risk of floppy iris syndrome (Alpha-1A).

## Alpha-Blockers and Anti-Muscarinic Combination

- Male LUTS often include a combination of voiding and storage symptoms.
- *Combination therapy:*
  - Results in a reduction of LUTS scores and

### Table 29.2 Comparison of Alpha-Blockers

| Drug | Half-life | Clinical Selectivity | Usual Daily Dose (mg) | Modified Release Formulation | Adverse Events |
|------|-----------|---------------------|----------------------|------------------------------|----------------|
| Terazosin | 12 h | Alpha1a=b=d | 1, 2, 5 or 10 | Yes | Mainly CV events (asthenia, dizziness, hypotension, impotence) |
| Alfuzosin | 10 h | Alpha1a=b=d | 7.5 or 10 | Yes | Mainly CV events (dizziness, headache, hypotension, dry mouth) |
| Doxazosin | 22 h | Alpha1a=b=d | 1 to 8 | Yes | Mainly CV events (dizziness, headache, hypotension, dyspnoea) |
| Tamsulosin* | 13–15 h | *Alpha1a=d>b* | 0.4 | Yes | Abnormal ejaculation, floppy iris syndrome, less CV AEs |
| Silodosin* | 13 h | *Alpha1a>d>b* | 4 or 8 | No | Abnormal ejaculation, floppy iris syndrome, less CV AEs |

\* Silodocin and Tamsulocin are Alpha1a selective.
*Abbreviations:* CV, cardiovascular; AEs, adverse events.

improvement of QoL after adding an anti-muscarinic.
- No acute urinary retention observed in urodynamically proven mild/moderate BOO.
- Does not affect urine flow or post-void residual (PVR) volume in patients with PVR at a baseline of <100 mL.
- *Fixed combination:*
  - Improves storage and voiding symptoms and QoL parameters.
- *EAU guidelines:* recommend anti-muscarinics in moderate-to-severe LUTS with mainly bladder storage symptoms.

## Alpha-Blockers and β3 Agonists Combination

- The rationale of using alpha-blockers with β3-AR is the same as the combination of alpha-blockers with anti-muscarinic drugs.
- Recent studies demonstrated the efficacy and safety of adding mirabegron in men taking tamsulosin in whom storage symptoms persist after an initial trial with an alpha-blocker.

## D) Intracellular Pathways Relevant to the Treatment of Lower Urinary Symptoms

### 1.   5-alpha-reductase (5AR) enzymes

- Two isoenzymes: type I and II.
- Type II is predominant in the prostate tissue.
- 5AR enzyme converts testosterone to dihydrotestosterone (DHT).
- DHT is a potent androgen that regulates prostate metabolism.
- 5AR inhibitors (5ARi) decreases DHT → reduces prostate volume and half PSA levels within six months to one year

### 5a-reductase inhibitors (5ARI)
- *Finasteride* inhibits preferentially type II 5α-reductase isoenzyme.
  - Prevents ~70% conversion of testosterone to DHT.
- *Dutasteride* inhibits both type I and II isoenzymes.
  - Prevent ~95% conversion of testosterone to DHT.
- No relevant clinical differences between them.
- Clinical effects are seen after a minimum period of 6–12 months.
- *After 2–4 years:*
  - IPSS reduces by 15–30%.
  - Qmax increases by 1.5–2.0 mL/s.
  - Prostate volume decreases by 18–28% within 6–12 months and remains stable thereafter.

- PSA decreases by 50% within 6–12 months.
- Little efficacy in prostates of <40 mL.
- Reduce the risk of long-term complications – acute urinary retention (AUR) by 57% and the need for surgery by 55% (PLESS study).
- *EAU guidelines* recommend 5ARi for men with moderate-to-severe LUTS and an increased risk of disease progression (e.g., prostate volume >40 mL, PSA >1.4 ng/mL).
- *Adverse effects:*
  - ~10% of men will report sexually related AEs:
    - Erectile dysfunction
    - Decreased libido
    - Decreased volume of ejaculate
    - Painful gynaecomastia (more common with dutasteride)

### Alpha-Blockers and 5ARi Combination for LUTS

- Supported mainly by two studies:
  - The Medical Therapy of Prostatic Symptoms Study (*MTOPS* – with placebo arm) compared the long-term efficacy of combination therapy with *finasteride* and *doxazosin* with either drug alone and with placebo in avoiding disease progression defined by one of these events: AUR, urinary incontinence, renal insufficiency, or recurrent urinary tract infection.
  - Combination of Dutasteride and Tamsulosin study (*CombAT* study) compared the long-term efficacy of combination therapy with *Avodart (dutasteride)* and *tamsulosin* with either drug alone (*no placebo arm*) in reducing the relative risk for AUR, BPH-related surgery, and BPH clinical progression over four years.
- The mean volume of the prostate included in CombAT study was superior to the mean prostate volume included in the MTOPS.
- As 5ARi are more effective in larger prostates, the effect of combined therapy was evident sooner in the CombAT than in the MTOPS study.
- Both studies demonstrated the superiority of combination therapy over alpha-blocker monotherapy in preventing:
  - Symptomatic progression.
  - Risk of AUR and benign prostate enlargement related surgery.
- The *EAU recommends* combination therapy in men with moderate-to-severe LUTS-BPH and who are at increased risk of disease progression (high prostate volume, high serum PSA, advanced age, high PVR, low Qmax).

### 2.   Phosphodiesterase 5 (PDE5) Enzyme

- Promotes the degradation of cyclic guanosine monophosphate (cGMP) → decreases SM relaxation

- PDE5 inhibitors (PDE5i) were developed for the treatment of erectile dysfunction (ED).
  - Act in cavernous tissue and increase the concentration of intracellular cGMP → lower calcium and reduce cavernous SM tone
- In the LUT, PDE5i promote SM relaxation of the bladder and prostate.
- Other potential effects in the bladder:
  - Increase bladder oxygenation.
  - Reduce collagen accumulation.
  - Decrease afferent nerve activity and inflammation.

## Phosphodiesterase 5 inhibitors (PDE5i)

- *Examples*: tadalafil, avanafil, vardenafil, sildenafil – all approved for ED.
- Tadalafil has the longest half-life of 17 hours (other PD5Ei ~3–5 hours) – ideal PDE5i for treatment of LUTS.
- Tadalafil 5 mg daily is the only PDE5i approved for male LUTS treatment.
- Improve the IPSS score and the International Index of Erectile Function (IIEF) score.
- Reduce both storage and voiding LUTS and improve quality of life (QoL).
- No change in Qmax.
- PDE5i and alpha-blockers combined are superior to alpha-blockers alone in improving IPSS score, IIEF score, and Qmax.
- *EAU guidelines* strongly recommend PDE5i in men with moderate-to-severe LUTS with or without ED.
- *Adverse effects:*
  - Flushing, gastroesophageal reflux, headache, dyspepsia, back pain (PDE11), and nasal congestion
- *Contraindications:*
  - *Drugs:* nitrates, potassium channel opener nicorandil or alpha1-blockers doxazosin, and terazosin (increases risk of hypotension).
  - *Medical conditions:* unstable angina pectoris, recent myocardial infarction (<3 months) or stroke (<6 months), myocardial insufficiency (New York Heart Association stage >2), hypotension, poorly-controlled blood pressure, significant hepatic or renal insufficiency (reduced metabolism and clearance of drug), anterior ischaemic optic neuropathy with sudden loss of vision.

## 3. Neurotransmitters

*Norepinephrine (NE) and serotonin (5-hydroxytryptamine, 5-HT) reuptake inhibitor*

- NE and 5-HT receptors are abundant in the spinal cord — particularly in the Onuf's nucleus from which innervation of the external sphincter has its origin.

- Increased activity of these neurons enhances the resting tone and contraction strength of the urethral striated sphincter.

## Selective noradrenaline and serotonin reuptake inhibitors (SNRi)

- *Duloxetine:* serotonin (5-HT) and norepinephrine (NE) reuptake inhibitor (SNRI).
  - Only approved drug to treat stress urinary incontinence (SUI) in females ineligible or waiting for surgical treatment.
- The cure rate for SUI with SNRI is ~10%.
- No improvement in QoL was found in the study using I-QoL as a primary endpoint.
- Duloxetine reduces SUI compared to pelvic floor muscle therapy or no treatment.
- Treatment discontinuation is due to the high incidence of AEs:
  - Nausea and vomiting (at least 40%)
  - Dry mouth, constipation, dizziness, insomnia, somnolence, and fatigue
- Speeds up the improvement of SUI after radical prostatectomy but does not increase the final number of patients clinically cured.

## 4. GABAergic drugs

- Baclofen and gabapentin have been used off-label to treat neurogenic bladder dysfunction in pilot studies.
  - GABA (Gamma aminobutyric acid) receptors exert an inhibitory tone on sensory fibres in the spinal cord, including those coming from the bladder.

# E) Plant Extracts: Phytotherapy

- Heterogeneous group of plant extracts – single plant or preparations obtained from ≥2 plants.
- *Examples:*
  - *Cucurbita pepo* (pumpkin seeds)
  - *Hypoxis rooperi* (South African star grass)
  - *Pygeum africanum* (bark of the African plum tree)
  - *Secale cereale* (rye pollen)
  - *Serenoa repens* (syn. *Sabal serrulata; saw palmetto*)
  - *Urtica dioica* (roots of the stinging nettle)
- Scientific rationale is unclear:
  - Anti-inflammatory properties or inhibit the conversion of testosterone into DHT.
  - Long-term studies do not show changes in prostate volume or serum PSA.

# Recommended Reading

1. Groat WC. Integrative control of the lower urinary tract: preclinical perspective. Br J Pharmacol. 2006;147(S2):S25–40.

2. Andersson KE, Wein AJ. Pharmacology of the lower urinary tract: basis for current and future treatments of urinary. Am Soc Pharmacol Exp Ther. 2004;56(4):581–631.

3. Chapple CR, Khullar V, Gabriel Z, et al. The Effects of antimuscarinic treatments in overactive bladder: an update of a systematic review and meta-analysis. Eur Urol. 2008;54(3):543–62.

4. Abrams P, Andersson K-E, Buccafusco JJ, et al. Muscarinic receptors: their distribution and function in body systems, and the implications for treating overactive bladder. Br J Pharmacol. 2006;148(5):565–78.

5. Matsumoto Y, Miyazato M, Furuta A, et al. Differential roles of M2 and M3 muscarinic receptor subtypes in modulation of bladder afferent activity in rats. Urology. 2010; 75(4):862–67.

6. Guay DR. Trospium chloride: an update on a quaternary anticholinergic for treatment of urge urinary incontinence. Ther Clin Risk Manag. 2005 Jun;1(2):157–67.

7. FC Burkhard, et al. Urinary incontinence in adults. EAU Guidelines. 2019;(March):1–100.

8. Igawa Y, Aizawa N. Incontinence: How do β3-adrenoceptor agonists work in the bladder? Nat Rev Urol. 2017;14(6):330–32.

9. Chapple CR, Cruz F, Cardozo L, et al. Safety and efficacy of mirabegron: analysis of a large integrated clinical trial database of patients with overactive bladder receiving mirabegron, antimuscarinics, or placebo. Eur Urol. 2020;77(1):119–28.

10. Gratzke C, van Maanen R, Chapple C, et al. Long-term safety and efficacy of mirabegron and solifenacin in combination compared with monotherapy in patients with overactive bladder: a randomised, multicentre phase 3 study (SYNERGY II). Eur Urol. 2018;74(4):501–09.

11. Drake MJ, Chapple C, Esen AA, et al. Efficacy and Safety of mirabegron add-on therapy to solifenacin in incontinent overactive bladder patients with an inadequate response to initial 4-week solifenacin monotherapy: a randomised Double-blind Multicentre Phase 3B Study (BESIDE). Eur Urol. 2016;70(1):136–45.

12. Herschorn S, Chapple CR, Abrams P, et al. Efficacy and safety of combinations of mirabegron and solifenacin compared with monotherapy and placebo in patients with overactive bladder (SYNERGY study). BJU Int. 2017;120(4):562–75.

13. Gravas S, et al. Management of neurogenic male lower urinary tract symptoms (LUTS). EAU guidelines. 2020. https://uroweb.org/guideline/treatment-of-non-neurogenic-male-luts/ online guidelines

14. Kakizaki H, Lee K-S, Yamamoto O, et al. Mirabegron add-on therapy to tamsulosin for the treatment of overactive bladder in men with lower urinary tract symptoms: a randomized, placebo-controlled study (MATCH). Eur Urol Focus. 2019;1–9.

15. Kaplan SA, Herschorn S, McVary KT, et al. Efficacy and safety of mirabegron versus placebo add-on therapy in men with overactive bladder symptoms receiving tamsulosin for underlying benign prostatic hyperplasia: a randomized, phase 4 study (PLUS). J Urol. 2020;201(Supplement 4).

16. Roehrborn CG, Siami P, Barkin J, et al. The effects of combination therapy with dutasteride and tamsulosin on clinical outcomes in men with symptomatic benign prostatic hyperplasia: 4-year results from the combat study. Eur Urol. 2010;57(1):123–31.

17. Nickel JC, Gilling P, Tammela TL, et al. Comparison of dutasteride and finasteride for treating benign prostatic hyperplasia: the enlarged prostate international comparator study (EPICS). BJU Int. 2011;108(3):388–94.

18. McConnell JD, Roehrborn CG, Bautista OM, et al. The long-term effect of doxazosin, finasteride, and combination therapy on the clinical progression of benign prostatic hyperplasia. N Engl J Med. 2003;349(25):2387–98.

19. Gacci M, Corona G, Salvi M, et al. A systematic review and meta-analysis on the use of phosphodiesterase 5 inhibitors alone or in combination with α-blockers for lower urinary tract symptoms due to benign prostatic hyperplasia. Eur Urol. 2012;61(5):994–1003.

20. Alan C, Eren AE, Ersay AR, et al. Efficacy of duloxetine in the early management of urinary continence after radical prostatectomy. Curr Urol. 2014;8(1):43–48.

# 30 Pharmacology of Male Sexual Function

*Andrei Kozan, Weida Lau, and Oliver Kayes*

## Erectile Dysfunction (see Chapters 12 and Chapters 22)

### Normal Physiology of Erection (Figure 30.1)

1. Sexual arousal → release of nitric oxide (NO) at nerve endings of the penis. Another source of NO is in the vascular endothelial cells.
2. NO diffuses into vascular smooth muscle cells in the penile corpus cavernosum → stimulate guanylyl cyclase (GC) and ↑ cyclic guanosine monophosphate (cGMP)
3. Activation of cGMP-dependent protein kinase (PKG) → phosphorylation of several proteins → lowering of cell calcium or reduction in sensitivity to calcium
4. Smooth muscle relaxation.
5. Accumulation of blood in the corpus cavernosum.

### Phases of Erection

- *Phase 0 – Flaccid phase*
  - Cavernosal smooth muscle contraction; sinusoids empty; minimal arterial flow.
- *Phase 1 – Latent (filling) phase*
  - Increased pudendal artery inflow; penile elongation.
- *Phase 2 – Tumescent phase*
  - Rising intracavernosal pressure with increasing engorgement.
- *Phase 3 – Full erection phase*
  - Increased cavernosal pressure (~100 mmHg) with full tumescence.
- *Phase 4 – Rigid erection phase*
  - Further increases in pressure (200–300 mmHg) plus ischiocavernosal muscle contraction.
- *Phase 5 – Detumescence phase*
  - Post-ejaculation driven by increasing sympathetic tone; smooth muscle contraction; vasoconstriction and reduced arterial flow; increased venous outflow.

## A) Pharmacology of Erectile Dysfunction (ED)

### Phosphodiesterase-5 Inhibitors (PDE5i)

#### Pharmacodynamics

- Enhance sexual function during sexual stimulation by penetrating the smooth muscle cells and inhibiting PDE5 enzyme.
- Deceased degradation of cGMP → maintains higher cellular levels of cGMP in both the corpus cavernosum and the vessels supplying it
- Increases relaxation of the smooth muscle → dilates the corporeal sinusoids → increases blood flow → erection

#### Pharmacokinetics (Table 30.1)

- Sildenafil and vardenafil peak absorption are each at ~30–60 min.
  - Serum half-life of 3–5 hours.
  - Absorption of these drugs is slowed by dietary lipids.
  - Should not be taken after a meal, particularly one high in fat content.
- Tadalafil is structurally distinct from vardenafil and sildenafil.
  - Peak absorption of 2–4 hours.
  - Half-life of 17.5 hours.
  - Tadalafil absorption is not affected by food intake.
- Avanafil – structurally distinct from other approved PDE5i.
  - Peak absorption at 20–30 minutes.
  - Half-life of ~6 hours.

#### Practical Prescribing

- PDE5i do not initiate an erection – sexual stimulation is required.
- The pathway may not work properly if the cGMP level in the corpus cavernosum smooth muscle cells is not elevated sufficiently, or if relaxation of the smooth muscle in the tissue is deficient/incomplete.

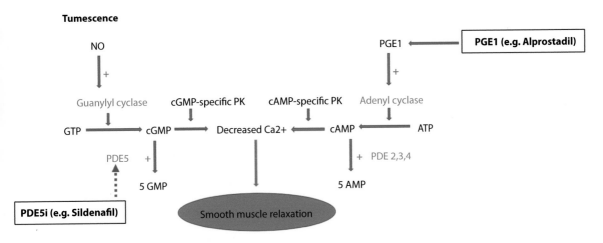

Figure 30.1 Physiology of normal penile erection and Therapeutic targets for erectile dysfunction. NO, nitric oxide; PDE, phosphodiesterase; PDE5i, phosphodiesterase 5 inhibitor; GTP, guanosine triphosphate; cGMP, cyclic guanosine monophosphate; PK, protein kinase; ATP, adenosine triphosphate; cAMP, cyclic adenosine monophosphate; $Ca^{2+}$, calcium; PG, prostaglandin.

**Table 30.1** Pharmacokinetics and Dosing Regimens of Phosphodiesterase 5 Inhibitors

| Pharmacokinetics | Tadalafil (20 mg) | Sildenafil (100 mg) | Vardenafil (20 mg) | Avanafil (200 mg) |
|---|---|---|---|---|
| Concentration max (ng/mL) | 378 | 560 | 18.7 | 5.2 |
| Time max (h) | 2 | 0.8–1 | 0.7–0.9 | 0.5–0.75 |
| Half-life (h) | 17.5 | 3–5 | 4–5 | 6–20 |
| Bioavailability (%) | | 40 | 15 | 8–10 |
| **Prescribing** | | | | |
| On demand (mg) | 10, 20 | 25, 50, 100 | 10, 20 | 50, 100, 200 |
| Daily dosing (mg) | 2.5, 5 | | | |

- At maximum doses, all three drugs improve the International Index of Erectile Function-Erectile Function (IIEF-EF) scores by 7–10 points compared with placebo treatment.
- Success rates with first-time prescription is ~60–75%.
- For patients who anticipate sexual activity at least twice a week, daily tadalafil can be considered.
- Daily tadalafil has also shown efficacy in the management of lower urinary tract symptoms (LUTS) from benign prostatic enlargement (BPE).
- Use each medication at maximum dose at least four times before declaring the drug a failure.
- For men who fail one PDE5i, a trial of an alternative PDE5i should be considered before advancing to second-line therapies.
- Up to 50% of PDE5i failures may be salvaged with re-education.

## Contraindications

- Princeton III Consensus.
- *Absolute contraindications*:
  - Unstable angina, active heart failure.
  - Concurrent nitrate use (sublingual nitroglycerin, isosorbide mononitrate or dinitrate).
  - Concurrent use of nitrates and PDE5i may lead to life-threatening hypotension.
  - If a PDE5i is taken and chest pain develops, organic nitrates should not be used for at least 24 hours for sildenafil (also vardenafil), 48 hours for tadalafil (due to its longer half-life), and at least 12 hours for avanafil.
- *Relative contraindication*:
  - Concurrent use of alpha-blocker for hypertension or LUTS (concern of orthostatic hypotension).
  - Vardenafil is not recommended in men with congenital QT syndrome and men taking

class IA or III antiarrhythmics (amiodarone, sotalol, quinidine).

## Side Effects

- Headaches (8–14%), flushing (4–6%), dyspepsia (5–18%), rhinitis (5%).
- Visual effects and blue vision (3%).
- Sildenafil and vardenafil cross-react with PDE6.
  - PDE6 predominates in the retina → visual disturbances
  - Tadalafil and avanafil have the lowest incidence of visual disturbances.
- Tadalafil has a significant association with myalgia (PDE11- back or girdle pain).
- Studies have failed to show a significantly increased risk of non-arteritic ischaemic optic neuropathy (NAION).

# Apomorphine

- Has a higher affinity for the D2-like receptors:
  - Thought to be the main site for the induction of erections in the paraventricular nucleus (PVN).
- Postulated to increase erectile responses by acting as a conditioner in the PVN, increasing the response to sexual stimuli → enhanced erections induced in the periphery
- Efficacious in the treatment of ED in the broad population at doses of 2 and 3 mg taken sublingually in an on-demand fashion.

## Side Effects

- Nausea, headache, and dizziness.

# Alprostadil

## Pharmacodynamics

- Prostaglandin-E1 (PGE1) analogue.
- Activation of prostaglandin receptors results in an increase in the intracellular concentration of cyclic adenosine monophosphate (cAMP) in the corpus cavernosum smooth muscles (Figure 30.1).
- Mediates relaxation of corpus cavernosum smooth muscle.
- Inhibits the release of noradrenaline from sympathetic nerves and suppresses angiotensin II secretion in the cavernosal tissues.

## Pharmacokinetics

- Metabolised by 15-hydroxydehydrogenase present in the corpus cavernosum.

## Practical Prescribing

- *Intracavernosal*
  - *Caverject* 10, 20, 40 mcg; viridal 10, 20, 40 mcg.

- First dose must be given by medically trained personnel.
- Self-administration is possible after appropriate training.
- *For ED:*
  - 2.5 mcg for one dose (first dose).
  - Followed by 5 mcg for one dose (second dose), to be given if there is some response to the first dose. Alternative 7.5 mcg for one dose (second dose), to be given if there is no response to the first dose.
  - Increase in steps of 5–10 mcg to obtain a dose suitable for producing an erection lasting not more than one hour.
- *For neurogenic ED:*
  - 1.25 mcg for one dose (first dose).
  - 2.5 mcg for one dose (second dose), then 5 mcg for another dose (third dose).
  - Increase in steps of 5–10 mcg to obtain a dose suitable for producing erection not more than one hour.
- Max frequency of injection is not more than three times per week with at least 24 h interval between injections.
- Max per dose: 60 mcg for Caverject and 40 mcg for Viridal.
- *Intraurethral suppository*
  - The medicated urethral system for erections (*MUSE*) is an intraurethral suppository of PGE1.
  - Administered via the urethral meatus.
  - The suppository dissolves → PGE1 diffusion across the urethra into the corpus spongiosum → enter corpora cavernosa via collateral vessels
  - Administration of the first dose should occur in the office to monitor the patient for hypotension (2% incidence at maximum dose).
  - 250, 500, 1000 mcg per dose.
- *Topical cream*
  - Vitaros 3 mg per 1 g – applied per urethra at the tip of the penis.
  - A starting dose with 3 mg can be considered especially in patients with serious ED, co-morbidity, or failure to PDE5i.
  - The maximum frequency is at 2–3 times per week and only once per 24-hour period.
- *Other intracavernosal injections therapy*
  - Two other agents are commonly used in erectogenic therapy.
  - Not FDA-approved for this indication, but are widely used:
  - *Papaverine* – non-specific phosphodiesterase inhibitor. Increases intracellular levels of both cAMP and cGMP.
  - *Phentolamine* – alpha1-adrenergic receptor blocker. Reduces sympathetic tone in the penis, thereby opposing vasoconstriction.

## Practical Prescribing

- Anatomical deformations of penis – follow up regularly to detect signs of penile fibrosis.
- Patients with Peyronie's disease should be carefully monitored because penile scarring may make injection technically difficult.
- The most serious adverse event is priapism (papaverine highest risk) – prevented by education and close monitoring of patients.

## Contraindications

- General contraindications:
  - Penile implants.
  - If sexual activity is medically inadvisable (e.g., orthostatic hypotension, myocardial infarction (MI), syncope).
- Not for use with other agents for ED, with predisposition to:
  - Prolonged erection
  - Thrombocythemia, polycythaemia, sickle cell anaemia
  - Multiple myeloma, leukaemia
- *Specific contraindication with intracavernosal use*:
  - Those with needle phobia.
  - Those unable to perform injection procedures.
- *Specific contraindication to intraurethral or topical use*:
  - Balanitis, severe hypospadias, urethral stricture, urethritis

## Side Effects

- *Intracavernosal*: penile pain (30%), ecchymosis, haematoma, priapism.
- *Intraurethral*:
  - Penile pain (32%), urethral burning (12%), minor urethral bleeding and irritations (5%), testicular pain (5%).
  - Female sexual partners reported vaginal burning/itching (6%).
  - Priapism (rare).
  - Dizziness caused by systemic absorption (rare).

# B) Pharmacology of Premature Ejaculation

## Dapoxetine

### Pharmacodynamics

- Short-acting selective serotonin reuptake inhibitor - (SSRI).
- SSRIs are typically prescribed for the treatment of depression.
  - Common side effects: delayed ejaculation and anorgasmia.
- Blocks the axonal reuptake of serotonin (5-hydroxytryptamine, 5-HT) from the synaptic cleft of central serotonergic neurons by 5-HT transporters → desensitise 5-HT1A and 5-HT1B receptors
- 5-HT acting on central postsynaptic receptors exerts an overall inhibitory control on the ejaculatory process.

## Pharmacokinetics

- Rapid distribution in the body.
- Readily absorbed after oral administration.
- Peak plasma concentration at ~1.5 hours after dosing.
- Half-life of dapoxetine 30 mg = 17.2 hours; 60 mg = 18.2 hours.
- Suitable for on-demand dosing.

## Practical Prescribing

- Dosing 30–60 mg.
- Taken 1–3 hours before sexual activity.
- Initial dose is at 30 mg, while subsequent doses are adjusted according to response.
- Increase in geometric mean intravaginal ejaculation latency time (IELT) at 12 weeks:
  - From baseline, 0.8 minutes (vs placebo, 1.2 minutes).
  - With 30 mg, 2.0 minutes; 60 mg, 2.3 minutes.
- Both doses demonstrate improved patient-reported outcome measures compared to placebo.
- Review treatment after four weeks or six doses, and at least every six months thereafter.
- Maximum of one dose per day; maximum 60 mg per day.

## Contraindications

- Bipolar disorder, mania, severe depression
- Syncope
- Significant cardiac disease, uncontrolled epilepsy

## Side Effects

- Nausea (17.3%), dizziness (9.4%), headache (7.9%), diarrhoea (5.9%), somnolence (3.9%), fatigue (3.9%), insomnia (3.8%), nasopharyngitis (3.1%)

# C) Pharmacology of Hypogonadism

- *Hypogonadism:* failure of the testes to produce physiological levels of testosterone (T).
- Low T levels can lead to physical and psychological symptoms.

- *Primary:* failure of the testes to produce enough T.
- *Secondary:* failure in hormonal stimulation of the testes – defect at the hypothalamic–pituitary axis.

# Testosterone Replacement Therapy (TRT)

- The different preparations, pharmacokinetics, side effects, advantages, and disadvantages are summarised in Table 30.2.

## Pharmacodynamics

- Treatment of T deficiency or hypogonadism is in the form of exogenous T.
- Available in various formulations:
  - Intramuscular (IM) injections
  - Subcutaneous pellets
  - Topical, intranasal, and oral formulations

## Practical Prescribing

- Choice of formulation:
  - *IM injections* – a cost-effective option. Fluctuations in libido and mood due to large variations in serum T level during the dosing interval.
  - *Transdermal patches* – a common side effect of skin irritation. Pre-treatment of the application site with 0.1% triamcinolone cream reduces the risk of irritation without reducing T absorption.
  - *Transdermal gel* – lower incidence of skin irritation than patches but result in variable increases in T levels. Patients should be counselled regarding the possible transfer of the drug to partners or children via direct skin contact.
  - *Oral therapies* – rarely used because of the need for multiple dosing regimens and fears of hepatotoxicity.

## Monitoring

- Baseline PSA test and digital rectal examination (DRE) recommended for men ≥40 years.
- Follow up visits at 3, 6, 12 months in the first year of treatment, followed by annual visits.
- Regular monitoring of T levels, haematocrit, PSA for prostate cancer, and cardiovascular risk factors.
- Total T target of 15–30 nmol/L.
- Consider phlebotomy for haematocrit at 50% or higher or change of medication/route of administration.

## Contraindications

- *Absolute contraindications*:
  - Locally advanced or metastatic prostate cancer
  - Male breast cancer
  - An active desire to father children
  - Haematocrit higher than 54%
  - Severe chronic heart failure (NYHA class IV)
- *Relative contraindications*:
  - Unevaluated prostate nodule or induration and PSA level higher than 4 ng/mL should be referred for urologic consultation before initiating T replacement.
  - Severe, untreated sleep apnoea.
  - Severe LUTS associated with BPE as indicated by IPSS >19.

## Side Effects

- *IM injections:* pain at the injection site, changes in mood, energy, and sexual desire.
- *Transdermal gels:* interpersonal transfer, skin irritation, fluctuations in absorption.
- *Other side effects:* polycythaemia, gynecomastia, oedema, acne, and other skin reactions.

## Testosterone Therapy and Cardiovascular (CV) Risk

- 2015 – T label change to include a warning for potential CV risk.
- Some studies have shown an associated risk; however, these studies have been criticised for methodological flaws.
- Other evidence supporting CV safety of TRT:
  - Coronary artery severity is inversely proportional to T.
  - TRT improves CV risk factors associated with metabolic syndrome (e.g., obesity and DM).
  - TRT facilitates reductions in inflammatory markers.
  - Other recent clinical trials on TRT have shown no increased risk of CV event or mortality.
- T therapy is based on evidence, effectiveness, and safety.
- Treatment-related sustained normalisation of serum T level is probably associated with lower mortality (British Society for Sexual Medicine, BSSM Guidance).

# D) Pharmacology of Male Infertility

## Gonadotoxins

- Drugs recognised with potential gonadotoxicity are summarised in Table 30.3.

**Table 30.2** Testosterone Replacement Options

| Common Formulation | Route | Dose | Pharmacokinetics | Advantages | Disadvantages |
|---|---|---|---|---|---|
| T enanthate or T cypionate | IM | 150–200 mg Q2w or 75–100 mg Q1w | Half-life 5–7 d | Short duration of action allows drug withdrawal if there are adverse side effects. | Levels fluctuate. |
| | | | Supraphysiologic T at first, hypogonadal at end of dosing period | Inexpensive, flexible dosing. | Supraphysiologic levels can cause a roller-coaster effect. |
| Sustanon 250 (T propionate 30 mg/mL, T isocaproate 60 mg/mL, T phenylpropionate 60 mg/mL, T decanoate 100 mg/mL) | IM | 250 mg Q3w | Peak levels reached at 24–48 h | Fast onset | Duration of action prevents drug withdrawal in event of adverse side effects. |
| | | | Plasma T levels return to the lower limit of normal range in 21 d | Freely available | Difficult to titrate. |
| T undecanoate (injection) | IM | 1000 mg Q10–14w | T maintained in normal range | Long-lasting | Long duration of action prevents drug withdrawal in the event of adverse side effects. |
| | | | | Lower frequency of administration improves compliance. | Pain at injection site. |
| | | | | | Large volume injection. |
| T undecanoate (oral) | Oral | 120–240 mg BD or TDS | Absorbed via lymphatics, bypasses portal system | Oral administration. | T variability in individual on different days and among individuals. |
| | | | | Flexible dose modification. | Multiple dosing daily. |
| | | | | Lymphatic absorption decreases liver involvement. | Must be taken with food. |
| T 1% and 2% gel | Top | 40–80 mg QDS | T maintained in normal range | Fast onset | Skin irritation at application site. |
| | | | | Flexible dose modification | Potential for interpersonal transfer – avoid contact with female, children, swimming for 4 h. |
| | | | | Normal serum levels for 24 h | Non-compliance long term. |
| T patch | Top | 5–10 mg OD | T maintained in normal range | Mimics circadian rhythm | Skin irritation |
| | | | | | Daily administration |

*Abbreviations:* T, testosterone; IM, intramuscular; Top, topical; Q, every; BD, twice a day; TDS, three times per day; OD, daily.

**Table 30.3** Agents Recognised with Potential Gonadotoxicity

| Class | Agents and Action |
|---|---|
| Cytotoxic and chemotherapeutics | Alkylating agents – **cyclophosphamide:** DNA damage during cell division. High chance of sustained gonadal dysfunction even after stopping. |
| | **Chlorambucil:** risk of azoospermia and oligospermia after cessation. |
| | Vinca alkaloids (**Vinblastine**), **Cisplatin** |
| Ionising radiation | **X-rays, Radiotherapy, Nuclear, Mining, Aviation** |
| | Dose-dependent. Mature spermatozoa cannot repair their own DNA. Minimum dose of radiation causing detectable DNA damage is 30 Gy. |
| Psychiatric medication | **Antipsychotics:** mainly by blocking CNS dopamine, inhibition of HPG axis and decreased libido. |
| | **Lithium:** decreases action of dopamine causing low libido and potency. |
| | **TCA:** hyperprolactinemia, ED, reduced libido, impaired ejaculation. |
| | **MAO inhibitors:** ED and ejaculatory dysfunction. |
| | **Valproic acid:** affects semen morphology and motility, small testicular volume. |
| Recreational | **Alcohol:** long-term/chronic consumption – low T, alteration in HPG axis, ED, reduced libido. |
| | **Marijuana:** affects spermatogenesis, sperm density and motility. |
| | **Cocaine:** reduced sperm count and motility. |
| | **Caffeine:** may cause sperm DNA defects. |
| | **Smoking:** affects sperm production, motility, and morphology. |
| Targeted therapy | IBD – **Sulfasalazine:** decreased sperm count, motility, and morphology, reversible after stopping. |
| | Epilepsy – **Phenytoin:** accelerates the breakdown and production of SHBG resulting in decreased levels of biologically active sex hormones. |
| Hormones | **Anabolic steroids:** suppress the HPG axis causing hypogonadotropic hypogonadism. High doses decrease sperm density, motility and increase morphologic anomalies. |
| | **Oestrogens, Diethylstilbestrol (DES):** testicular atrophy, ED, low libido. |
| Cardiovascular medication | **Aspirin** in large doses: low semen volume and concentration, decreased motility, DNA fragmentation. |
| | **Calcium channel blockers:** impair acrosome reaction. |
| | **Spironolactone:** inhibits production of T, ED, low sperm count. |
| Poisons | **Arsenic:** high levels inhibit sensitivity of gonadotroph cells to GnRH and decrease gonadotropin secretion. |
| | **Lead:** oligospermia, low motility and viscosity. |
| | **Pesticides:** herbicides, heavy metals. |
| Antibiotics | **Nitrofurantoin:** safe at low doses, high-doses cause maturation arrest. |
| | **Erythromycin:** reduces sperm motility and density. |
| | **Tetracyclines:** affect sperm motility by binding to mature spermatozoa. |
| Other | **Chronic heat:** reduces testicular weight and sperm production and results in more morphologically abnormal sperm. |
| | **Cimetidine:** blocks DHT receptors in the pituitary gland, hypothalamus. Causes loss of libido, ED and low sperm. |

*Abbreviations:* CNS, central nervous system; HPG, hypothalamic-pituitary-gonadal; TCA, tricyclic antidepressants; ED, erectile dysfunction; MAO, monoamine oxidase inhibitor; T, testosterone; IBD, inflammatory bowel disease; SHBG, sex hormone-binding globulin; DHT, dihydrotestosterone.

# Retrograde Ejaculation (RE)

## Sympathomimetics (e.g., Ephedrine/Pseudoephedrine)

### Pharmacodynamics

- Release of stored norepinephrine from sympathetic nerve endings, and also direct binding to alpha and beta receptors.
- Stimulation of alpha-adrenergic receptors of smooth muscle cells located at the bladder neck leads to increased tone and aiding full closure of internal bladder sphincter during ejaculation → promotes antegrade emission

### Pharmacokinetics

- Half-life for ephedrine: 3–6 hours.
- Half-life for pseudoephedrine varies by urinary pH.
  - 9–16 hours in alkaline urine.
  - 3–6 hours in acidic urine.
- Metabolised in the liver and excreted in the urine.

### Practical Prescribing

- Dosing: ephedrine 10–15 mg QDS, pseudoephedrine 60 mg QDS.
- Given 7–10 days prior to planned ejaculation.
- Use is unlicensed in the UK.
- Pseudoephedrine has been illegally used to produce methamphetamine; therefore it comes under pharmacy medications.
- Recommendation – induce antegrade ejaculation in the absence of spinal cord injury, anatomical abnormalities, or pharmacological agents.

### Contraindications

- Hypersensitivity, severe hypertension.
- Within 14 days of monoamine oxidase inhibitor (MAO).
- Benign prostate hyperplasia.

### Side Effects

- Sleep disturbance, urinary retention, angle-closure glaucoma, anxiety, arrhythmias, palpitations, impaired circulation, dry mouth, hallucination, headache, hypertension, irritability, nausea, vomiting.

### Monitoring

- Continuous therapy leads to tolerance and should not be recommended.
- If it fails, proceed to sperm collection from post-orgasmic urine.
- Acidic urine can be toxic to sperm; therefore, alkalinisation can be used with sodium bicarbonate 650 mg QDS.

### Efficacy

- Medical treatments for RE are successful in up to 50% of patients.

## Alpha$_1$ Agonist (e.g., Midodrine)

### Pharmacodynamics/Kinetics

- Alpha-1-selective adrenergic agonist.
- Undergoes extensive enzymatic hydrolysis in the systemic circulation.
- Midodrine is converted to desglymidodrine (active agent, 15x more potent).
- Half-life for midodrine: 25 minutes (c.f. desglymidodrine is 3–4 hours).
- Excretion is mainly in the urine, minimal in faeces.

### Practical Prescribing

- 7.5–17.5 mg TDS oral daily.
- May cause marked elevation in blood pressure.
- Use is unlicensed in the UK.
- Titrate dose in increments of 2.5 mg per dose (e.g., increase from 5 mg TDS to 7.5 mg TDS) every 24 hours whilst monitoring blood pressure.

### Contraindications

- Aortic aneurysm, blood vessel spasm, bradycardia, cardiac conduction disturbances, cerebrovascular occlusion, congestive heart failure, MI, hypertension
- Hyperthyroidism, narrow-angle glaucoma, phaeochromocytoma

### Side Effects

- Hypertension, paraesthesia, piloerection, scalp pruritus, urinary retention, chills, flushing, gastrointestinal discomfort, headache, nausea, skin reactions, stomatitis, anxiety, arrhythmias.

### Monitoring

- Treatment must be stopped if supine hypertension is not controlled by reducing the dose.

### Recommendation/Guidelines and Efficacy

- As with ephedrine/pseudoephedrine.

# Tricyclic Antidepressants (e.g., Imipramine)

## Pharmacodynamics

- Inhibit the neuronal reuptake of norepinephrine and serotonin into the presynaptic nerve terminals.
- It may also downregulate beta-adrenergic and serotonin receptors.

## Pharmacokinetics

- Metabolism is in the liver by CYP450.
- Half-life: 6–18 hours.
- Excreted in the urine.

## Practical Prescribing

- 25 mg BD.
- Limited quantities of tricyclic antidepressants should be prescribed.
- Effects of alcohol are enhanced.
- Use is unlicensed in the UK.
- It is unclear if higher doses up to 300 mg daily are more effective.

## Contraindications

- Acute recovery post-MI.
- Co-administration with serotoninergic drugs as risk of serotonin syndrome (MAO inhibitors, linezolid, methylene blue).

## Side Effects

- Fatigue, anxiety, depression, suicidal thoughts, sedation, decreased appetite, confusion, arrhythmias, dizziness

## Monitoring

- Monitor for changes in behaviour and suicidal tendencies.

## Recommendation/Guidelines and Efficacy

- As with ephedrine/pseudoephedrine.

# Gonadotrophin Therapy (Including Oral Adjunctive Treatments) for Correcting Hypogonadism in Male Infertility

## Gonadotrophins

- Strongly recommended in the treatment of secondary hypogonadism resulting from pituitary deficiency.

- *Human chorionic gonadotropin* (HCG):
  - Injected subcutaneously 500–2,000 IU 2–3 times per week until normal T levels are reached.
  - If there is a failure of stimulation of spermatogenesis, then FSH can be added at 75 IU three times per week, increasing to 150 IU three times per week if indicated.

# Selective Oestrogen Receptor Modulators (e.g., Clomiphene)

- Clomiphene acts at the level of the hypothalamus, occupying cell surface and intracellular oestrogen receptors (ERs) for longer durations than oestrogen.
- Interferes with receptor recycling, effectively depleting hypothalamic ERs and inhibiting normal testosterone negative feedback.
- Impairment of the feedback signal → increased pulsatile GnRH secretion from the hypothalamus → pituitary gonadotropin (FSH, LH) release

# Aromatase Inhibitors (e.g., Anastrozole)

- An enzyme of the cytochrome p450 – present in the prostate, testes, adipose tissue of men, brain, and bone.
- Converts T and androstenedione to estradiol and estrone.
- Through negative feedback on the hypothalamus–pituitary axis, estradiol will act to reduce gonadotropic secretions, ultimately affecting spermatogenesis.
- *Anastrozole:* potent and selective non-steroidal aromatase inhibitor.
  - Prevents the conversion of T to estradiol.
  - Improves serum and intratesticular T levels.

# E) Pharmacology of Penile Deformity (Peyronie's Disease)

## Oral Medication

- Contemporary clinical guidelines do not support the routine use of oral medication for Peyronie's disease (PD) due to a lack of robust controlled clinical trials.

# Vitamin E (Alpha-Tocopherol)

## Pharmacodynamics

- An antioxidant that has protective effects against free radicals.

- Prevents the oxidation of vitamin A and C.
- Protects the cell membranes' polyunsaturated fatty acids from attack by free radicals and protects red blood cells against haemolysis.

## Pharmacokinetics

- Absorption is reduced in patients with a history of malabsorption.
- Metabolised by the liver and excreted in the faeces.

## Practical Prescribing

- 400 IU OD or BD.
- In high doses (such those used by urologists), it can cause a warfarin-like effect; therefore, adjustments of warfarin doses might be necessary.

## Contraindications

- Hypersensitivity.

## Side Effects

- Fatigue, headaches, flatulence, diarrhoea, blurred vision, risk of haemorrhagic stroke, and it can suppress the action of other antioxidants

## Monitoring

- Duration of treatment: 3–6 months and patients should be warned about the anticoagulant/thrombolytic effects.

# Potassium Para-Aminobenzoate (Potaba)

## Pharmacodynamics/Kinetics

- A member of the vitamin B group.
- Increases oxygen uptake by the tissues, inducing an anti-fibrotic effect and enhancing the activity of MAO.

## Practical Prescribing

- 3 g QDS.
- Poorly tolerated due to gastrointestinal side effects, volume, and frequency of dosing.
- Low food intake such as fasting can lead to hypoglycaemia.

## Contraindications

- Hyperkalaemia, severe liver damage, avoid with sulphonamides antibiotics

## Side effects

- Nausea, anorexia, fever, rash, hepatitis, pruritus, confusion.

## Monitoring

- Monthly liver function tests – discontinue if elevated.
- Avoid if GFR <45 mL/min.
- Increased risk of hyperkalaemia.

# Tamoxifen

## Pharmacodynamics

- Non-steroidal oestrogen receptor antagonist.
- Known to the urologist for the prevention of gynecomastia mainly when taking non-steroidal anti-androgens for prostate cancer.
- Mainly used in breast cancer.
- In PD, it regulates transforming growth factor $\beta1$ (TGF-$\beta1$) secretion by fibroblasts.

## Pharmacokinetics

- Binds to proteins, 99% in plasma.
- Half-life: 7–14 hours.
- Metabolised in the liver by the P450 enzymes and excreted mainly in the faeces but also in the urine.

## Practical Prescribing

- 20 mg BD daily.
- 6–12 weeks in the early, painful phase of the disease.

## Contraindications

- Genetic predisposition to venous thromboembolism (VTE) or significant family history of VTE.

## Side Effects

- Hot flashes, nausea, oedema, fatigue, anaemia, alopecia, embolism and thrombosis, muscle complaints, musculoskeletal pain

## Monitoring

- Patients should be aware of the risk of VTE and report a sudden onset of pain in the calf of one leg or breathlessness.

# Colchicine

## Pharmacodynamics

- Anti-inflammatory properties.
- Disrupts spindle cell fibres and inhibits cell mitosis.
- Blocks the lipoxygenase pathway of arachidonic acid.
- Inhibits mobility and adhesion of leucocytes and wound contracture by binding tubulin and causing depolymerisation.
- Interference with transcellular movement of protocollagen.

## Pharmacokinetics

- Half-life: ~30 hours.
- Metabolised by the liver and excreted in the urine.

## Practical Prescribing

- 0.6 mg TDS daily.
- Caution must be exercised since evidence comes only from uncontrolled studies.
- Not in the British National Formulary (BNF).

## Contraindications

- Blood disorders.
- Use with caution in hepatic impairment, cardiac disease, the elderly, and gastrointestinal disease.

## Side Effects

- Nausea, vomiting, abdominal pain, diarrhoea, agranulocytosis, bone marrow disorders

# Acetyl Esthers of Carnitine (Acetyl- and Propionyl-L-Carnitine)

## Pharmacodynamics

- L-carnitine is biosynthesized in the liver and kidneys from amino acids lysine and methionine. It is a naturally occurring, non-protein amino acid.
- Inhibits acetyl coenzyme A, resulting in an antiproliferative response eventually. It is thought to suppress fibroblast activity and collagen production, thus reducing fibrosis.

## Practical Prescribing

- 1 g BD for three months.
- Not licensed.

## Contraindications

- Nil significant

## Side Effects

- Abdominal cramps, diarrhoea, nausea, abnormal skin odour.

# Pentoxifylline

## Pharmacodynamics/Kinetics

- Increases tissue oxygenation, downregulates TGF β1, and increases fibrinolytic activity.
- Additional weak PDE5 inhibitor effect.
- Binds to red blood cells, then extensively metabolised in the liver, and excreted in urine.

## Practical Prescribing

- 400 mg TDS daily.
- Unlicensed and mainly used in liver conditions and peripheral vascular disease and venous ulcers (adjunct).
- Gastrointestinal side effects lessened by administrations with food.

## Contraindications

- Patients previously exhibiting intolerance to pentoxifylline, xanthines (e.g., caffeine, theophylline), or any component of the formulation.
- Recent cerebral and/or retinal haemorrhage or acute MI.
- Severe coronary artery disease.

## Side Effects

- Mainly gastrointestinal, nausea, vomiting, agitation, angina, haemorrhage, headache, hot flushes

## Monitoring

- Caution in patients with risk of haemorrhage, renal, or hepatic impairment.

# Intralesional Treatment

## Steroids

- Inhibit phospholipase A2, decrease collagen synthesis, and suppress immune response.
- Treatment is not associated with a significant reduction in plaque size, penile curvature, or pain.
- Guidelines do not recommend its clinical use.

# Verapamil

## Pharmacodynamics

- A calcium channel blocker.

- Inhibit the exocytosis of collagen, fibronectin, and glycosaminoglycan.
- Inhibit the ultimate formation of scar.

## Practical Prescribing

- 10 mg/10 mL or 10 mg/20 mL injections given once every two weeks for a total of 12 injections.
- Not licensed in the BNF.
- Improvement might not be noted immediately.

## Contraindications

- Acute MI

## Side Effects

- Nausea, light-headedness, ecchymosis, pain.

## Interferon Alpha-2b

### Pharmacodynamics

- Inhibits collagen synthesis, decreases fibroblast proliferation and extracellular matrix production, and improves the wound healing process.

### Practical Prescribing

- $5 \times 10^6$ units in 10 mL of saline, twice weekly for 12 weeks.
- Not licensed in the BNF.
- Non-steroidal anti-inflammatories (NSAIDS) can manage side effects before injection.

### Side Effects

- Flu-like symptoms, rash, myalgia, arthralgia, fever.

## Clostridium Collagenase Histolyticum (CCH, Xiapex®)

### Pharmacodynamics

- Chromatographically purified bacterial enzyme.
- Selectively attacks and hydrolyses collagen (primary constituent of PD plaques), breaking its build-up in the plaque.

### Practical Prescribing

- The original treatment protocol in all studies – two injections of 0.58 mg of CCH 24–72 hours apart every six weeks for up to four cycles, with penile modelling procedure.
- Alternative dosing regimens – 0.9 mg injections four weeks apart for 12 weeks with similar safety and efficacy.
- *Delivery*:
  - Induce an erection via prostaglandin injection or vacuum device to mark the target area.

- Plaques injection (+/− fracture) when the penis is flaccid.
- Indicated in men with penile curvature of >30° and practice cautionary use if there is concomitant anticoagulation.

## Contraindications

- Avoid injecting into structures containing collagen (urethra, nerves, corpora cavernosa).
- Hypersensitivity

## Side effects

- Penile pain, swelling, ecchymosis, and — rarely — corporal rupture.

# Topical Therapy

- Currently, there is no evidence to demonstrate that topical agents achieve sufficient penetration from the skin into the tunica albuginea.
- Transdermal electromotive drug administrations (EMDA) have been used to overcome this impediment.
- Medicines studied in this setting include verapamil/dexamethasone and H-100 gel.
- The evidence is not sufficient to recommend their use in a clinical setting.

# F) Pharmacology of Priapism

- *Priapism* – abnormally prolonged and often painful erection (>4h).
- This erection may not be related to sexual desire or stimulation.
- It often will not be relieved by orgasm.
- Categorised as ischaemic/non-ischaemic or acute/stuttering/chronic.
- Drugs that can induce priapism are summarised in Table 30.4.

# Acute Priapism

## Phenylephrine

### Pharmacodynamics/Kinetics

- Selective alpha1-adrenergic receptor agonist without beta related cardiac effects (ionotropic/chronotropic).
- It's metabolised in the intestinal wall and excreted in the urine.

### Practical Prescribing

- 200-250 mcg every 5–10 min until detumescence at a maximum of 1 mg within one hour.
- The vial is 10 mg in 1 mL and needs to be diluted with 19 mL of saline such that the concentration becomes 0.5 mg/mL.

**Table 30.4** Medicines Recognised as Increasing the Risk of Priapism

| Medicine Class | Examples |
| --- | --- |
| Antipsychotics/Antidepressants | Trazodone, Fluoxetine, Sertraline, Lithium, Clozapine, Risperidone, Chlorpromazine, Olanzapine, Thioridazine |
| Recreational drugs | Alcohol, Cocaine, Marijuana, Crack Cocaine |
| Vasoactive erectile agents | Prostaglandin E1 (Alprostadil), Phentolamine, Papaverine |
| Alpha-adrenergic receptor antagonists | Tamsulosin, Doxazosin, Prazosin, Terazosin |
| Antihypertensives | Propranolol, Hydralazine, Guanethidine |
| Anticoagulants | Warfarin, Heparin |
| Hormones | Testosterone, Gonadotrophin-releasing hormone |
| Medicines used in ADHD | Methylphenidate, Atomoxetine |
| Phosphodiesterase type 5 inhibitors | Sildenafil, Tadalafil, Vardenafil Avanafil |
| Poisons/Toxins | Scorpion bites, Spider bites |

*Abbreviations:* ADHD, attention deficit hyperactivity disorder.

- Inject intracavernous aliquots of 0.5 mL.
- Drug of choice if aspiration alone fails.

## Contraindications

- Malignant or poorly controlled hypertension or MAO inhibitors.

## Side Effects

- Hypertension, headache, tachycardia with palpitations, reflex bradycardia, cardiac arrhythmias, dizziness
- Very rarely, subarachnoid haemorrhage

## Monitoring

- Ensure adequate BP and pulse monitoring in a controlled environment.

## Efficacy

- 43–81%.

## Alternative Treatment Options

- Etilefrine (and norephedrine) is the second most used sympathomimetic according to EAU guidelines.
- Not licensed in the UK.
- Methylene blue and adrenaline have also been reported as alternatives.
- Oral terbutaline (5 mg) or pseudoephedrine may be used as oral alternatives particularly in drug-induced priapism (e.g., following pro-erectile penile injections).

- Mixed beta-agonist ($\beta2>\beta1$) with moderate alpha-agonist activity causing relaxation of the smooth muscle with less effect on heart rate.
- Terbutaline's mechanism of action in erection is not fully understood.
- Terbutaline's beta-2-agonist and smooth muscle relaxant effect into the corpus cavernosum is limited by the stagnant blood in priapism, suggesting alternate means of effect, if any.

## Stuttering Priapism

- Pseudoephedrine, Etilefrine, Terbutaline (as above).
- Medications used to manage stuttering priapism are summarised in Table 30.5.

## Hormone Therapy

### Pharmacodynamics

- Suppress action of androgens on penile erection by down-regulating testosterone.

### Practical Prescribing

- GnRH agonists or antagonists
- Anti-androgens (e.g., finasteride, ketoconazole)
- Oestrogens
- No specific consensus on dose or duration, so use standard regimes.

### Contraindications

- Prepubertal/adolescent men who have not reached sexual maturation.

**Table 30.5** Pharmacological Treatments Used in the Management of (Ischaemic) Stuttering

| Drugs | Mechanism of Action | Side Effects | Comments |
|---|---|---|---|
| GnRH agonists | Suppresses LH by receptor down-regulation | Hot flashes, gynecomastia, loss of sexually-induced erections, asthenia | Not advised for prepubertal men or those seeking fertility |
| DES (oestrogen) | Suppresses pituitary function by feedback inhibition | Cardiovascular side effects, ED, loss of libido, gynecomastia, VTE | Not advised for prepubertal men or those seeking fertility |
| Anti-androgens | Suppression of androgen receptors | Hot flashes, gynecomastia, diarrhoea, loss of libido, oedema and rash | Liver function should be monitored |
| Ketoconazole | Reduction of T levels | Adrenal suppression, drug interactions, QT syndrome, hepatotoxicity | Must be given daily prednisone. Needs monitoring |
| 5α-reductase inhibitors | Inhibits conversion of T to DHT | Decreased libido, impotence, ED, ejaculatory dysfunction, and gynecomastia | Check for prostate cancer prior |
| Gabapentin | Inhibits voltage-gated calcium channels; reduces T and FSH levels | Anorgasmia, decreased potency | Dizziness, drowsiness, and peripheral oedema. In children: hyperactivity and mood swings |
| Digoxin | Inhibits the sodium-potassium pump, cardiac glycoside | Decreased libido, anorexia, nausea, vomiting, confusion, blurred vision, headache, gynecomastia, rash, arrhythmia | Blood levels checked. Needs monitoring |
| PDE5 Inhibitors | Increases PDE5 function | Headache, dizziness, flushing, dyspepsia, nasal congestion and rhinitis | Nitrates, severe cardiac issues are contraindicated |
| Baclofen | Inhibits penile erection and ejaculation through GABA activity; γ-aminobutyric acid agonist | Drowsiness, confusion, dizziness, weakness, fatigue, headache, hypotension, and nausea | Relieves muscle spasm and may help treat priapism, but its use is limited by associated risk of sedation and increase seizure risk. |
| Terbutaline | β2-agonist (oral) | Nervousness, tremor, drowsiness, heart palpitation, headaches, dizziness, hot flashes, nausea and weakness | Diabetes, hypertension, hyperthyroidism, history of seizure are contraindicated |
| Metaraminol | Vasoconstriction; α1 and β1 adrenergic receptor agonist | Hypertension, coronary ischaemia, cardiac arrhythmias, death | Tachycardia, abscess formation, tissue necrosis, or sloughing at injection site |
| Phenylephrine | Vasoconstriction; Selective α1 and β1 adrenergic receptor agonist | Headache, hypertension, bradycardia, palpitations, sweating, insomnia, worsening BPH | Recommended as initial preferred agent above other sympathomimetics. History of epilepsy or on anticonvulsant medication is contraindicated. |
| Etilefrine | Vasoconstriction; α1-selective agonist, | Tachycardia; increases stroke volume | Drug availability and manufacturing problems |

*Source:* Adapted from Levey et al. [1].

All prevent ischaemic and stuttering priapism episodes except, Baclofen – prevents recurrent reflexogenic erections, and in patients having prolonged erections from neurological disease; Terbutaline/Metaraminol/Phenylephrine – treats acute ischaemia and stuttering episodes; Etilefrine – treats and prevents acute ischaemia and stuttering episodes.

*Abbreviations:* BPH, benign prostatic hyperplasia; DHT, dihydrotestosterone; ED, erectile dysfunction; FSH, follicle-stimulating hormone; GABA, γ-aminobutyric acid; GnRH, gonadotrophin-releasing hormone; LH, luteinizing hormone; PDE5, phosphodiesterase 5; T, testosterone; VTE, venous thromboembolism.

### Side Effects

- Hot flushes, erectile dysfunction, gynecomastia, loss of libido, fatigue.

### Monitoring

- Cardiovascular toxicity of oestrogens limits their use.

## PDE5 Inhibitors

### Pharmacodynamics

- Paradoxical effect.
- Increase the concentration of cGMP in the smooth muscle in a NO dysfunctional state.
- The change in NO pathway with downregulation of cavernosal PDE5 prevents the complete degradation of cGMP in the corpora cavernosa.

### Practical Prescribing

- Sildenafil 25–50 mg/day, tadalafil 5–10 mg three times per week.
- Initiated only when the penis is flaccid.
- Not licensed.

## Digoxin

### Pharmacodynamics/Kinetics:

- Inhibits the sodium-potassium pump.
- Decreases the $Na^+$ concentration gradient and prevents efflux of $Ca^{2+}$ from the smooth muscle cell.
- Increases intracellular calcium → penile detumescence
- Half-life: 1–3 days.

### Practical Prescribing

- 0.25–0.5 mg daily.
- Not licensed in the BNF.

### Contraindications

- Severe cardiac dysfunctions.

### Side Effects

- Decreased libido, blurred vision, headache, anorexia, nausea, vomiting, gynecomastia, rash, confusion, arrhythmia

### Monitoring

- Monitor levels in renal impairment.

### Efficacy

- Levey et al. in 2012 reported a reduced number of hospital visits and improved life quality.

## Recommended Reading

1. Levey HR, Kutlu O, Bivalacqua TJ. Medical management of ischemic stuttering priapism: a contemporary review of the literature. Asian J Androl. 2012; 14(1): 156–163.
2. European Association of Urology (EAU), EAU guidelines on sexual and reproductive health 2020.
3. Wein A, Kavoussi L, Partin A, Peters C. Campbell-Walsh Urology. 11th edition, China: Elsevier; 2016.
4. Whalen K (ed), Finkel R, Panavelil TA. Lippincott Illustrated Reviews: Pharmacology. 6th edition. Philadelphia, United States of America: Wolters Kluwer; 2014.
5. The British National Formulary. Available from https://bnf.nice.org.uk.

# 31 Antimicrobial Agents

*Thomas E. Webb, Karl H. Pang, and Ased Ali*

## Introduction

- An antimicrobial agent is a natural or synthetic substance that kills or inhibits the growth of microorganisms.
- Three main types of antimicrobials are used in urology: *antibiotics, anti-fungals,* and *anti-parasitics.*

## A) Antibiotics

- Most commonly used group of antimicrobials.
- Term was derived from the Greek *anti-* (against) and *bios* (life) – first suggested in 1942 by Dr Selman A. Waksman, a soil microbiologist.
- The first antibiotic was discovered by Alexander Fleming in 1928.
- Antibiotics kill or slow the growth of bacteria.
- Consist of chemicals produced by/derived from microorganisms (typically bacteria or fungi).
- Antibiotics are commonly classified into their:
  - *Type of action:*
    - Bactericidal: work by killing bacteria.
    - Bacteriostatic: work by stopping the bacteria from multiplying.
  - *Mechanism of action:*
    - Inhibitors of cell wall synthesis.
    - Inhibitors of nucleic acid synthesis.
    - Inhibitors of protein acid synthesis (including anti-metabolites).
- A summary of antibiotic mechanism of action and resistance is shown in Figure 31.1 and Table 31.1.

### 1. Inhibitors of cell wall synthesis

- The peptidoglycan cell wall is unique to all bacteria.
- Comprised of polysaccharide chains cross-linked by D-amino containing peptides.
- Two main classes of antibacterial drugs target the cell wall synthesis:
  1. Beta-lactams (also beta-lactamase inhibitors)
  2. Glycopeptides (only active against gram-positive bacteria)

### Beta-Lactam Antibiotics

- *Examples:* penicillins, cephalosporins, carbapenems, monobactams.
- The beta-lactam ring (Figure 31.2) is common to all these antibiotics and must be intact for antibacterial action.
- The different groups are distinguished by structures attached to the ring and the shape of the second ring.

### Mechanism of Action

- All contain a beta-lactam ring – mimics the D-ala-D-ala peptide sequence that serves as the substrate for bacterial cell wall transpeptidases.
- Irreversibly bind to the Penicillin-Binding Protein (PBP) – transpeptidase is responsible for the peptidoglycan crosslinking and cell wall formation.
- By blocking peptidoglycan crosslinking, they inhibit cell wall synthesis during replication → build-up of precursor molecules → activation of the bacterial cell's autolytic system and cell lysis

### Metabolism

- Primarily renal excretion.
- Exceptions:
  - Nafcillin – biliary
  - Anti-staphylococcal penicillins (e.g., oxacillin, dicloxacillin)
  - Ceftriaxone – both renal and biliary

### General Adverse Effects

- Hypersensitivity reactions.
- Jarisch–Herxheimer reaction (important when treating syphilis).

### Resistance

- *Alteration of target site*
  - MRSA and MRSE synthesise a second PBP with much lower affinity for beta-lactam

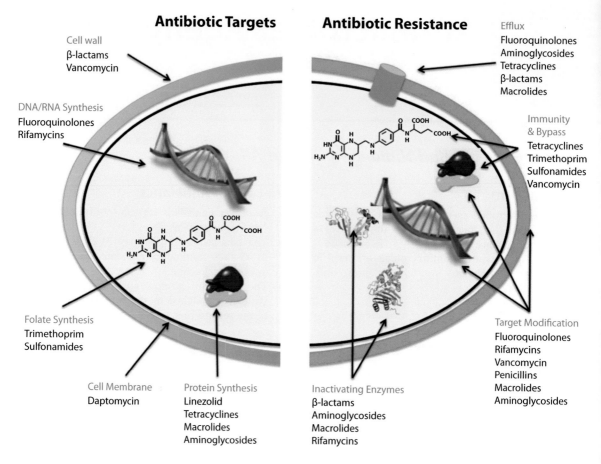

**Figure 31.1** Antibiotic targets and mechanisms of resistance. (Adapted from Wright et al. [3])

**Figure 31.2** Beta-lactam ring.

antibiotics → able to continue with cell wall synthesis
- *S. Pneumonia, N. gonorrhoeae, and H. Influenzae* are also able to utilise PBP changes.
- *Alteration in access to target*
  - Altered bacterial porins in the outer membrane reduces its permeability to beta-lactams, gaining access to PBPs.
- *Beta-lactamases*
  - Split beta-lactam rings.
  - Commonly produced by gram-negative and anaerobic organisms.

- Some specifically target certain subclasses of beta-lactams (e.g., penicillins or cephalosporins).
- Others (e.g., Extended Spectrum Beta-lactamases [ESBLs]) are active against the majority of the class.

## Beta-Lactamase Inhibitors

- *Beta-lactamase inhibitors* are processed by beta-lactamase but act as *'suicide substrates'* which lead to beta-lactamase degradation. Examples include:
  - Clavulanic acid (combined Amoxicillin – Co-Amoxiclav)
  - Tazobactam (combined with piperacillin – Tazocin)

## I. Penicillins

- Have a bicyclic penam structure and share structural features with the cephalosporins.
- *Key features*
  - Bactericidal.

**Table 31.1** Characteristic of Antibiotics Used to Treat Urinary Tract Infection

| Mechanism | Agent | Common Side Effects/ Cautions | Safety in Pregnancy |
|---|---|---|---|
| Inhibition of cell wall synthesis | *Beta-lactam:* bactericidal (e.g., Penicillin, Cephalosporin) | Hypersensitivity, diarrhoea | Safe |
| | *Glycopeptides:* bactericidal (e.g., Vancomycin) | Ototoxicity, nephrotoxicity | Unsafe |
| Inhibition of nucleic acid synthesis and anti-metabolites | *Quinolones:* bactericidal (inhibits DNA gyrase) (e.g., Ciprofloxacin) | Tendon damage, interaction with warfarin | Unsafe |
| | *Nitroimidazoles:* bactericidal (e.g., Metronidazole) | Gastrointestinal, metallic taste | Unsafe |
| Inhibition of protein synthesis | *Tetracycline:* bacteriostatic (e.g., Doxycycline) | Hepatoxicity, deposition in growing bones and teeth | Unsafe |
| | *Macrolides:* bacteriostatic (e.g., Erythromycin) | Gastrointestinal | Unsafe |
| | *Aminoglycosides:* bactericidal (e.g., Gentamicin) | Ototoxicity, nephrotoxicity | Unsafe in the 2nd and 3rd trimesters |
| Others | *Trimethoprim:* bacteriostatic (inhibits dihydrofolate reductase) | Folate antagonist – neural tube defect | Unsafe in the 1st trimester |
| | *Nitrofurantoin:* bactericidal (metabolites disrupt DNA/RNA) | Hepatotoxicity, peripheral neuropathy, pulmonary fibrosis | Unsafe in the 3rd trimester |
| | *Fosfomycin:* bactericidal (inhibits the formation of *N*-acetylmuramic acid) | Hyponatraemia, hypokalaemia | Unsafe |

- Regarded as safe in pregnancy.
- Rarely can cause immediate/delayed allergic reactions, which manifest as skin rashes, fever, angioedema, and anaphylactic shock.
- *Adverse effects*: hypersensitivity, haemolytic anaemia, seizures, interstitial nephritis diarrhoea, pseudomembranous colitis, drug-induced rash when treating patients with infectious mononucleosis using aminopenicillins.
- *Urological uses*: upper and lower urinary tract infections (UTI), genital skin infections, and gonorrhoea.

- *Four types:*
  - **Natural**
    - Based on the original penicillin-G structure.
    - Active against gram-positive *Streptococci, Staphylococci,* and some gram-negative bacteria (e.g., *meningococcus*).
    - *Examples*: penicillin-G (IM/IV), penicillin V (oral).
    - *Urological uses*: gram-positive aerobes, gram-negative cocci, spirochaetes, branching gram-positive anaerobes.

- **Penicillinase-resistant**
  - Intrinsically active against beta-lactamase, producing bacteria through the addition of bulky side chains.
  - Resistance is still possible due to alteration of the binding site of PBP, resulting in reduced affinity (one of the main virulence factors in MRSA).
  - *Examples*: nafcillin, dicloxacillin, oxacillin, methicillin.
  - *Urological uses*: gram-positive aerobes, especially *Staphylococcus aureus* (non-MRSA).

- **Aminopenicillins**
  - Broader spectrum.
  - Better oral absorption.
  - Structures are similar to penicillin (susceptible to beta-lactamase degradation).
  - *Examples*: ampicillin and amoxicillin.
  - *Urological uses*: some gram-positive aerobes and gram-negative bacilli including *E. coli, Proteus,* and Enterococci.

- **Extended spectrum**
  - Intrinsically beta-lactamase resistant.
  - *Examples*: IV piperacillin (+ tazobactam), IV ticarcillin, IV carbenicillin.

- *Urological uses*: extended spectrum gram-negative bacilli, especially *Pseudomonas,* but also *E.coli, Proteus,* and anaerobes (e.g., bacteroides, gram-positive aerobes).

## II. Cephalosporins

- Action is similar to that of penicillins due to the presence of a beta-lactam ring, but other parts of the chemical structure are different.
- *Key features*
  - Bactericidal.
  - Regarded as safe in pregnancy.
  - Rarely can cause immediate/delayed allergic reactions.
  - *Adverse effects:* hypersensitivity, autoimmune haemolytic anaemia, thrombocytopenia, neutropenia, vitamin K deficiency increasing bleeding tendency. Some cephalosporins may cause flushing, tachycardia, or hypotension when consumed with alcohol (disulfiram reaction). They can lower seizure threshold and can increase nephrotoxicity of aminoglycosides.
  - *Urological* uses: upper and lower UTIs, genital skin infections, and gonorrhoea.
- Grouped into 'generations' by their antimicrobial properties; latter generations tend to have greater gram-negative activity than earlier generations.

### First Generation

- Excellent coverage against most gram-positive pathogens.
- *Examples:* cephalexin, cephradine, cefazolin (IV/IM).
- *Urological uses:* gram-positive cocci, *Proteus mirabilis, E. coli, Klebsiella.*

### Second Generation

- Expanded gram-negative spectrum in addition to the gram-positive spectrum of the first-generation cephalosporins.
- *Examples:* cefaclor (oral), cefuroxime (oral and IV), cefoxitin, Ccfotetan (IV).
- *Urological uses:* gram-positive cocci, *E. coli, Klebsiella, Proteus mirabilis, Gonorrhoea,* and *Serratia.*

### Third Generation

- Much greater gram-negative activity and decreased gram-positive activity.
- *Examples:* cefixime (oral), ceftriaxone, cefotaxime, ceftazidime, cefoperazone (IV).
- *Urological uses:* severe gram-negative infections that are resistant to other beta-lactams (particularly Enterobacteriaceae). Ceftazidime and cefoperazone are effective against *Pseudomonas.* Ceftriaxone can be used in gonorrhoea and for perioperative prophylaxis against wound infection.

## Fourth Generation

- Extended-spectrum agents with similar activity against gram-positive organisms as first-generation cephalosporins.
- Have a greater resistance to beta-lactamases. Many can cross the blood brain barrier.
- *Example:* cefepime (IV).
- *Urological uses:* may rarely be used for severe UTI and intra-abdominal infections, but they work well against *Pseudomonas* and *Staphylococcus.*

## III. Carbapenems

- Powerful intravenous-only agents usually reserved for treatment of severe bacterial infections — typically where bacteria are known/suspected to be multidrug-resistant (MDR).
- *Key features*
  - Bactericidal.
  - Broad-spectrum.
  - Intrinsic beta-lactamase resistance.
  - *Examples:* imipenem (+ cilastatin), meropenem, ertapenem, doripenem.
  - *Urological uses:* gram-positive cocci, gram-negative bacilli, and anaerobes.
  - Considered a 'last resort' drug because of its significant adverse effects.
  - *Adverse effects:* secondary fungal infections, can lower seizure threshold (especially imipenem), gastrointestinal (GI) upset, rash, thrombophlebitis.
  - Best avoided during pregnancy but may be used if potential benefit outweighs the risk.

## IV. Monobactams

- Monocyclic, bacterially-produced beta-lactam antibiotics.
- The beta-lactam ring is not fused to another ring, giving it intrinsic beta-lactamase resistance.
- *Key features*
  - Bactericidal.
  - Highly effective only against gram-negative bacilli, including *Pseudomonas.*
  - Useful alternative for penicillin-allergic patients and an alternative to aminoglycosides for patients with renal insufficiency.
  - *Example:* aztreonam.
  - Considered a 'last resort' drug because of its significant adverse effects.
  - Best avoided during pregnancy but animal studies have failed to reveal evidence of embryotoxicity, fetotoxicity, or teratogenicity.

- *Urological uses:* severe aerobic gram-negative bacilli infection in patients who have a serious beta-lactam allergy.
- *Adverse effects:* secondary fungal infections, can lower seizure threshold, GI upset, rash, thrombophlebitis.

## Glycopeptides

- Composed of either glycosylated cyclic or polycyclic non-ribosomal peptides.
- Synthesised from a family of gram-positive, spore-forming soil bacteria organisms that form a true mycelium known as actinobacteria.

### Mechanism of Action

- Bactericidal – inhibit cell wall synthesis by binding the terminal D-ala-D-ala moiety of cell wall precursor peptides; therefore, it is only effective against gram-positive bacteria.
- *Metabolism: renal.*
- *Resistance*: alteration/mutation of peptidoglycan receptors leading to reduced antibiotic affinity.

### Key Features

- *Examples:* vancomycin (IV & Oral, although not absorbed) and teicoplanin (IV).
- Increased risk of toxicity when administered with aminoglycosides, loop diuretics, or ciclosporin.
- *Urological uses:* MRSA and Staphylococcal wound infections, implant related prophylaxis and infection, Enterococcus infection, *C. difficile* infection.

### Adverse Effects

- Ototoxicity and nephrotoxicity, *'red man syndrome'*, and hypotension due to histamine release if administered too quickly (Vancomycin).
- Concentrations need to be monitored

## 2. Inhibitors of nucleic acid synthesis

### Quinolones and Fluoroquinolones

- Fluoroquinolones (fluoridated quinolones) are synthetic compounds (Figure 31.3).
- The earliest first-generation agents are *quinolones,* which are poorly absorbed and are rarely used now.
- Newer agents are fluoroquinolones – well tolerated broad-spectrum agents, but recently have some new MHRA warning regarding adverse effects.

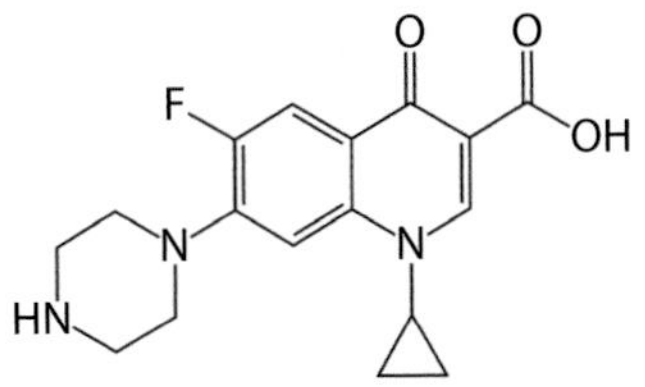

Figure 31.3 A Quinolone is a 2-ringed nitrogen containing system with a ketone.

### Mechanism of Action

- Bactericidal – kill bacteria by inhibiting bacterial enzyme *DNA gyrase.*
- *Metabolism: mostly renal but biliary for moxifloxacin.*
- *Resistance:* alteration to the target enzymes (*DNA gyrase* and *topoisomerase IV* enzyme).

### Key Features

- Excellent oral bioavailability with absorption of oral agents often equivalent to intravenous.
- *Four generations* of agents (mild differences).
- *First* generation (e.g., oxlonic acid, rosoxacin) – no longer used.
- *Second* generation (e.g., Ciprofloxacin, Norfloxacin, Ofloxacin) – most commonly used in urology.
- *Third* generation (e.g., Levofloxacin) – has activity against *Streptococci.*
- *Fourth* generation (e.g., Moxifloxacin) – acts on DNA gyrase and topoisomerase IV making it more useful in resistant strains. May be used in refractory urethritis.
- Not safe in pregnancy and should be avoided in children.
- *Urological uses:* UTI, prostatitis, urethritis, epididymo-orchitis, and skin infections.

### Adverse Effects

- GI upset, central nervous system disturbances (headache, confusion, dizziness, tremor), phototoxicity.
- Prolongation of the QT interval.
- Reduced seizure threshold.
- Tendinopathy and tendon rupture.
- Small increased risk of aortic aneurysm and dissection.

## Nitroimidazoles

- Share similar chemical structure with the organic compound 5-Nitroimidazole (Figure 31.4).

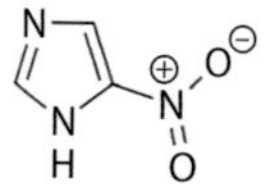

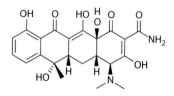

**Figure 31.4** 5-Nitroimidazole.

- May be used to combat both anaerobic bacterial and parasitic infections.

### Mechanism of Action

- Bactericidal – inhibits nucleic acid synthesis by disrupting the DNA of microbial cells.
- *Metabolism:* renal.

### Resistance

- Still being elucidated, likely based around enhanced activity of DNA repair enzymes.

### Key Features

- Useful against anaerobes and facultative anaerobes (e.g., Clostridium, Bacteroides, Gardnerella vaginalis) and some protozoal infections.
- *Examples:* metronidazole (oral and IV) used for both bacterial and protozoal infections; tinidazole (oral) only used for protozoal infections.
- Contraindicated in the *first trimester* and should be used with caution in the *second* and *third trimester*.
- *Urological uses:* bacterial vaginosis, *Trichomonas vaginalis*, prevention of post-operative infections due to anaerobic bacteria, particularly with species of bacteroides and anaerobic streptococci.

### Adverse Effects

- Nausea, a metallic taste, loss of appetite, and headaches.
- Disulfiram-like reaction when consumed with alcohol (flushing, tachycardia, hypotension).

## 3. Inhibitors of protein synthesis

### Tetracyclines

- An old class of antibiotics derived from a species of *Streptomyces* bacteria.
- Their name is derived from their chemical structure containing four hexagonal rings (Figure 31.5).

### Mechanism of Action

- Bacteriostatic – inhibit bacterial protein synthesis via interaction with the 30S subunit of the bacterial ribosome.

**Figure 31.5** Tetracycline containing four hexagonal rings.

### Metabolism

- GI (doxycycline)
- Renal (oxytetracycline, tetracycline, minocycline)

### Resistance

- Tetracycline efflux pumps found in gram-negative enteric bacteria actively pump out antibiotic.
- Ribosomal protection proteins stabilise the ribosome, maintaining protein synthesis.

### Key Features

- Effective against a wide variety of microorganisms, including spirochetes, atypical bacteria, rickettsia, and amoebic parasites.
- *Examples:* doxycycline, oxytetracycline, tetracycline (oral), minocycline (oral or IV).
- Should not be used in children under the age of eight, specifically during periods of tooth development.
- Should not be used in pregnancy.
- *Urological uses:* UTI, epididymo-orchitis, and sexually transmitted infections (STIs) including *chlamydia* and *mycoplasma*.

### Adverse Effects

- GI upset, oesophageal ulceration, sore mouth or tongue.
- May cause skin photosensitivity, increasing the risk of sunburn under exposure to UV light.
- Very rarely causes severe headache and vision problems, which may be signs of dangerous secondary intracranial hypertension.

### Macrolides

- Derived from a type of Streptomyces bacteria.
- Name based on the macrocyclic lactone ring in their chemical structure (Figure 31.6).
- Spectrum and uses are similar to penicillins.

### Mechanism of Action

- Bacteriostatic – target bacterial ribosomes and prevent protein production.
- *Metabolism:* biliary.

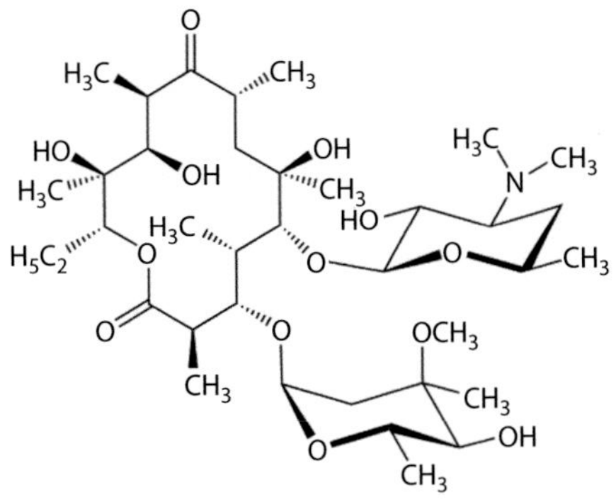

Figure 31.6 Macrocyclic lactone ring. The lactone (cyclic ester) at upper-left is the macrolide ring.

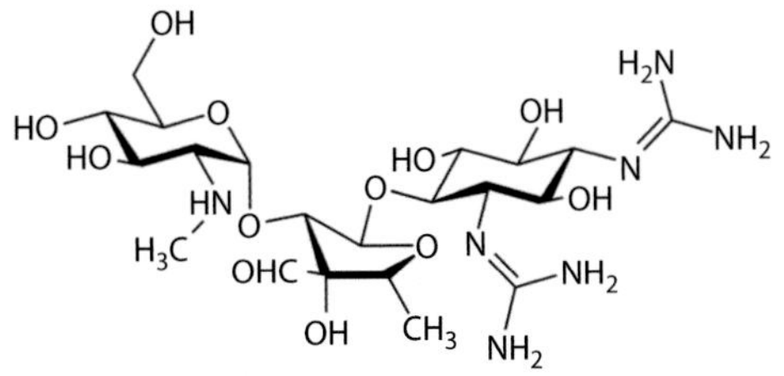

Figure 31.7 Streptomycin containing an amino-modified glycoside (sugar) molecule.

- Some *Pseudomonas aeruginosa* and other gram-negative bacilli have decreased membrane cell permeability to aminoglycosides, leading to moderate resistance.

### Resistance

- Target site modification/mutation to prevent antibiotic binding.
- Macrolide efflux pumps actively pump out antibiotic.

### Key Features

- *Examples:* erythromycin, clarithromycin (oral and IV), azithromycin (oral only).
- Erythromycin is safe during pregnancy.
- Azithromycin may be used if other alternatives are not possible.
- Clarithromycin should not be used in pregnancy.
- *Urological uses:* urethritis, epididymo-orchitis, and STIs including *Neisseria gonorrhoeae*.

### Adverse Effects

- GI upset. It is rarely associated with reversible deafness and allergic reactions.

## Aminoglycosides

- Derived from various species of Streptomyces and Acinetobacter bacteria.
- Named based on the molecule containing an amino-modified glycoside (Figure 31.7).

### Mechanism of Action

- Bactericidal – binds to the 30S subunit of the bacterial ribosome.
- *Metabolism: renal.*

### Resistance

- Alteration/mutation of the ribosomal binding site.
- Direct enzymatic inactivation of the antibiotic.

### Key Features

- Treat infections caused by gram-negative bacteria.
- Often used in combination with beta-lactams to ensure better antimicrobial coverage.
- Broken down in the stomach – cannot be given orally and must be injected/instilled.
- *Examples:* gentamicin, amikacin, neomycin, kanamycin.
- Should not be used during pregnancy unless the benefits outweigh the risks of the medication.
- *Urological uses:* UTIs, gram-negative sepsis.

### Adverse Effects

- Ototoxicity.
  - Vestibulotoxic (gentamicin)
  - Cochleotoxic (amikacin, neomycin, and kanamycin)
- Nephrotoxicity related to the accumulation of high concentrations of aminoglycoside antibiotic in the renal cortex.
- Concentrations commonly monitored using the *Hartford* nomogram:
  - Based on ideal body weight, height, gender, and creatinine clearance of >30 mL/min.

## 4. Others

- Three antibiotics commonly used in urology fall into classes of their own.
  - Nitrofurantoin
  - Trimethoprim
  - Fosfomycin

### Nitrofurantoin

- Low resistance and few interactions with other medications make it a popular choice for lower UTIs.

- Sometimes referred to as a *'urinary tract antiseptic'* because it has very poor tissue penetration and low plasma concentrations, which are not suitable for treating upper UTIs.

## Mechanism of Action

- Bactericidal – activated inside bacteria to unstable metabolites → disrupt ribosomal RNA, DNA, and other intracellular components.

## Metabolism

- Renal.
- Not suitable for patients with poor renal function who are unlikely to produce therapeutic concentrations of drug in their urine.

## Resistance

- Relatively uncommon due to multiple target sites.
- Resistance is likely associated with efflux pumps.

## Key Features

- Concentrates in urine and works best on bacteria present in acidic urine.
- Active against most gram-positive cocci and *E.coli*, but has poor activity against *Proteus* and *Klebsiella*, which are naturally resistant.
- Avoid during the *third trimester* of pregnancy because it may produce neonatal haemolysis.
- *Urological uses:* lower UTI.
- Adults and children that have been prescribed with it long-term require therapy monitoring.
  - Monitor liver function and pulmonary symptoms, especially in the elderly (discontinue if lung function deteriorates).

## Adverse Effects

- GI disturbances, hypersensitivity.
- Rarely: hepatotoxicity, peripheral neuropathy, and pulmonary fibrosis.

## Trimethoprim

- In use since the 1960s and is originally synthesised to potentiate activity of sulphonamides (a pre-penicillin antimicrobial) by sequential inhibition of folic acid synthesis.
- May be combined with sulphonamide, sulfamethoxazole as *Co-Trimoxazole* (Septrin), which is rarely used in the UK due to adverse effects.

## Mechanism of Action

- Bacteriostatic – inhibits *dihydrofolate reductase* (the enzyme required for folate production in bacteria).
- Folate action leads to interaction with methotrexate.
- *Metabolism: renal – need to reduce dose in renal failure.*

## Resistance

- Increased production or alterations in the dihydrofolate reductase binding site.

## Key Features

- Well absorbed when administered orally.
- Reaches high concentrations in the kidney.
- Active against gram-positive and gram-negative bacteria.
- Increasing resistance due to previously frequent usage as 1st line for treatment for UTI in the community.
- Teratogenic risk during the *first trimester* (folate antagonist).
- *Urological uses:* UTI, epididymo-orchitis, some types of urethritis.
- Trimethoprim inhibits tubular creatinine secretion leading to rapid but reversible rise in serum creatinine, particularly in the elderly and those with chronic kidney disease.

## Adverse Effects

- GI disturbance, rashes, hyperkalaemia, blood disorders

## Fosfomycin

- Old antibiotic from the 1960s.
- Phosphoenolpyruvate (PEP) analogue that is produced by Streptomyces.

## Mechanism of Action

- Bactericidal – inhibits cell wall synthesis by impeding the formation of *N*-acetylmuramic acid (a component of bacterial cell wall).
- This mechanism is a step prior to that inhibited by beta-lactam antibiotics.
- *Metabolism: Renal*

## Resistance

- Relatively low resistance.
- Target site mutation.
- Membrane transporter modification leading to decreased uptake.

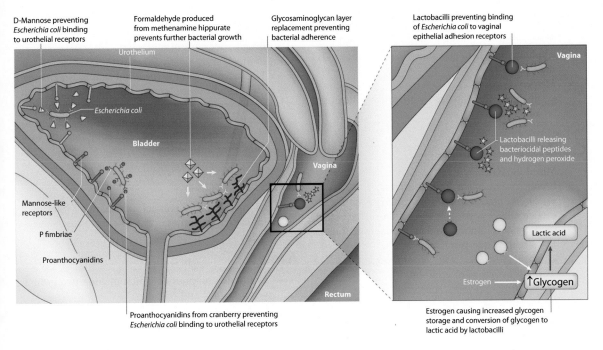

**Figure 31.8** Non-antibiotic interventions for urinary tract infection. (Reprinted by permission from Springer Nature [4])

## Key Features

- Active against a range of gram-positive and gram-negative bacteria, including *Staphylococcus aureus* and *Enterobacteriaceae.*
- Only to be used in pregnancy if the potential benefits outweigh the risks.
- *Urological uses:* lower UTIs.

## Adverse Effects

- Mild electrolyte imbalances (e.g., hypernatremia, hypokalaemia), diarrhoea.

# Non-Antibiotic Treatments for Cystitis and Recurrent UTIs

- With increasing levels of bacterial resistance, there is a drive to reduce the quantity of antibiotics used particularly in the prophylaxis of UTIs.
- Figure 31.8 summarises the current non-antibiotic interventions.

## D-Mannose

- Naturally occurring sugar found in many foods (e.g., cranberries).
- Reduces the adherence of bacteria to the urothelium.
  - Competes for and blocks FimH adhesin.

- Inhibits Type 1 fimbria of uropathogenic bacteria to the uroepithelial cells.
- *Preparation:* tablets or powder sprinkled over food/tea.

## Methenamine Hippurate

- Methenamine Hippurate acts as a urinary tract *antiseptic.*
- The *methenamine* component is hydrolysed to formaldehyde in acidic urine, which is highly bactericidal.
- The *hippuric acid* component has some antibacterial activity and helps keep the urine acidic.
- Often taken in conjunction with *ascorbic acid* to further help acidify the urine.
- *Adverse effects* are uncommon but include epigastric discomfort and skin reactions.

## Oestrogens

- Vaginal use has been shown to reduce UTI recurrence in postmenopausal women.
- Oestrogen receptors are found in the urinary bladder and vagina.
- *Mechanisms:*
  - Increase the proportion of glycogen-producing vaginal epithelial cells.

## Intravesical Glycosaminoglycans (GAG)

- Intravesical hyaluronic acid and chondroitin sulphate have been shown to reduce UTI recurrence rates.
- *Mechanisms:*
  - Replaces the GAG layer to prevent bacterial adherence.

## Cranberry

- Mixed evidence.
- Cranberry is a plant from the family Ericaceae – *Vaccinium macrocarpon/oxycoccos/erythocarpum.*
  - Contains water, fructose, ascorbic acid, flavonoids, anthocyanidins, proanthocyanidins, catechins, triterpenoids.
  - *Anthocyanidins* and *proanthocyanidins* are the most relevant components.
- *Mechanism:* prevents bacterial adherence to urothelium.
  - *Fructose* – mannose-specific type 1 fimbriae.
  - *Proanthocyanidins* – type p pili.

## Probiotics

- Live microorganisms.
- Augments normal flora.
- *Lactobacillus* – predominant commensal organisms in the vaginal/periurethral areas.
- *Mechanisms:*
  - Competitive inhibition of uropathogens binding to vaginal epithelial cells.
  - Conversion of glycogen into bacteriocins, hydrogen peroxide, and lactic acid (acidic environment).

## B) Anti-Fungals

- In urology, anti-fungals/anti-mycotics are most frequently used to treat *Candida* infections.
- Other fungi may also be encountered particularly in immunocompromised patients.
- Candida commonly affects genital tissues but can also be found in the urine, particularly in the presence of a urological devices (e.g., a catheter or stent).
- Treatment can be used systemically or locally.
- Two classes of anti-fungals are primarily used in urological practice:
  - Polyenes and azoles

## Polyenes

- Bind to ergosterol in the fungal cell membrane → form pores that disrupt electrolyte balance

### Key Features

- Broad spectrum of efficacy.
- *Route of elimination:* GI (largely unabsorbed).
- This topical agent is regarded safe in pregnancy.
- *Urological uses:* treatment of vaginal and oropharyngeal candidiasis, chemical dermatitis ('nappy rash'), prophylactic administration in immunosuppression or in conjunction with long term antibiotic prophylaxis.

### Adverse Effects

- GI symptoms, contact dermatitis (Stevens–Johnson syndrome).

## Azoles

- Synthetic compounds which include two groups – imidazoles and triazoles.

### Mechanism of Action

- Inhibition of lanosterol 14-alpha-demethylase – an enzyme required for the synthesis of ergosterol (main component of fungal cell membranes).

## Imidazoles

### Key Features

- Used primarily as local preparations to treat vulvovaginal and penile Candidiasis.
- *Examples:* topical clotrimazole, econazole, miconazole, ketoconazole (oral), and miconazole (IV for systemic therapy).
- *Route of elimination:* mostly biliary, slightly renal.
- Ketoconazole has poor renal excretion and low urinary levels, limiting urological usage.
- Oral agents are not recommended in pregnancy.

## Triazoles

### Key Features

- Used systemically to treat a variety of fungal infections, including vulvovaginal and penile Candidiasis plus urinary tract fungal infections.
- *Examples:* itraconazole and fluconazole (oral and IV).
- *Route of elimination:* renal.
- Not recommended in pregnancy.
- *Urological uses:* fluconazole for the treatment of UTIs caused by Candida, Torulopsis, and

Cryptococcus; Itraconazole for infections caused by Candida, Aspergilla, Blastomyces, Coccidioides, Histoplasma, and Sporotrichosi. Itraconazole is used for vulvovaginal candidiasis but not commonly for urinary tract fungal infections.

# C) Anti-Parasitics

## Anthelmintics

### I. Praziquantel

- Used to treat infections caused by parasitic worms.
- Also used as 'preventive chemotherapy' programmes, distributing the drug to school-aged children/at-risk population.

#### Key Features

- Increases the permeability of the membranes of schistosome cells towards calcium ions which results in contraction of the parasites, resulting in paralysis in the contracted state.
- *Route of elimination:* renal (but metabolised in liver).
- Believed to be safe during pregnancy.
- *Urological uses:* schistosomiasis.

#### Adverse Effects

- Poor coordination, abdominal pain, vomiting, headache, and allergic reactions.

### II. Albendazole

- Used to treat infections caused by parasitic worms.
- Broad spectrum.

#### Key Features

- Causes degenerative alterations in the intestinal cells of the worm by binding to the colchicine-sensitive site of β-tubulin, preventing assembly into the microtubules. Also results in impaired uptake of glucose by the larval and adult stages of the susceptible parasites.
- *Route of elimination:* biliary.
- Should be avoided in pregnancy.
- *Urological uses:* lymphatic filariasis and elephantiasis caused by Wuchereria bancrofti. Hydatid disease of the urinary tract by Echinococcus granulosus.

#### Adverse Effects

- GI upset, headache, dizziness, reversible hair loss, elevated liver enzymes.
- Rarely leukopenia, hepatitis, acute liver failure and acute kidney injury, irreversible bone marrow suppression.

## Anti-Protozoals

- Metronidazole and tinidazole (see nitroimidazoles).

## Recommended Reading

1. Goering R, Dockrell HM, Zuckerman M, Chiodini P. Mim's Medical Microbiology and Immunobiology, 6th Edition. Elsevier. 2018.
2. Mulvey MR, Simor AE. Antimicrobial resistance in hospitals: how concerned should we be? CMAJ. 2009;180(4) 408–15.
3. Wright GD. Q&A: Antibiotic resistance: where does it come from and what can we do about it? BMC Biol. 2010.8:123.
4. Sihra N, Goodman A, Zakri R et al. Nonantibiotic prevention and management of recurrent urinary tract infection. Nat Rev Urol. 2018; 15(12)750–76.

# 32 Blood Products and Antithrombotic Agents

*Karl H. Pang and Michael Laffan*

## Blood Products

- Blood products are obtained from volunteer donors.
- Whole blood donations: ~405–495 mL (mean 470 mL) collected into 63 mL of citrate phosphate dextrose (CPD) anticoagulant.
- Processed into components: red blood cells, platelets, plasma, cryoprecipitate (Table 32.1).
- Some components — mainly platelets in the UK — are also collected by pheresis.
- *Indications:*
  - *Red blood cells* - blood loss, anaemia
  - *Platelets* - thrombocytopenia, platelet dysfunction, or reversal of antiplatelet treatment
  - *Plasma* - used primarily for coagulation components
    - Disseminated intravascular coagulation (DIC)
    - Major haemorrhage to avoid dilutional coagulopathy
    - Some clotting factor deficiency disorders (e.g., Factor V deficiency).
    - Liver disease (multiple factor deficiency)
  - *Cryoprecipitate* - Von Willebrand factor (VWF), Fibrinogen, FVIII, FXIII
    - Primarily used for fibrinogen replacement
- Blood is filtered to remove white blood cells to leave $<1 \times 10^6$ in the pack.
  - Reduces vCJD infection.
  - Reduces the incidence of febrile transfusion reactions and alloimmunisation to white cell antigens and HLA.
- *Tested for:*
  - HIV, Hepatitis B/C/E, HTLV
  - Syphilis
  - ABO and RhD
  - Some donations are also tested for CMV, malaria, West Nile Virus, Trypanosoma cruzi

## Pharmacology of Antithrombotic Agents

### Antiplatelet Agents (Table 32.2)

- Prevent platelet adhesion, activation, and aggregation.
- *Uses:* prevent thrombotic events in high-risk groups (e.g., coronary artery disease, cerebral vascular disease, peripheral vascular disease).
- Increases the risk of bleeding in high-risk surgery.
- Mechanism of action is shown in Figure 32.1.

### Cyclooxygenase (COX) Inhibitor

- *Example:* acetylsalicylic acid (aspirin)
- *Uses:*
  - Secondary prevention of cardiovascular disease
  - Management of acute coronary syndrome (ACS)
  - Transient ischaemic attack (TIA)
  - Ischaemic stroke (not secondary to atrial fibrillation or AF)
- Low dose aspirin inhibits COX-1 in platelets in the portal circulation. It is then metabolised in the liver and very little enters the systemic circulation.
- Inhibition of COX prevents platelets from synthesising *thromboxane A2.*
- Platelets cannot synthesise COX and so remain inhibited for the rest of their life span.
- High dose aspirin enters the circulation and inhibits both COX-1 and COX-2 in other tissues producing anti-inflammatory and analgesic effects.

### P2Y12 Receptor Antagonists

- *Examples:* clopidogrel, prasugrel, ticagrelor
- *Uses:*
  - TIA
  - Ischaemic stroke
  - Peripheral arterial disease
  - ACS, myocardial infarction
- Inhibit P2Y12 receptor (G-protein receptor for ADP).
- Inhibiting ADP results in reduced intracellular signalling and platelet activation.
- *Thienopyridines* (clopidogrel, prasugrel) need biotransformation to become active.
  - Hydrolysed by esterases and undergo oxidation by hepatic cytochrome P450 isoenzymes to form the active metabolite.

**Table 32.1** Characteristics of blood components

| Characteristics | Red Cells | Pooled Platelets | Plateletpheresis | Fresh Frozen Plasma |
|---|---|---|---|---|
| Number of donor | 1 | 4 | 1 | 1 |
| Volume (mL) | 220–340 | mean 300 | mean 199 | mean 274 |
| Content | Hb >40 gHct 0.5–0.7 | $308 \times 10^9$ per unit | $280 \times 10^9$ per unit | mean 83 IU/mL Factor VIIIc |
| Additions | SAG-M, CPD | CPD | ACD | CPD |
| Storage temperature | 2–6 °C | 20–24 °C | 20–24 °C | under −25 °C |
| Shelf life from donation | up to 35 days | 5 days | 5 days | 36 months (24 h at 4 °C after thawing) |

*Abbreviations:* Hb, haemoglobin; Hct, haematocrit; CPD, citrate phosphate dextrose; SAG-M, saline, adenine, glucose, mannitol additive solution; ACD, acid citrate dextrose.

- The metabolite binds covalently and irreversibly to the P2Y12 receptor.
- Ticagrelor-cyclopentyltriazolopyrimidine (non-thienopyridine).
  - Reversible, non-competitive antagonist of the ADP receptor.

## Glycoprotein IIb/IIIa Antagonists

- *Examples:* abciximab, tirofiban, eptifibatide
- *Uses:* ACS
- Glycoprotein IIbIIIa is the most abundant protein on the platelet surface.
- Prevents platelet aggregation.

## Other Antiplatelet Agents

- *Phosphodiesterase inhibitors*
  - Cilostazol and dipyridamole
  - Interfere with the degradation of cyclic adenosine monophosphate and cyclic guanosine monophosphate in platelets and on endothelial cell (EC) surface.
- *Antiplatelet side effects*
  - Bleeding
  - Gastrointestinal irritation
- *Antiplatelet reversal*
  - The most commonly used antiplatelet agents are clopidogrel and aspirin, both are irreversible.
  - After discontinuation, it takes 5-7 days for normal platelet function to occur via the synthesis of new, uninhibited platelets.
  - Platelet transfusion may be used if urgent, but in a major study of intracerebral haemorrhage, this resulted in poorer outcomes.
  - Tranexamic acid (anti-fibrinolytic): amino acid lysine → bind plasminogen lysine receptors → reduces conversion to plasmin → prevents fibrin degradation.

## Anticoagulants (Table 32.3)

- Target the coagulation cascade to reduce thrombin generation.

### Vitamin K Antagonist (VKA)

- *Example:* warfarin
- *Uses:* Prophylaxis of thromboembolism
  - AF
  - Prosthetic heart valves
  - Venous thromboembolism (VTE, prophylaxis, and/or treatment)
  - Arterial thrombosis, including left ventricular thrombus
- Disrupts the formation of clotting factors II, VII, IX, X, and Proteins C and S.
- Mean plasma half-life ~40h.
- It is an indirect anticoagulant and the onset of action depends on fall in levels of II, VII, IX, and X according to their half-lives.
- Inactivation and metabolism via CYP2C9, CYP1A1, CYP3A4. No renal dependence.
- The dose-response varies widely between patients and from time to time in any individual patient. Therefore, it is essential to monitor the achieved anticoagulant effect using the INR.
- *Reversal:*
  - Coagulation will take approximately five days to return to normal after discontinuation of warfarin.
  - Vitamin K (takes ~6h if given IV and ~24h if given orally).
  - Prothrombin complex concentrate (PCC) - contains factors II, VII, IX, X. This has an immediate effect but of limited duration; therefore, it is usually combined with Vitamin K.

**Table 32.2** Characteristics of a) oral and b) intravenous (IV) antiplatelets

| a) Characteristic | Aspirin | Clopidogrel | Prasugrel | Ticagrelor |
|---|---|---|---|---|
| Mechanism | COX-1 inhibitor | P2Y12 receptor antagonists | | |
| Bioavailability | 68% | 50% | 80% | 36% |
| Time to plasma peak concentration | 30–40 min | 1 h | 30 min | 1.5 h |
| Time to plasma steady-state | | 2–8 h | 30 min to 4 h | 30 min to 2 h |
| Plasma half-life | 15–30 min | 8 h, active metabolite ~30 min | 7 h | 7 h |
| Plasma protein binding | Strong | Strong | Strong | Strong |
| Time from last dose to offset | 7–10 days | 7–10 days | 7–10 days | 5 days |
| Reversibility of platelet inhibition | No | No | No | Yes |
| Discontinuation before surgical intervention | 0–5 days | 7 days | 10 days | 7 days |

| b) Characteristic | Cangrelor | Abciximab | Eptifibatide | Tirofiban |
|---|---|---|---|---|
| Mechanism | P2Y12 receptor antagonist | Glycoprotein IIb/IIIa inhibitor | | |
| Plasma peak concentration | Seconds | Dose-dependent | Dose-dependent | Dose-dependent |
| Time to plasma steady-state | Seconds | Initial bolus and continuous application | Initial bolus and continuous application 4–6 h | Initial bolus and continuous application 10 min |
| Plasma half-life | 2–5 min | 10–15 min | 2.5 h | 2 h |
| Time from last dose to offset | 60 min | 12 h | 2–4 h | 2–4 h |
| Reversibility of platelet inhibition | Yes | Yes | Yes | Yes |
| Discontinuation before surgical intervention | 1–6 h | 48 h | 8 h | 8 h |

## Non-VKA Oral Anticoagulants

- Also known as novel oral anticoagulants (NOAC) or direct oral anticoagulants (DOAC).
- *Uses:*
  - Treatment of VTE
  - Prophylaxis of recurrent or postoperative VTE
  - Prophylaxis of stroke and embolism from atrial fibrillation
  - Prophylaxis of atherothrombotic events in combination with aspirin
    - ACS, coronary artery disease
    - Peripheral artery disease
- Directly inhibit factor IIa/thrombin (dabigatran) or Xa (rivaroxaban, apixaban, edoxaban).
- Faster onset and offset of action than warfarin.
- Routine blood monitoring not necessary.
  - Specific assays are available if needed.
- All DOACs are dependent on renal excretion to some degree (unlike warfarin). Caution and dose adjustment may be needed.
- *Reversal:*
  - Only dabigatran (IIa inhibitor) has a reversal agent — *idarucizumab*.
  - Xa inhibitors are not easily reversed, but fortunately, have a short half-life.

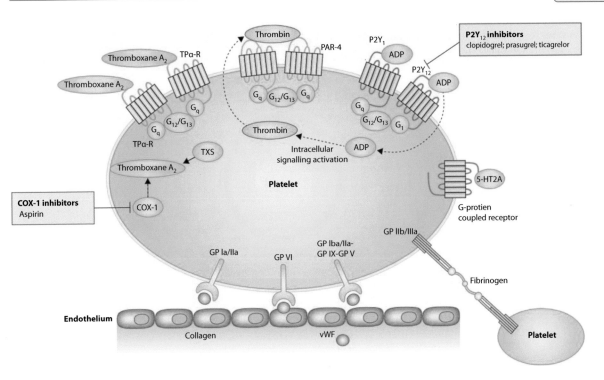

Figure 32.1 Platelet pathways and commonly used oral antiplatelet treatments. Disruption of the endothelium exposes adhesive proteins of the subendothelial matrix (collagen and von Willebrand factor [vWF]) that interact with platelet-receptor glycoproteins (GP). Intracellular signalling pathways result in the release of robust platelet activators such as ADP, adrenaline, serotonin, thrombin, and thromboxane A2. These agonists bind to G-protein-coupled receptors and further potentiate the process. Ultimately, GP IIb/IIIa binds to fibrinogen and results in platelet aggregation. ADP, adenosine 5'-diphosphate; 5-HT2A, serotonin receptor 2A; COX-1, cyclooxygenase 1; PAR, protease-activated receptor; TP-R, thromboxane prostanoid receptor; TXS, thromboxane A2 synthase; G, G-protein. Dotted arrows show the movement of molecules. (Reprinted with permission from Elsevier [2])

- *PCC* or *recombinant factor VIIa* may be considered.
- A specific reversal agent — 'Andexanet' — has been licensed in the USA and Europe and is approved by NICE only for major GI haemorrhage.

## Parenteral Anticoagulants

- *Examples:* unfractionated heparin (UFH) and low molecular weight heparin (LMWH).
- *Uses of UFH:*
  - Therapeutic doses of UFH given by intravenous infusion require intensive monitoring. It is used when renal failure precludes LMWH use or when rapid reversal may be needed.
  - Almost any high-risk thrombotic situation
  - Treatment of VTE
  - Acute peripheral arterial occlusion
  - Prosthetic valves
- *Problems with UFH:*

- Complicated pharmacokinetics
- Requires intensive monitoring
- Heparin-induced thrombocytopenia and thrombosis
- *Uses of LMWH:*
  - Has a more reliable dose-response than UFH and is given subcutaneously in a therapeutic weight-adjusted dose without the need for monitoring.
  - Prophylactic dose may be fixed, but adjustments according to renal function and weight are being introduced.
  - Therapeutic doses require adequate renal function. If this is not adequate, then monitoring or switching to UFH is required.
  - Used in VTE treatment and prophylaxis.
- *Problems of LMWH:*
  - Renal dependent excretion.
  - Only partially reversible by protamine.
  - Heparin-induced thrombocytopenia (HIT) and thrombosis, although less than UFH.

**Table 32.3** Characteristics of a) oral and b) parenteral anticoagulants.

| a) Characteristic | Warfarin | Dabigatran | Apixaban | Edoxaban | Rivaroxaban |
|---|---|---|---|---|---|
| Mechanism of action | Vitamin K antagonist | Direct inhibition IIa | Direct inhibition Xa | | |
| Bioavailability (%) | 80 | 6 | 66 | 62 | 80 |
| Plasma half-life | 20–60 h | 12–14 h | 8–15 h | 10–14 h | 7–10 h |
| Duration of action from last dose | 48–96 h | 48 h | 24 h | 24 h | 24 h |
| Tmax | Variable | 2 h | 2.5–4 h | 1–2 h | 1–3 h |
| Elimination | Metabolism | 80% renal | 25% renal | 50% renal | 50% renal, 50% hepatic |
| Drug interaction | CYP2C9, CYP3A4, CYP1A2 | P-glycoprotein inhibitors | CYP3Y4, P-glycoprotein inhibitors | P-glycoprotein inhibitors | CYP3A4 inhibitors or inducers and P-glycoprotein inhibitors |
| Discontinuation before surgical intervention (depends on bleeding risk and renal function) | 3-5 d (+/- bridge with LMWH) | 48–72 h | 48–72 h | 48–72 h | 36–72 h |

| b) Characteristic | UFH (s.c./i.v) | LMWH (s.c) | Fondaparinux (s.c) | Argatroban (i.v) | Bivalirudin (i.v) |
|---|---|---|---|---|---|
| Mechanism of action | Indirect inhibition Xa = IIa | Indirect inhibition Xa > IIa | Indirect inhibition Xa | Direct inhibition IIa | |
| Bioavailability (%) | 30 (sc) | 90 | 100 | 100 | 100 |
| Plasma half-life | 1 h | 4 h | 17 h | 50 min | 24 min |
| Duration of action from last dose | Dose-dependent (s.c.) | Dose-dependent | 48–96 h | 2–4 h | 1 h |
| Peak plasma concentration | 4 h (s.c.) | 3 h | 2 h | | 0.25–2 h |
| Elimination | Reticulo-endothelial system and renal | Hepatic metabolism, renal excretion 10% | Renal | 65% faeces, 22% urine | 20% renal |

*Abbreviations:* s.c, subcutaneous; i.v, intravenous; UFH, unfractionated heparin; LMWH, low molecular weight heparin, Tmax, time taken to reach maximum concentration

- A longer half-life than UFH and subcutaneous administration gives the extended duration of effect.
- LMWH contains shorter polymers than UFH.
- Heparins bind to and potentiate antithrombin.
  - Antithrombin inactivates clotting factors IIa, IXa, Xa, XIa, XIIa

- *Reversal:*
  - UFH has a short half-life of 60–90 minutes and can be completely reversed using protamine (1 mg neutralises 100 u).
  - LMWH are only partially reversible with protamine (on average ~50%) plus the subcutaneous administration acts as a depot.

## Anticoagulants Side Effects:

- Bleeding
- Gastrointestinal
- HIT (heparin) - an immune-mediated highly thrombotic condition requiring immediate cessation of all heparin exposure and use of an alternative anticoagulant (e.g., argatroban).

# Thromboprophylaxis Pre- and Post-Surgery

- Surgery induces a hypercoagulable state, increasing the risk of VTE (see Virchow's triad) and of bleeding. The challenge is to achieve the optimum balance between these two opposing risks.
- Cumulative risk during the first four weeks post-surgery:

**(DH) Depaetment of Health**

## RISK ASSESSMENT FOR VENOUS THROMBOEMBOLISM (VTE)

| Mobility - all patients (tick one box ) | Tick | | Tick | | Tick |
|---|---|---|---|---|---|
| Surgical patient | | Medical patient expected to have ongoing reduced mobility relative to normal state | | Medical patient NOT expected to have significantly reduced mobility relative to normal state | |
| **Assess for thrombosis and bleeding risk below** | | | | **Risk assessment now complete** | |

| **Thrombosis risk** | | | |
|---|---|---|---|
| **Patient related** | Tick | **Admission related** | Tick |
| Active cancer or cancer treatment | | Significantly reduced mobility for 3 days or more | |
| Age > 60 | | Hip or knee replacement | |
| Dehydration | | Hip fracture | |
| Known thrombophilias | | Total anaesthetic + surgical time > 90 minutes | |
| Obesity (BMI >30 kg/m$^2$) | | Surgery involving pelvis or lower limb with a total anaesthetic + surgical time > 60 minutes | |
| One or more significant medical comorbidities (eg heart disease; metabolic, endocrine or respiratory pathologies; acute infectious diseases; inflammatory conditions) | | Acute surgical admission with inflammatory or intra-abdominal condition | |
| Personal history or first-degree relative with a history of VTE | | Critical care admission | |
| Use of hormone replacement therapy | | Surgery with significant reduction in mobility | |
| Use of oestrogen-containing contraceptive therapy | | | |
| Varicose veins with phlebits | | | |
| Pregnancy or < 6 weeks post partum (see NICE guidance for specific risk factors) | | | |

| **Bleeding risk** | | | |
|---|---|---|---|
| **Patient related** | Tick | **Admission related** | Tick |
| Active bleeding | | Neurosurgery, spinal surgery or eye surgery | |
| Acquired bleeding disorders (such as acute liver failure) | | Other procedure with high bleeding risk | |
| Concurrent use of anticoagulants known to increase the risk of bleeding (such as warfarin with INR >2) | | Lumber puncture/epidural/spinal anaesthesia expected within the next 12 hours | |
| Acute stroke | | Lumber puncture/epidural/spinal anaesthesia within the previous 4 hours | |
| Thrombocytopaenia (platelets< 75x10$^9$/l) | | | |
| Uncontrolled systolic hyperyension (230/120 mmHg or higher) | | | |
| Untreated inherited bleeding disorders (such as haemophilia and von Willebrand's disease) | | | |

Figure 32.2 Department of health risk assessment for venous thromboembolism tool. (Adapted from NICE Guidelines [7])

- ~50% of major bleeds occur between surgery and the next morning, and ~90% during the first four postoperative days.
  - The risk of VTE is almost constant during the first four postoperative weeks.
- LMWH reduces the relative risk of VTE by ~50% and increases the relative risk of major bleeding by ~50%.
- The Department of Health Risk Assessment for Venous Thromboembolism Tool is frequently used in the UK (Figure 32.2) and all patients should be risk assessed on admission to the hospital.
- The *NICE 2018* (updated August 2019, https://www.nice.org.uk/guidance/ng89) guidelines include:
  - Offer VTE prophylaxis to those undergoing abdominal (including urological) surgery who are at risk of VTE.
  - Consider 28 days postoperative pharmacological VTE prophylaxis for major cancer surgery (e.g., cystectomy).
  - Prophylaxis should usually comprise
    - Mechanical prophylaxis: anti-embolism stockings or intermittent pneumatic compression.
    - Pharmacological prophylaxis: usually LMWH.
- Patients already on therapeutic anticoagulation before surgery will need to have this discontinued and may require bridging according to the estimation of risk (British Society for Haematology guidelines).

## Recommended Reading

1. Blood products, Transfusion handbook. Joint United Kingdom blood transfusion and tissue transplantation services professional advisory committee.
2. Mega JL and Simon T. Pharmacology of antithrombotic drugs: an assessment of oral antiplatelet anticoagulant treatments. Lancet. 2015;386(9990)281–291.
3. Koenig-Oberhuber V and Filipovic M. New antiplatelet drugs and new oral anticoagulants. Br J Anaesth. 2016;117 Suppl 2:ii74–ii84.
4. Ellis G, Camm AJ, Datta SN. Novel anticoagulants and antiplatelet agents; a guide for the urologist. BJU Int. 2015;116(5):687–696.
5. Tikkinen KAO et al. Systematic review of observational studies of risk of thrombosis and bleeding in urological surgery (ROTBUS): introduction and methodology. Syst Rev. 2014;3:150.
6. Tikkinen KAO et al. Thromboprophylaxis in Urological Surgery. EAU Guidelines. 2017.
7. Venous thromboembolism in over 16s: reducing the risk of hospital-acquired deep vein thrombosis or pulmonary embolism. NICE Guidelines (NG89). Updated Aug 2019.
8. Violette PD et al. Guideline of guidelines: thromboprophylaxis for urological surgery. BJU Int. 2016;118(3): 351–358.
9. Keeling D, Campbell Tait R, Watson H. Peri-operative management of anticoagulation and antiplatelet therapy. Br J Haematol. 2016;175(4):602–613.

# 33 | Urological Anti-cancer Agents

*Bernadett Szabados and Thomas Powles*

## A) Cytostatic Agents

- Cytostatic agents are plant-derived or synthetic substances that intervene during the cell cycle and inhibit cell growth or cell division.

## Cell Cycle

- DNA replication and division of cytoplasm and organelles.
- Production of two separate daughter cells.
- *Four phases:*
  - G1 phase
  - S phase (synthesis)
  - G2 phase (G1 + S + G2 collectively known as interphase)
  - M phase (mitosis)
- *Interphase* = cell growth.
  - *G1 phase* (Post mitotic gap phase). The cell growth begins after mitosis, with the production of cytoplasm and extra organelles.
  - *S phase* = DNA replication.
  - *G2 phase* = preparation for mitosis; production of microtubules.
  - *M Phase* (Mitotic phase) = active cell division.

## Classification of Cytostatic Agents

- Classified based on their mechanisms of action (Figure 33.1).

### Alkylating Agents (Ifosfamide, Cyclophosphamide, Estramustine)

- Disruption of the G1 phase.
- Attachment of an alkyl group to the guanine base of DNA → DNA strands are unable to separate and duplicate

### Platinum Analogues (Cisplatin, Carboplatin, Oxaliplatin)

- Disruption of G1 phase.
- Creation of extra bonds between two DNA bases → crosslink inhibits DNA repair and/or DNA synthesis in cells

### Antimetabolites (Gemcitabine, Methotrexate)

- Disruption of S phase.
- Incorporation of chemically altered nucleotides in DNA or RNA.
- *Subgroups:*
  - Anti-folates (Methotrexate and Pemetrexed)
  - Purine analogues (Azathioprine)
  - Pyrimidine analogue (Gemcitabine, 5-Fluorouracil)

### Anti-Microtubule Agents (Paclitaxel, Vinblastine)

- Disruption of mitosis.
- Subgroups:
  - *Vinca alkaloids* (Vinblastine, Vincristine)
    - Prevent the formation of microtubules → inhibition of cell division
  - *Taxanes* (Paclitaxel, Docetaxel)
    - Prevent microtubule disassembly → prevents completion of mitosis

### Topoisomerase Inhibitors I (Topotecan) and II (Etoposide)

- Disruption of G2 phase.
- Topoisomerase produces single- or double-strand breaks in DNA.
- Its spontaneous reassembly allows the normal unwinding of DNA.

### DNA Intercalation (Anthracyclines: Doxorubicin, Adriamycin)

- Disruption of the G1, G2, and M phases.
- Insertion of ligands between two strands of DNA → prevent DNA polymerases binding

### Cytotoxic Antibiotics (Bleomycin, Mitomycin-C)

- Disruption of the G1, G2, and M phases.

**Table 33.1** Overview of Urological Cancer Drugs and NICE Approved First-Line Treatment Regimens

| Cancer | Therapeutic Agents | NICE Approved First-Line Treatment Regimens In The Metastatic Setting |
|---|---|---|
| Urothelial Carcinoma | Intravesical chemotherapy: MMC, gemcitabine | Gemcitabine/Cisplatin (for cisplatin eligible) |
| | Intravesical immunotherapy: BCG | |
| | Intravenous chemotherapy:<br>• Gemcitabine – Cisplatin/Carboplatin<br>• MVAC: Methotrexate, Vinblastine, Adriamycin, Cisplatin<br>• MVEC: Methotrexate, Vinblastine, Epirubicin, Cisplatin<br>• Paclitaxel<br>• Vinflunine | Gemcitabine/Carboplatin (if PD-L1 negative and cisplatin-ineligible) |
| | Immune Checkpoint inhibitors: PD-1, PD-L1 inhibitors | PD-1 or PD-L1 if PD-L1 positive |
| Renal Cell Carcinoma | Immunotherapy:<br>• Interferon-α, Interleukin-2<br>• Checkpoint inhibitors: PD-1, PD-L1 inhibitors | Ipilimumab/Nivolumab (IMDC intermediate or poor risk); Axitinib/Avelumab (IMDC good, intermediate and poor risk) |
| | Targeted therapy<br>• TK inhibitors: Sunitinib, Pazopanib, Axitinib, Cabozantinib, Lenvatinib, Tivozanib.<br>• Monoclonal antibody against circulating VEGF: Bevacizumab<br>• mTOR Inhibitors: Everolimus, Temsirolimus | Sunitinib or Pazopanib (IMDC good risk) Cabozantinib (IMDC intermediate and poor risk) |
| Prostate Cancer | Chemotherapy: docetaxel, cabazitaxel<br>Androgen Deprivation Therapy (ADT)<br>• LHRH – agonist: Buserelin, Goserelin, Leuprorelin<br>• LHRH – antagonist: Degarelix<br>• Non-steroidal anti-androgens: Bicalutamide, Flutamide, Abiraterone, Darolutamide<br>• Steroidal anti-androgens: Cyproterone acetate, Enzalutamide, Apalutamide | **Castration-naïve + M0**: observation or ADT<br>**Castration-naïve + M1**: ADT/Abiraterone or ADT/Docetaxel<br>**Castration-resistant + M0**: Enzalutamide or apalutamide<br>**Castration-resistant + M1**: Abiraterone or Enzalutamide or Docetaxel |
| | Oestrogens | |
| Testicular cancer | Chemotherapy:<br>• Carboplatin adjuvant setting BEP: Cisplatin, Etoposide, Bleomycin<br>• PEI: Cisplatin, Etoposide, Ifosfamide<br>• TIP: Paclitaxel, Ifosfamide, Cisplatin<br>• VIP: Vinblastine, Ifosfamide, Cisplatin | 3–4 cycles BEP |
| Penile cancer | Chemotherapy:<br>• Paclitaxel, Ifosfamide, Cisplatin<br>• Paclitaxel, Cisplatin, 5-FU<br>• CMB: Cisplatin, Methotrexate, Bleomycin<br>• VBM: Vincristine, Bleomycin, Methotrexate | Paclitaxel, Ifosfamide, Cisplatin |

*Abbreviations:* MMC, Mitomycin-C; BCG, Bacillus Calmette-Guérin; PD-1, programmed cell death protein 1; PD-L1, programmed cell death ligand 1; TK, tyrosine kinase; VEGF, vascular endothelial growth factor; ADT, androgen deprivation therapy; LHRH, luteinising hormone-releasing hormone; 5-FU, 5-fluorouracil.

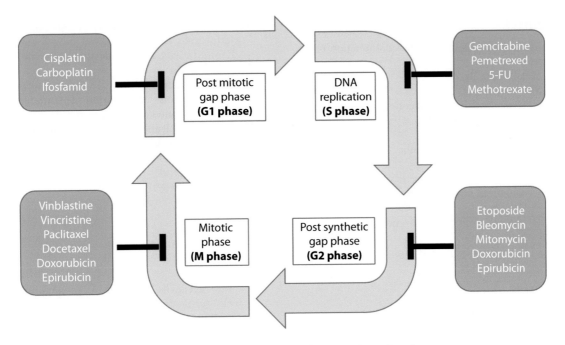

Figure 33.1 Effect of cytostatic drugs on the cell cycle.

- Various mechanisms of action including:
  - DNA intercalation
  - Topoisomerase inhibition
  - DNA alkylation (Mitomycin-C)

## Substance Profiles of Cytostatic Drugs

### Bleomycin

- Mechanism: production of free radicals that cleave DNA.
- Excretion: renal (60–70%).
- *Side effects:*
  - Pulmonary fibrosis and impaired lung function (regular lung function tests and chest x-ray advised)
  - Fever, rash, urticaria, hyperpigmentation, hair loss, Raynaud's phenomenon

### Carboplatin

- Mechanism: crosslinking of DNA between two DNA bases.
- Excretion: renal.
- *Side effects:*
  - Bone marrow suppression, especially thrombocytopenia
  - Nausea and vomiting
  - Neurotoxicity and ototoxicity in high doses
  - Nephrotoxicity

### Cisplatin

- Mechanism: crosslinking of DNA between two DNA bases.
- Excretion: renal (adjust the dose according to creatinine clearance).
- *Side effects:*
  - Ototoxicity (cumulative, dose-dependent)
  - Nephrotoxicity (hypomagnesaemia – first sign of tubulointerstitial nephropathy)
  - Cardiotoxicity: especially in combination with etoposide and bleomycin (PEB regimen for testicular cancer), arrhythmias, myocardial infarction
  - Nausea and vomiting
  - Neurotoxicity
  - Hair loss
  - Bone marrow suppression

### Doxorubicin (Adriamycin)

- Mechanism: DNA intercalation inhibits the progression of topoisomerase II.
- Metabolism: liver.
- *Side effects:*
  - Dilated cardiomyopathy – congestive heart failure (cumulative dose-dependent)
  - Nausea and vomiting
  - Hair loss
  - Hepatotoxicity
  - Dermatitis and stomatitis

## Docetaxel

- Mechanism: disrupts the normal function of the microtubules.
- Metabolism: liver.
- *Side effects:*
  - Hypersensitivity reactions (hypotension, bronchospasm) – accompany with dexamethasone therapy
  - Fluid retention syndrome – accompany with dexamethasone therapy
  - Nail changes and onycholysis – reduce with cooling of fingers and toes during infusion
  - Hair loss
  - Mucositis – reduce with mouthwashes
  - Neutropenia
  - Neurotoxicity (palmar and plantar)

## Etoposide

- Mechanism: topoisomerase inhibitor.
- Excretion: renal.
- *Side effects:*
  - In combination with cisplatin and bleomycin – increased cardiotoxicity (myocardial infarction, arrhythmias)
  - Blood pressures drop after etoposide infusion
  - Nephrotoxicity
  - Neurotoxicity
  - Hepatotoxicity
  - Hair loss

## Gemcitabine

- Mechanism: antimetabolite – pyrimidine analogue.
- Excretion: renal.
- *Side effects:*
  - Flu-like symptoms – myalgia, limb pain, headache – therapy with NSAIDs
  - Bone marrow suppression (neutropenia and thrombocytopenia)
  - Peripheral oedema
  - Pulmonary toxicity (Acute respiratory distress syndrome)
  - Rash, shortness of breath
  - Mouth sores, diarrhoea
  - Neuropathy
  - Hair loss
  - Hepatotoxicity with elevated transaminases

## Methotrexate

- Mechanism: antimetabolite of the antifolate type.
- Excretion: renal.
- *Side effects:*

- Pneumonitis and pulmonary fibrosis (Monitor with regular lung function and chest X-rays)
- Nephrotoxicity; contraindication if creatinine is ≥2 mg/dL
- Hepatotoxicity
- Bone marrow suppression (neutropenia, thrombocytopenia)
- Diarrhoea, ulcerations of the stomach and intestinal mucosa
- Stomatitis
- Dermatological reactions (rash, itching, photosensitivity)

## Paclitaxel

- Mechanism: anti-microtubule agent.
- Metabolism: liver.
- *Side effects:*
  - Hypersensitivity reaction – premedication with dexamethasone or ranitidine
  - Cardiotoxicity – monitoring of cardiac function
  - Hypotonic shock – blood pressure control
  - Neurotoxicity (paraesthesia)
  - Arthralgia and myalgia
  - Hepatotoxicity
  - Bone marrow suppression (neutropenia)

## Vinblastine

- Mechanism: anti-microtubule, which inhibits the assembly of microtubules.
- Excretion: biliary and renal.
- *Side effects:*
  - Ileus – consider spasmolytic and prokinetics
  - Sensorimotor and autonomic neurotoxicity
  - Bone marrow suppression (neutropenia)
  - Hepatotoxicity
  - Dermatitis, stomatitis
  - Myocardial ischaemia, myocardial infarction (coronary spasm).

# Most Common Chemotherapy Regimens in Urological Cancer

## Urothelial Cancer

- Neoadjuvant treatment for muscle-invasive urothelial cancer of the bladder.
  - 3–4 cycles of gemcitabine/cisplatin.
  - One cycle = three weeks
  - W1 day one of each infusion: gemcitabine/cisplatin combined infusion.
  - W2 day one of each infusion: gemcitabine only (booster).
  - W3: treatment break.

- Other common regimens: MVAC
- Metastatic transitional cell carcinoma of the urothelium:
  - Treatment naive, cisplatin eligible: Six cycles of gemcitaine/cisplatin
  - Treatment naive, cisplatin ineligible, PD-L1 negative: Six cycles of gemcitabine/carboplatin (if performance status is poor, GFR <60 mL/min, previous neuropathy, hearing loss or NYHA > 2).
- Other treatment regimens for chemotherapy-refractory patients
  - Weekly paclitaxel
  - Combination of carboplatin/ paclitaxel
  - Participation in clinical trial

## Prostate Cancer

- Castration-naive metastatic prostate cancer.
  - Six cycles of Docetaxel every three weeks.
- Castration-resistant metastatic prostate cancer treated with previous docetaxel.
  - Six cycles of Cabazitaxel every three weeks.

## Testicular Germ Cell Tumours

- High-risk stage I seminoma.
  - One cycle adjuvant, single-agent high-dose carboplatin.
- Advanced testicular germ cell tumours.
  - 3–4 cycles of Bleomycin/Etoposide/Cisplatin (BEP); or
  - Four cycles of Etoposide/cisplatin (EP) if concerned about Bleomycin toxicity.
- Relapsed disease following post-orchiectomy chemotherapy.
  - Etoposide, ifosfamide, and cisplatin (VIP).
- Platinum-refractory disease.
  - Second or subsequent relapse; or
  - Progression during or immediately after initial platinum-based chemotherapy.
  - Paclitaxel/ifosfamide are used followed by high-dose carboplatin plus etoposide with autologous hematopoietic cell transplantation.

## Penile Cancer

- First-line systemic therapy for metastatic/recurrent disease.
  - Paclitaxel, Ifosfamide, Cisplatin every 3–4 weeks.

# B) Intravesical Chemotherapy and Immunotherapy

- The current gold standard treatment:

- Intermediate-risk non-muscle invasive bladder cancer (NMIBC) – intravesical chemo-therapy.
- High-risk NMIBC – intravesical immuno-therapy.

# Intravesical Chemotherapy Instillation

## A Single, Immediate, Post-Operative Instillation

- Mitomycin-C (MMC), epirubicin, gemcitabine or pirarubicin: equivocal effect.
- Destroys circulating tumour cells.
- Significantly reduces the rate of recurrence (~40%) compared to transurethral resection of bladder tumour (TURBT) alone in patients with NMIBC.
- Administered within 24 hours (ideally within six hours) after TURBT.
  - After this period, tumour cells are firmly implanted and are covered by the extra-cellular matrix, making the instillation therapy ineffective.
- Contraindicated if bladder perforation is suspected.

## Additional, Adjuvant Instillations

- Continuation depends on the patient's relapse or progression risk according to the EORTC risk calculator.
- *Intermediate-risk* NMIBC benefit from a course of intravesical chemotherapy.
  - Reduce the risk of recurrence.
  - NICE recommend six MMC instillations.

## Intravesical Mitomycin-C

- Cytotoxic antibiotic is the most commonly used intravesical chemotherapy.
- High molecular weight – risk of systemic absorption and side effects are small (Table 33.2).

## Intravesical Bacillus Calmette–Guérin (BCG) Immunotherapy

- Recommended for *high-risk NMIBC*.
  - Commence at least two weeks after TURBT.
  - Induction course: once weekly for six weeks.
  - Maintenance: three times, once weekly at 3, 6, 12, 18, 24, 30, 36 months (Lamm's protocol).
  - Total duration: three years (27 doses).
- *Mechanism of action.*

**Table 33.2** Toxicity Profile of Intravesical Mitomycin-C

| Frequency of Side Effects | |
|---|---|
| **1–10%** | **<1%** |
| Lower urinary tract infection | Necrotising cystitis |
| Local irritative voiding symptoms (dysuria, increases frequency, nocturia) | Allergic (eosinophilic) cystitis |
| Haematuria | Stenosis of the urinary tract |
| Allergic skin reaction (exanthem, contact dermatitis, palmar/plantar erythema) | Reduction of bladder capacity |

**Table 33.3** Toxicity Profile of Intravesical BCG

| Frequency of Side Effects | | |
|---|---|---|
| **>10%** | **1–10%** | **<1%** |
| Nausea | Fever >38°C | Miliary tuberculosis |
| Urinary tract infection | | Reiter's syndrome (reactive arthritis), conjunctivitis, arthritis, cystitis |
| Pollakisuria, dysuria | | Hepatitis |
| Asymptomatic, bacterial prostatitis | | Skin lesions (exanthema, abscess) |
| Fever <38°C, flu-like symptoms | | Orchitis, epididymitis, symptomatic granulomatous prostatitis |
| General malaise | | Sepsis |

- Infiltrates the bladder mucosa (fibronectin) → granuloma formation with invasion of granulocytes and T lymphocytes (interleukins, TNF-alpha, interferon-gamma) → inflammatory reaction destroying mycobacteria and tumour cells
- Tumours break down → components are recognised by the immune system as foreign body → provokes antibody formation against tumour cells
- Side effects and management of toxicity are shown in Tables 33.3 and 33.4.

# C) Hormonal Therapies

## Androgen Synthesis (Testosterone and 5α-Dihydrotestosterone [DHT])

### Testis

- Testosterone – synthesised from cholesterol in Leydig cells (Figure 33.2).
- Controlled by the luteinising hormone (LH) produced by the pituitary gland.
  - LH is controlled by the hypothalamic gonadotropin-releasing hormone (GnRH).
  - LH is inhibited by testosterone via a negative feedback mechanism.

### Adrenal Glands

- de novo steroidogenesis from cholesterol to DHEA (Figure 33.2).
  - Can be converted by enzymatic processes to testosterone.
- Free testosterone is transported into the cytoplasm of target tissue cells.
  - Binds to the androgen receptor (AR).
  - Testosterone/AR or DHT/AR complex undergoes a structural change.
  - Enters the cell nucleus and binds directly to specific DNA nucleotide sequences.
  - Influences transcriptional activity of certain genes.
- Anti-androgen drugs are summarised in Table 33.5.

### Oestrogens

- Induce a negative feedback on the pituitary gland → decreases LH/FSH secretion
- Stimulate sex hormone-binding globulin (SHBG) synthesis → decrease levels of circulating free testosterone in the blood
- Direct suppression of Leydig cell function → reduce testosterone production
- *Side-effects:* increased risk of thromboembolic events.

**Table 33.4** Management of Localised and Systemic BCG Toxicity

**Management of Localised Side Effects**

| Symptomatic cystitis | *<48 h:* |
|---|---|
| | Symptomatic treatment with pain killers or NSAIDs |
| | If symptoms improve, continue instillations |
| | *>48 h:* |
| | Postpone instillation |
| | Perform urine culture |
| | Start empirical antibiotic treatment |
| | *If symptoms persist while on antibiotic treatment* |
| | With positive culture: adjust antibiotic treatment according to sensitivity |
| | With negative culture: start quinolones |
| | *If symptoms persist after 10 d* |
| | Anti-tuberculosis drugs: isoniazid for three months |
| | Discontinuation of BCG treatment |
| Haematuria | Perform urine culture to exclude haemorrhagic cystitis<br>Perform cystoscopy to exclude the presence of bladder tumour |
| Symptomatic granulomatous Prostatitis, epididymo-orchitis | Discontinuation of BCG treatment |
| | Perform urine culture |
| | Start treatment with quinolones |
| | If quinolones are not effective – isoniazid and rifampicin for three months |

**Management of Systemic Side Effects**

| Fever (<38.5°C) < 48 h | Generally resolve within 48 hours, with or without antipyretics. |
|---|---|
| Flu-like symptoms | |
| Fever > 38.5°C > 48 h | Permanent discontinuation of BCG instillations. |
| Without signs of sepsis | TB work up with urine culture, blood tests, chest X-ray. |
| | Prompt treatment with >2 antimicrobial agents while diagnostic evaluation is conducted. |
| | Consultation with an infectious disease specialist. |
| BCG sepsis | Permanent discontinuation of BCG instillations. |
| | Immediate treatment with isoniazid, rifampicin, and ethambutol daily for six months |
| Rash, arthralgia and/or arthritis, Reiter's Syndrome (reactive arthritis) | Rare complication and considered autoimmune reaction. |
| | Discontinuation of BCG treatment |
| | Treatment with antihistamines or NSAIDs |
| | If no improvement: proceed to corticosteroids, high-dose quinolones, or anti-tuberculosis drugs (isoniazid for three months) |
| Allergic reactions | Antihistamines and anti-inflammatory agents. |
| | Consider high-dose quinolones or isoniazid and rifampicin for persistent symptoms. |
| | Delay therapy until reactions resolve. |

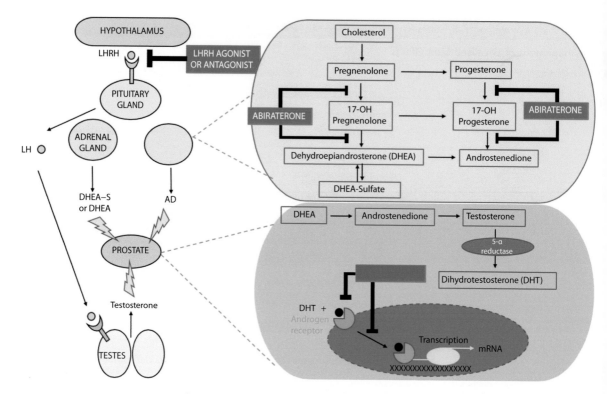

**Figure 33.2** Pathways and current drugs in prostate cancer. AD, androstenedione; LH, luteinising hormone; LHRH, luteinising hormone-releasing hormone.

## Luteinising-Hormone-Releasing Hormone Agonists

- Medical castration.
- Chronic exposure to GnRH agonists → overstimulation of pituitary GnRH receptors → number of GnRH receptors decreases → decreased LH and FSH in the hypophysis → lack of stimulation of Leydig cells → reduced production of testosterone in the testes → reduced testosterone release to the periphery
- Castration level is reached within 2–4 weeks.
- Side effects and management are summarised in Table 33.6.
- 'Flare-up' phenomenon: first injection of LHRH agonist induces a transient rise in testosterone levels.
  - Starts 2–3 days after injection – lasts for ~1 week.
  - May lead to increased clinical symptoms such as:
    - Increased bone pain, acute urinary retention, skeletal events
  - Concomitant androgen receptor antagonist – bicalutamide/flutamide is administered during the first four weeks.

## Luteinising-Hormone-Releasing Hormone Antagonists

- Competitive receptor blockade of the pituitary LHRH receptor.
- Castration level at day three.
- No initial testosterone flare-up, so concomitant anti-androgens is not necessary.
- Similar toxicity profile to the LHRH antagonists.
  - Immediate allergic reactions within the first 30 minutes of injection.
  - Possible QT prolongation.

## Steroidal Anti-Androgens

- *Cyproterone acetate*
  - Dual mechanism of action:
    - Inhibition of prostate cells AR.
    - Negative feedback effect on the hypothalamus and pituitary gland.
  - *Side effects:* similar to LHRH antagonists:
    - Depressed mood, dyspnoea, fatigue, gynaecomastia, hepatic disorders, hot flush, hyperhidrosis, nipple pain, restlessness, weight change
- *Abiraterone acetate*

**Table 33.5** Anti-androgen Drugs

| Anti-androgen Types | Agents |
| --- | --- |
| Oestrogens | Oestradiol diethylstilboestrol (DES) |
| LHRH – Agonist | Buserelin |
| | Goserelin |
| | Leuprorelin |
| LHRH – Antagonist | Degarelix |
| Non-steroidal anti-androgens | Bicalutamide |
| | Flutamide |
| | Enzalutamide |
| | Apalutamide |
| Steroidal anti-androgens | Cyproterone acetate |
| | Abiraterone acetate |

**Table 33.6** Side Effects of LHRH Antagonists and Their Management

| Side Effects | Management |
| --- | --- |
| Hot flashes (55–80%) | Medroxyprogesterone, cyproterone acetate |
| Fatigue | Exercise |
| Gynaecomastia, mastalgia (10–20%) | Prophylactic radiotherapy (8 Gy), mastectomy, tamoxifen |
| Increase in body fat, decrease in muscle mass | Exercise |
| Anaemia | Blood transfusions |
| Decrease in bone density | Physical training, bisphosphonates, calcium + vitamin-D, denosumab |
| Erectile dysfunction and loss of libido | PDE5i, MUSE®, cavernosal injection, vacuum device, penile implant |
| Depression | Antidepressants, psycho-oncological support |
| Sleep disorders | |
| Cognitive degradation | |

*Abbreviations:* PDE5i, phosphodiesterase 5 inhibitor; MUSE, medicated urethral system for erection (Prostaglandin E1, Alprostadil).

- Selective and irreversible blockage of 17α-hydroxylase and C17,20 lyase.
- Inhibition of androstenedione synthesis in the testes and adrenal glands.
- Decreased systemic levels of testosterone and cortisol.
- Increased levels of mineralocorticoid steroids
- Used in combination with prednisone/prednisolone to prevent drug-induced hyper-aldosteronism (high sodium, low potassium).
- *Side effects*: hypertension, hypokalaemia, increased transaminase levels.
- *Current uses*:
  - Castration-sensitive metastatic prostate cancer combined with ADT.
  - Castration-resistant prostate cancer (CRPC) in chemotherapy – naïve and pre-treated setting.

## Non-Steroidal Anti-Androgens

- *Bicalutamide*
  - Competitive inhibition of AR on the surface of prostate cells.
  - Serum level of testosterone remains within the normal physiological range.

- Monotherapy usually preserves libido and potency.
- *Side effects:*
  - Lower incidence of diarrhoea and liver dysfunction.
  - Maintenance of bone mineral density.
- *Enzalutamide*
  - Second-generation AR antagonist.
  - Higher affinity for the AR receptor than bicalutamide.
  - Prevents translocation of AR from the cytoplasm to the nucleus.
  - Within the nucleus, it inhibits AR binding to the chromosomal DNA.
  - *Side effects:* fatigue, diarrhoea, hot flushes, headache.
  - Used in CRPC in chemotherapy-naïve and pre-treated setting.
- *Apalutamide*
  - Novel anti-androgen that is closely related to enzalutamide.
  - Binds to the same ligand-binding site as bicalutamide.
    - But has a 7–10-fold higher affinity for the AR.
  - *Side effects:* rash, hypothyroidism, increased risk of pathological bone fracture.

# D) Targeted Therapies
## Cellular Communication

- Interaction of tyrosine kinase (TK) receptors on the cell surface with extracellular messengers, such as the following growth factors:
  - Epidermal growth factor (EGF)
  - Transforming growth factor alpha (TGF-α)
  - Platelet-derived growth factor (PDGF)
  - Vascular endothelial growth factor (VEGF)
- Activation of one of two important signalling cascades:
  - RAS / RAF / MEK / ERK signalling pathway; or
  - PI3K / AKT / mTOR signalling cascade.
  - Both trigger pro-mitogenic activity for cell proliferation and neoangiogenesis.

## Development of Renal Cancer

- Loss of function of the von Hippel-Lindau (*VHL*) gene → VHL disease
  - Chromosome 3p.
  - Most common cause for inherited clear cell renal cell carcinoma (RCC).
- Absence of VHL → accumulation of hypoxia-inducible factor (HIF) → production of growth

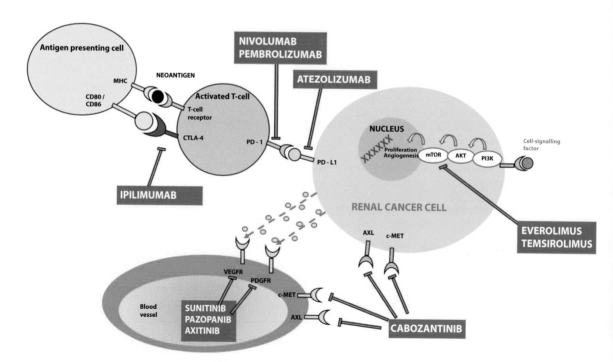

Figure 33.3 Pathways and current drugs in renal cell carcinoma. PD-1, programmed death protein 1; PD-L1, programmed death ligand 1; CTLA-4, cytotoxic T-lymphocyte-associated protein 4.

factors (VEGF, PDGF, erythropoietin, tumour growth factor) → promotion of neoangiogenesis
- Inhibition of intracellular signalling pathways = targets for anti-angiogenic drugs.

## Tyrosine Kinase Inhibitors (TKI)

### Sunitinib, Pazopanib, Sorafenib, and Axitinib

- Inhibition of all receptors for PDGF and VEGF receptors (Figure 33.3).
- Reduces tumour vascularization and triggers cancer cell apoptosis – tumour shrinkage.
- *Sunitinib:* (50 mg per day, four weeks on, two weeks off), median progression-free survival 11 months with a response rate of 31%.
- *Pazopanib:* (800 mg once daily), median

progression-free survival 8.4 months, with a response rate of 33%.
- *Side effects* of VEGF-targeted agents are shown in Table 33.7.

### Cabozantinib and Lenvatinib

- Targets VEGF receptors + other signalling enzymes (e.g., c-MET, AXL, fibroblast growth factor receptor [FGFR]).
- Cabozantinib: (60 mg once daily), median progression-free survival 8.2 months, with a response rate of 46%.

### Bevacizumab

- Monoclonal antibody – blocks circulating VEGF-A.
- 10 mg/kg IV given every two weeks.

**Table 33.7** Side Effects of VEGF-targeted Agents

| Frequency of Toxicity all Grades | |
|---|---|
| >10 % | 1–10 % |
| **Bone marrow toxicity** | |
| Thrombocytopenia | Leukopenia |
| Anaemia | Lymphopenia |
| Neutropenia | |
| **Metabolic toxicity** | |
| Hypothyroidism | Dehydration |
| Anorexia | Elevation of transaminase |
| | Elevation of lipase and amylase |
| **Neurological toxicity** | |
| Dysgeusia | Paraesthesia |
| **Cardiac toxicity** | |
| High blood pressure | |
| **Gastrointestinal toxicity** | |
| Stomatitis, mucositis | Dysphagia |
| Dry mouth | Ulcerations in the mouth |
| Nausea, vomiting | Bleeding gums |
| Diarrhoea | Proctalgia, rectal bleeding |
| **Dermatological toxicity** | |
| Palmar-plantar erythrodysesthesia (hand-foot syndrome) | Erythema |
| | Peeling of the skin |
| Yellow discolouration of the skin | Dermatitis |
| Changing of the hair colour | Acne, hyperkeratosis |
| Hair loss | Itching |

## Mammalian Target of Rapamycin (mTOR) Inhibitors

- Temsirolimus, everolimus.
- External cell growth factors/cancer cells activate the intracellular signalling pathway via - phosphoinositide-3-kinase (PI3K) and rapamycin → induces cell growth and angiogenesis
- mTOR inhibitors induce G1 arrest and apoptosis (Figure 33.3).

# E) Cancer Immunotherapy

## Immunotherapy in Renal Cancer in the Pre-Targeted Therapy Era

- Interferon alpha (IFN-α) monotherapy or, in combination with bevacizumab as well as interleukin-2 (IL-2), were frequently used in metastatic RCC.
- Response rate of 25% and 7.5% durable complete response with high-dose bolus IL-2.
- But it has high toxicity rates:
  - Capillary leak syndrome, myocardial infarction, respiratory failure, vomiting, diarrhoea, mortality rate (4%)

## Immune Checkpoint Inhibition

- Cancer exploits a series of immune escape mechanisms that were developed initially to avoid autoimmunity, like:
  - Hijacking of the immune-cell–intrinsic checkpoints that are induced on T-cell activation (Figure 33.4).

- Immune checkpoint inhibitors are monoclonal antibodies targeting and blocking:
  - The inhibitory T-cell receptor programmed death-1 (PD-1);
  - The cytotoxic T-lymphocyte associated antigen 4 (CTLA-4)-signalling; and
  - Restores tumour-specific T-cell immunity.
- *PD-1* receptor inhibitors: pembrolizumab and nivolumab.
- *PD-L1* receptor inhibitors: atezolizumab, durvalumab, avelumab.
- *CTLA-4* receptor inhibitor: ipilimumab, tremelimumab.

- *Toxicities* (Table 33.8):
  - Delayed onset – inflammatory/autoimmune in nature.
  - Any-grade immune-related side effects ~30% (severe grade ~6%).
  - Occur within weeks to three months after treatment initiation.
  - Can occur up to six months after the completion of treatment.
  - *Management*: oral/intravenous high-dose corticosteroids (1 mg/kg).

## Most Common Immune Checkpoint Inhibitor Regimens Used in Urological Cancer

- Given until disease progression or loss of clinical benefit.

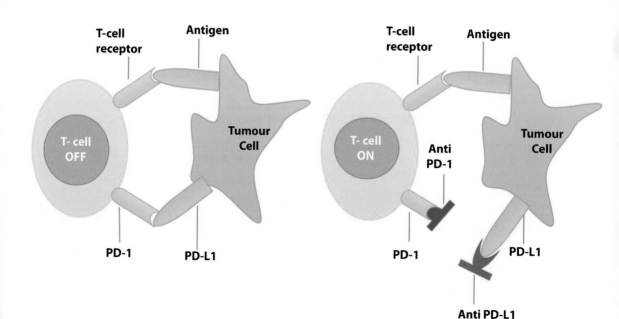

Figure 33.4 Mechanism of action of immune checkpoint inhibitors.

**Table 33.8** Treatment-related Toxicities

| Organ System | Symptoms |
|---|---|
| Dermatological | Maculopapular rash<br>Pruritus |
| Endocrine | Hyper/hypothyroidism |
| | Hyperglycaemia – diabetes |
| | Adrenal insufficiency |
| Gastrointestinal | Diarrhoea/colitis |
| Hepatic | Raised liver enzymes (ALT, AST) |
| Pancreatic | Elevation of amylase/lipase |
| | Pancreatitis |
| Pulmonary | Pneumonitis |
| Renal | Elevated serum creatinine/acute renal failure |
| Nervous system | Myasthenia gravis |
| | Guillain–Barré syndrome |
| | Peripheral neuropathy |
| | Encephalitis |
| Cardiovascular | Myocarditis |
| Musculoskeletal | Inflammatory arthritis<br>Myositis |

## Metastatic Urothelial Cancer

- *First-line, cisplatin-ineligible, PD-L1 positive:*
  - Atezolizumab (PD-L1i) or pembrolizumab (PD-1i): IV every three weeks.
- *After platinum-containing chemotherapy:*
  - Atezolizumab: IV every three weeks.

## Metastatic Renal Cell Carcinoma

- *First-line, IMDC intermediate, or poor risk:*
  - Four cycles of Nivolumab (PD-1i) with ipilimumab (CTLA-4i) every three weeks.
  - Followed by Nivolumab monotherapy.
  - Nivolumab + ipilimumab compared to sunitinib in first-line metastatic RCC:
    - Higher response rate (42% vs 27%).
      - Higher overall survival.
- *Previously treated RCC (previous VEGF-TKI therapy):*
  - Nivolumab monotherapy.
- *Combination treatments in RCC previously investigated*
  - With VEGF, mTOR – most develop treatment resistance within 12 months.
  - Hence, the development of combination treatments.
    - Keynote-426 phase III trial comparing the combination pembrolizumab + axitinib to sunitinib.
      - 12-months overall survival of 90% vs 78%.
      - Response rate of 59% vs 36%.
- Immune checkpoint inhibitors are currently under investigation in further settings:
  - NMIBC with BCG.
  - Neoadjuvant/adjuvant treatment for MIBC.
  - Neoadjuvant/adjuvant treatment after high-risk RCC.

## Recommended Reading

1. Price P, Sikora K, Illidge T. Treatment of Cancer 5th Edition. London: CRC Press; 2008.
2. James ND, de Bono JS, Spears MR et al. Abiraterone for prostate cancer not previously treated with hormone therapy. N Engl J Med. Massachusetts Medical Society; 2017;377(4):338–51.
3. Ryan CJ, Smith MR, Fizazi K et al. Abiraterone acetate plus prednisone versus placebo plus prednisone in chemotherapy-naive men with metastatic castration-resistant prostate cancer (COU-AA-302): final overall survival analysis of a randomised, double-blind, placebo-controlled phase 3 study. Lancet Oncol. Elsevier; 2015;16(2):152–60.
4. Hussain M, Fizazi K, Saad F et al. Enzalutamide in men with nonmetastatic, castration-resistant prostate cancer. N Engl J Med. Massachusetts Medical Society; 2018;378(26): 2465–74.
5. Motzer RJ, Tannir NM, McDermott DF et al. Nivolumab plus ipilimumab versus sunitinib in advanced renal-cell carcinoma. N Engl J Med. Massachusetts Medical Society; 2018 Apr 5;378(14):1277–90.
6. Rini BI, Plimack ER, Stus V et al. Pembrolizumab plus axitinib versus sunitinib for advanced renal-cell carcinoma. N Engl J Med. 2019; 380:1116–27.

# 34 External Beam Radiotherapy and Brachytherapy

*Sophia C. Kamran and Jason A. Efstathiou*

## Radiation Physics

- *Radiation*: emission/transmission of energy in the form of waves or particles.
  - Diagnostic or therapeutic.
- Includes electromagnetic radiation:
  - Radio waves, microwaves
  - Infrared, visible light, ultraviolet
  - X-rays
  - Gamma radiation
- *Ionising radiation:* travels as a particle or electromagnetic wave.
  - Carries energy to detach electrons from atoms – '*ionising*' an atom.
- The radioactive decay of an atomic nucleus results in:
  - *Alpha radiation: emission* of alpha particles (two protons, two neutrons).
  - *Beta radiation:* emission of beta particles.
    - beta$^-$ = electrons
    - beta$^+$ = protons
  - *Gamma radiation:* emission of electromagnetic energy (photon).

## Therapeutic Ionising Radiation

- Creation of free radicals, causing irreparable DNA damage in cancer cells.
- DNA damage leads to cell death in actively dividing cells, while normal tissues can regenerate and heal.
- Radiation dose is measured in Gray (Gy).
- Dose *fractionation:* total radiation dose is divided into a higher dose per treatment for fewer total treatments (hypofractionated radiotherapy, HFX).
  - Reduces toxicity to healthy cells.
  - Utilises the differences in the DNA repair capacity of normal and tumour cells.
  - Allows efficacious tumour killing through the '5 Rs'.
- *5 Rs:*
  - *Recovery/Repair:* allows normal cells time to recover from the damage. More efficient in normal cells compared with cancer cells.

Fractionation allows more cells to be in the sensitive phase.
  - *Reoxygenation:* allows more oxygen-dependent killing because tumour cells have hypoxic cores (radioresistant). As cells die, more oxygen becomes available for free radical formation.
  - *Reassortment:* radiotherapy at time intervals allows cells to redistribute themselves over all phases of the cell cycle. Radiation is most effective in cells about to divide.
    - M > G2 > G1> early S > late S
  - *Repopulation:* allows normal rapidly dividing cells (bowel) to repopulate.
  - *Intrinsic radiosensitivity:*
    - Squamous cell carcinoma and adenocarcinoma – radiosensitive.
    - Seminoma and lymphoma – radiosensitive.
    - Melanoma, glioma, sarcoma – radioresistant.

## Basic Principles About External Beam Radiation

- The production and delivery of ionising radiation using an external beam radiation therapy (EBRT) machine is based on either:
  1. Radioactive decay of a nuclide; or
  2. Production due to the electrical acceleration of electrons or other charged particles.
- Historically (1950s), EBRT machines were based on cobalt, $^{60}$Co, decay.
  - Largely replaced by linear accelerators which produce high energy x-rays.
- *Linear accelerator machines:*
  - Much more versatile than $^{60}$Co machines.
  - Produce x-rays or electrons and allow multiple energies for treatment.
  - *Photon* radiation.

## Conformal Radiation

- EBRT has evolved over the years – *conformal planning involves*:
  - Creation of a high-dose target volume shaped to '*conform*' to the tumour/target.

- Maximally spares high dose to critical/normal structures. Planning involves:
  - *Contouring* (or drawing) of treatment and normal structure volumes on 3D images.
  - Using *multiple beams* to result in higher doses where beams overlap — individual beams shaping to *'conform'* to the target — while incorporating other components of treatment delivery to ensure treatment accuracy, including image-guidance, motion management, and reproducible patient set-up.
- 3D conformal radiation therapy (3d-CRT) is the first type of conformal therapy developed.
- Still commonly used in many disease sites and for different treatment goals (including palliation).
- IMRT is a newer technique.

## Intensity Modulated Radiation Therapy (IMRT)

- Involves inverse planning and mathematical optimisation.
- Complex beam intensity distribution across the beam.
- Precise radiation to a specific area.
- Can alter the dose depending upon the shape of the target.
- Ideal when the target volume abuts a critical structure that is necessary to avoid.
  - Example: in *prostate cancer (PCa)*, the rectum is posterior, the bladder is anterior and superior, and the hips are lateral to the gland.
- Organ movement becomes an issue with dose escalation.
  - Therefore, it is combined with image-guided RT (IGRT).
- 3D-CRT and IMRT allow for dose escalation to the tumour and targets.
  - Improves biochemical control.
  - Allows novel delivery methods (e.g., moderate hypofractionation and stereotactic body radiation therapy).

## Complications of Radiotherapy

- Desquamation:
  - Temporary cessation in epithelial cell production
  - Skin thinning/ulceration (~2 weeks following RT)
- Cystitis and haematuria, small capacity bladder
- Proctitis – diarrhoea/bleeding
- Infertility (pelvic/testicular RT)
- Obliterative endarteritis
- Lymphoedema
- Urethral stricture
- Urinary incontinence

- Late malignancy

## Relative Contraindications to Radiotherapy

- Severe lower urinary tract symptoms (LUTS)
- Inflammatory bowel disease
- Previous pelvic irradiation

## Basic Principles About Brachytherapy

- Brachytherapy (Greek 'short-distance' therapy).
- Sealed radioactive sources are placed inside/next to areas which require treatment.
- Irradiates a localised area, sparing healthy tissues further away from the source.
- Delivered using *low-dose*-rate (LDR) or *high-dose*-rate (HDR) sources.
- *LDR* sources:
  - Permanent brachytherapy or seed brachytherapy (prostate cancer).
  - Seeds are placed within a tumour permanently to decay and deliver radiation.
  - Once fully decayed, the seeds remain in place inert.
- *HDR* brachytherapy:
  - Delivered using placement of temporary catheters.
  - The source is directed to an area (sec to mins) before removal.
- The dose distribution from LDR or HDR depends on the physical properties of the radioactive isotope used, as well as other characteristics such as source activity.
- *Side effects:* LUTS, prostatitis, proctitis.

## Radiation for Genito-Urinary Malignancies

### Prostate Cancer

- Dose-escalattion to 79.2 Gy improves biochemical control and rates of distant metastases compared to 70.2 Gy (RTOG 0126, NCT00033631) (Figure 34.1).
- Conventional fractions: 1.8–2 Gy.
- Moderate HFX: 2.4–3.4 Gy per fraction.
- Ultra (extreme) HFX: >5 Gy per fraction.
- $\alpha/\beta$ ratio: characterise tissue and/or tumour sensitivity to radiation dose per treatment.
- PCa harbours a lower $\alpha/\beta$ ratio compared to the normal surrounding tissues.
  - HFX RT may improve cancer control outcomes, increase convenience, and offer better resource utilisation.

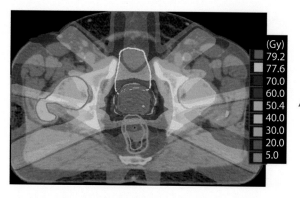

**Figure 34.1** Dose distribution radiation plan for IMRT of the prostate. Cross-sectional image demonstrates the prostate (red), rectum (light blue/green), bladder (yellow), right femoral head (dark blue) and left femoral head (pink). The prostate was treated to 79.2 Gy.

## PSA Bounce

- Benign PSA rise following EBRT/brachytherapy.
- Usually <1.5 ng/mL.
- Mean time to PSA bounce is ~9 months (later with brachytherapy).
- Recurrent disease following RT is indicated by a PSA >2 ng/mL above nadir.

## Extreme Hypofractionation

- Also known as stereotactic body radiotherapy (SBRT).
- Emerging treatment option for localised PCa.
- Requires image-guidance.
- Early data have demonstrated low toxicities and excellent control.

## NICE Guidelines 2019: Radiation Options

- Conventional RT – 74 Gy in 37 fractions over 7.5 weeks;
- HFX RT using image-guided IMRT – 60 Gy in 20 fractions over four weeks; or
- Brachytherapy (Table 34.1).
- *Low-risk:* EBRT or LDR brachytherapy alone (Figure 34.2).
- *Intermediate- and high-risk:*
  - Six months of androgen deprivation therapy (ADT) before EBRT; or
  - Brachytherapy in combination with EBRT.
- *High-risk:* consider continuing ADT up to three years with EBRT.
- Men with LUTS are at risk of deterioration.
- *EAU guidelines* recommend the following for LDR:

- International prostatic symptom score (IPSS) of ≤12.
- Maximum flow rate of >15 mL/min.
- Prostate volume of <50 cm$^3$.

## Adjuvant/Salvage Radiation

- Following radical prostatectomy.
- Risk of recurrence increases with adverse pathology:
  - Extraprostatic extension
  - Seminal vesicle invasion
  - Positive surgical margins
- Upfront adjuvant or salvage RT when there is evidence of PSA recurrence (>0.1 ng/mL).
- Clinical target – *prostatic fossa* + pelvic nodal fields) as defined by CT or MRI.
- *Recommended dose:* 64–72 Gy in standard fractionation.
- Addition of ADT in the salvage setting improves overall, metastasis-free, and progression-free survival compared with RT alone.

## Proton Beam Therapy

- *Proton* – positively charged particles found in an atomic nucleus.
- Deposit radiation at the *end* of the particle's path in the tissue (the Bragg peak).
  - *Note: photons* deposit radiation *along* their path.
- Cost considerations.
- Limited rigorous evidence on toxicity and cancer control benefits compared to IMRT.

# Bladder Cancer

- Organ-preservation with trimodality therapy (TMT) is an accepted alternative to radical cystectomy (RC) for the treatment of muscle-invasive bladder cancer.
- RT *does not* treat carcinoma in situ.
- *TMT* involves:
  - Transurethral resection of the bladder tumour (TURBT).
  - Followed by radiation and concurrent radiosensitising chemotherapy.
- No completed randomised trials compared RC to TMT.
  - Many studies demonstrate comparable cancer outcomes in selected patients.

## Radiation Fields

- Small pelvic field or not.
- If a small pelvic field is *used,* boost fields may include the whole bladder, the bladder tumour alone, or both.

**Table 34.1** Comparison of Low and High-dose Rate Brachytherapy

| Characteristics | LDR | HDR |
|---|---|---|
| Source | Permanent | Temporary |
| Isotope | Iodine-125 (I-125) most common<br>Half-life: 59.4 days | Iridium-192 (IR-192) Half-life: 74 days |
| | Palladium-103 (Pd-103)<br>Half-life: 17 days | |
| | Cesium-131<br>Half-life: 9.7 days | |
| Dose delivery | Over weeks and months | In minutes |
| Side effects | Resolve over months | Resolve over weeks |
| Radiation protection issues for patient/ carers. | Yes | No |

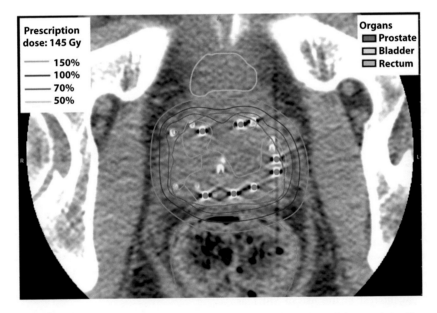

**Figure 34.2** Dose distribution radiation plan for LDR brachytherapy treatment of the prostate. Cross-section image demonstrates the prostate (red), rectum (green), bladder (yellow). The lime green dots indicate where the radioactive seeds are placed within the prostate gland. This prostate was treated with iodine- 125 seeds to a total dose of 145 Gy.

- If a small pelvic field is *not used,* either the entire bladder or the bladder tumour can be treated alone, or both can be treated.

## Radiation Dose

- Radiation dose: 60–66 Gy range using standard fractionation.

- Moderate HFX: 2.75 Gy/fraction to a total of 55 Gy.
- Radiation can be delivered either once or twice a day.
- Built-in treatment break can allow for restaging cystoscopy and biopsies.
  - Complete response – consolidative chemoradiation is delivered.

- Poor treatment response – salvage RC is recommended.

## NICE Guidelines 2015

- *Radiosensitiser* (e.g., mitomycin combined with fluorouracil (5-FU) or carbogen combined with nicotinamide).
- 64 Gy in 32 fractions over 6.5 weeks; or
- 55 Gy in 20 fractions over four weeks.

## Testicular Cancer

- Seminomas are radiosensitive.
- *Stage I seminoma:* adjuvant radiotherapy following radical orchidectomy.
  - Field:
    - Paraaortic lymph nodes alone extending from T11/12 to L5/S1
    - 20 Gy in 10 fractions (MRC trial showed *non-inferiority* compared with 30 Gy in 15 fractions).
    - Reduces relapse rate to 1–3% (from ~15–20% with orchidectomy alone).
- *Alternatives:* active surveillance or adjuvant chemotherapy with carboplatin.
- *Stage II seminoma*
  - Radiation to the paraaortic and ipsilateral pelvic nodes is effective.
  - Recommended for non-bulky tumours (stage IIA-B).
  - Chemotherapy is recommended for more bulky, advanced tumours (select IIB and IIC).

## Renal Cell Carcinoma (RCC)

- Radiation has been evaluated in the post-operative, adjuvant setting without a definitive consensus on its role.
- It is generally reserved mostly for the palliative setting.
- RCC is relatively radioresistant.
- There is recent interest in the use of SBRT as primary therapy, particularly for non-surgical candidates.
  - Early data demonstrates good local control rates and relatively low toxicity.
- *Intraoperative EBRT* delivered at the time of surgery with electrons can be considered for patients who are found to have more advanced disease invading into local tissues that cannot be fully resected at the time of nephrectomy.
- *Metastatic RCC*
  - SBRT to a metastatic lesion can result in improved systemic response durability to targeted therapy or immunotherapy.

- In responders to systemic therapy except for one or two lesions, consolidation with SBRT to the non-responding lesion(s) can be considered.

## Penile Cancer

- Brachytherapy or EBRT.
- Achieves high local control rates with penile preservation.
- *T-stage 1-3, tumour size <4 cm:*
  - EBRT $\geq$60 Gy (daily fraction $\geq$2 Gy) with brachytherapy; or
  - Brachytherapy alone.
- *Brachytherapy:* penile preservation rates of 87% in five years and 70% in 10 years.
- *Specific complication:*
  - *EBRT:* urethral stenosis (20–35%), glans necrosis (10–20%), late fibrosis.
  - *Brachytherapy:* meatal stenosis (6.6–40%).
- Follow-up is needed as local failures can be surgically salvaged with high cure rates.
- *Locally advanced tumours*
  - It is recommended for nodes to be resected and any multiple positive nodes or extranodal extension should receive post-operative EBRT.

## Recommended Reading

1. Gunderson LL, Tepper JE. Clinical Radiation Oncology. 3rd edition. Philadelphia, PA, USA: Saunders Elsevier; 2012.
2. Michalski JM, Moughan J, Purdy J, Bosch W, Bruner DW, Bahary JP, et al. Effect of standard vs dose-escalated radiation therapy for patients with intermediate-risk prostate cancer: The NRG Oncology RTOG 0126 Randomized Clinical Trial. JAMA Oncol. 2018;4(6):e180039.
3. Greco C, Vazirani AA, Pares O, Pimentel N, Louro V, Morales J, et al. The evolving role of external beam radiotherapy in localized prostate cancer. Sem Oncol. 2019; 46(3): 246–53.
4. Carrie C, Hasbini A, de Laroche G et al. Salvage radiotherapy with or without short-term hormone therapy for rising prostate-specific antigen concentration after radical prostatectomy (GETUG-AFU 16): a randomised, multicentre, open-label phase 3 trial. Lancet Oncol. 2016;17(6): 747–756.
5. Shipley WU, Seiferheld W, Lukka HR et al. Radiation with or without antiandrogen therapy in recurrent prostate cancer. N Engl J Med. 2017;376(5):417–28.
6. Zaorsky NG, Davis BJ, Nguyen PL et al. The evolution of brachytherapy for prostate cancer. Nat Rev Urol. 2017;14(7):415–39.
7. James ND, Hussain SA, Hall E et al. Radiotherapy with or without chemotherapy in muscle-invasive bladder cancer. N Engl J Med. 2012;366(16):1477–88.

# Index